TRUSTING DOCTORS

TRUSTING DOCTORS

The Decline of Moral Authority in American Medicine

JONATHAN B. IMBER

PRINCETON UNIVERSITY PRESS *Princeton and Oxford*

Copyright © 2008 by Princeton University Press
Published by Princeton University Press, 41 William Street, Princeton, New Jersey 08540

In the United Kingdom: Princeton University Press, 6 Oxford Street, Woodstock, Oxfordshire
OX20 1TW

Library of Congress Cataloging-in-Publication Data
Imber, Jonathan B., 1952–
    Trusting doctors : the decline of moral authority in American medicine / Jonathan B. Imber.
        p.   cm.
    Includes bibliographical references and index.
    ISBN 978-0-691-13574-8 (hardcover : alk. paper)   1. Medical ethics.   2. Medical policy—
Moral and ethical aspects.   I. Title.
    R724.I5446 2008
    174.2—dc22   2008005153

British Library Cataloging-in-Publication Data is available

This book has been composed in Minion

Printed on acid-free paper. ∞

press.princeton.edu

Printed in the United States of America

10   9   8   7   6   5   4   3   2   1

To Amy, Elizabeth, and David

And to the blessings of family

אשתך כגפן פריה בירכתי ביתך בניך כשתלי זיתים סביב לשלחנך

All in all there are two things, two remedies—both for internal use—which, regrettably enough, physicians nowadays forget or neglect to prescribe. —Alas, it is all the more regrettable that neither one nor the other is particularly easy to manage, even though the physician did remember to prescribe it. One of these, used when everything is safely over—a small dose, a drop is sufficient; too much is detrimental and may even elicit the opposite effect —is jesting, a timely jest, a felicitous fancy, a priceless, surprising something, a droll, jesting incident, a turn of phrase that all of a sudden turns everything upside down. . . . In other words, jesting is one; the other, which physicians nowadays do not prescribe either, is the pastor.

—Søren Kierkegaard to Julie Thomsen, January 1849

Hence too probably the fact that transactions of healing are so closely connected, the world over, with sentiments of religion. Perhaps the fact is due, in part, to some latent association that connects diseases with sin and, to much the same extent, connects the hope of healing with some possibility of a divine medication. However this may be, the mystery of healing, as we are constituted, stands in close affinity with God and the faith of his supernatural operation.

—Horace Bushnell, *Nature and the Supernatural*, 1858

CONTENTS

A Sociological Perspective

I began research on this book with the assumption that not only is trusting doctors one of life's necessities, but that doing so is connected to the essential meaning of professional character. A profession that is not a conspiracy against the laity must demonstrate through each one of its practitioners a consistency in character that is not exclusively based on intelligence and technical skills. The capacity to deal adequately with other human beings, which is certainly one element of competence, also reflects the cultural expectations that link together professionalism, character, and trust.

The very notion of character, and a focus on the individual practitioner, may at first appear to challenge the standard sociological perspective on medicine. That perspective, both in terms of personal accountability and social epidemiology, has established beyond question the importance of structural considerations with regard to the organization and delivery of medical services. But the bases for trusting a doctor within these dimensions have always required more than professional competence and more than institutional efficiency. Over the decades at the end of the twentieth century, doctors in America were compelled to adapt to the demands of the financial and corporate architects of managed care, just as at the beginning of that century they needed to adapt to the clinical expectations of scientific medicine.[1] Something of lasting consequence must be at stake in the fact that physicians today think about issues in new ways and that their practices are organized very differently from those of their predecessors, yet we continue to call them doctors even as we reconsider what our trust in them entails.

After World War II, social science (with the exception of economics) and medicine worked largely in collaboration. Throughout most of the 1950s, the sociological study of medicine was conducted within the systems of medical education and allied medical services in an effort to inform and transform them. The emergence of an adversarial social science critique within medicine never amounted to much during this period, largely because of a rapid transformation in who was seen to be working within rather than outside the system. Within this context, the chief success of the new field of medical ethics during the past three decades or so has been institutional—that is, where social science and social work once were in medical schools, philosophers, ethicists, lawyers, and their publicists now are. (If a physician of any serious reputation in medical ethics has a degree in addition to an M.D., it is typically in philosophy or law.) Meanwhile, beyond attempts to observe and document the motives and behavior of "corrupt," "impaired," or "deviant" doctors, little attention has been paid in recent decades to basic questions about the definition and development of professional character in general.[2]

Despite the existence of overdetermined conceptualizations of professional dominance and deviant practitioners, overintellectualized celebrations of physician virtues, and overgeneralized despair about a starved medical system, the practicing physician is still expected to clarify and help resolve the many difficulties of those who seek medical attention. I, too, seek to clarify difficulties. For the sociologist, there are principally two approaches, which are not mutually exclusive: (1) to conduct empirical research in whatever present one finds oneself, in order to report as honestly and as clearly as possible what is currently the case, and (2) to search the historical record for material that enhances our understanding present circumstances. In my book *Abortion and the Private Practice of Medicine,* I combined these two approaches to examine the historical and social sources of the medical profession's intellectual and moral ambivalence about abortion. Despite the fact that courts and social movements have entirely usurped public discourse on this issue, physicians have their own stories to tell about the meanings of their work, whether or not the courts or partisans in the abortion wars want to hear them.[3]

At certain points in this new book, by using both historical and more contemporary examples of the evolving nature of medical morality, I will consider the topic of abortion again, here to illustrate what I consider a central aspect of the challenge of medical vocation and public trust in the profession, that is, how the culture of medical practice intersects with the demands of historical change, in particular around that cluster of issues now called bioethical. My argument is intended to be straightforward: the stances taken about medical morality by Catholic writers, which included centrally the matter of abortion and which were largely marginal to public interest and attention during the nineteenth century, have reappeared with remarkable public salience over the last few decades. Today questions about abortion, end-of-life care, and new medical technologies have so profoundly affected public consciousness that it is impossible to write a history of American judicial and legislative developments without understanding how the politics of these issues arose out of specific cultural changes in both medicine and the larger society.

One of these changes pertains to the ways in which public trust in the character and person of the physician has been diminished in the face of challenges to both the triumphs of medical progress and a perceived arrogance on the part of individual practitioners. The morally marginal issues of the nineteenth century acquired a public and political urgency at the end of the twentieth century that neither physicians nor anyone else was fully prepared to resolve. As people's trust in professionals and institutions in general declined, in medicine a new realm of thought—bioethics—arose as the public face of medical morality, no longer bound to the religious roots that had nourished it historically but also not completely indifferent to those roots as sources to be acknowledged and considered. This process continues to the present moment, as illustrated in the voluminous and mostly ignored (at least from the standpoint of widespread publicity) reports of the President's Council on Bioethics.[4] For more than thirty years, successive presidential commissions and advisory groups have offered counsel about politically charged and ethically complex matters, with the matter of abortion in one respect or another always claiming a place for attention as emblematic of questions about the value of human life.

End-of-life dilemmas are also much debated, including how we might understand the extraordinary pressures put on physicians first, and courts finally, to settle contentious disagreements over the new possibilities for extending life—but to what purpose, and who will decide?—and over the moral acceptability of euthanasia or physician-assisted suicide. Thorny ethical questions have also been raised by new scientific possibilities, including DNA analysis, cloning, and stem-cell research.

In addressing the distinctively Protestant and Catholic sources that have heavily influenced what I describe here as medical morality in the past—encompassing a range that extends from the nature of the moral character of the physician to the ethical conundrums that have shaped and challenged that character—I do not mean in any way to neglect the significant question of the ethnic composition of the medical profession itself. For decades, until the middle of the twentieth century, the majority of physicians in this country, and their allies, were Christian Protestants. The discrimination against the entry of Jews and Catholics into the profession before then has been well documented in recent years, and for a time Jews in particular were singled out as characterologically unfit to practice medicine.[5] But even as this aspect of what was then meant by "character" had its malicious effects in promoting prejudice and injustice, the kinds of medical-ethical matters taken up by Catholics in particular ran parallel to similar concerns raised by Jewish physicians. And even though Jewish and Catholic physicians generally conformed to established standards of medical practice—which confirms how the culturally predominant norms of law, etiquette, and reputation form the bases of professionalism of all kinds—they brought different perspectives into play.

The relative emphasis I give in this book to a growing focus on women's health as a crucial, if not *the* crucial, factor in the profound realignment of the physician-patient relationship should not be taken as any indication of the lesser importance of many other factors related to the question of trust more generally. The story of the historic discrimination against African Americans in terms of access to both medical care and medical education contains many lessons about the transformative actions taken by African Americans themselves, through local and national associations, in order to break down barriers of entry to the profession that were even greater than those that faced Jews and Catholics.[6] I will consider all these factors, but my main intention is to highlight how multiple critiques of physician authority have led to a diminution of that authority even as the profession—once predominantly white, male, and Protestant—has come to accept into its ranks for training and practice not only Catholics, Jews, women, and African Americans, but also people who come from every other part of our increasingly diverse society.

The role of science, having served more than a century in defining the professional thought and practice of medicine, has opened a terrain of seemingly endless vistas of possible causes and effects in the onset and treatment of disease. In chapter 3 I will describe the implications of how nineteenth-century champions of the mission of science sought clearer pathways between cause and effect when they initiated a discussion about the efficacy of prayer. Less an attack on prayer than on the religious establishment that promoted it as an effective means of influencing nature or the outcome of illness, their arguments form a background for the theme I will take up in chapter 7, in an account of how the development of social epidemiology, which came about as the result of concerns about the dangers of cigarette smoking, offered a new, scientific way of demonstrating cause and effect statistically rather than individually. In the nineteenth century, the claim that science could not verify that prayer had any real effect on improving health offended religious believers on several counts. In the twentieth, early claims that cigarettes had real and demonstrable negative effects on health stimulated extraordinary scientific interest and research, while at the same time they provoked others (including, of course, the manufacturers of tobacco products) into questioning the new science of epidemiology. In both cases, a peculiar and important displacement of the physician as a mediator between a patient's behavior and a patient's health was at stake. If prayer worked, what did that mean for trust in scientific medicine? If tobacco seemed to harm some and not others, what did that mean for trusting a particular physician's guidance about one's own personal health? The answers, as these chapters illustrate, were never straightforward, nor have they been completely resolved as of the present moment.

Every attempt to characterize medicine as a profession must face this irreducible fact: persons practice medicine. A physician, and thus physician-hood, is more than the sum total of medical degree, license, and professional specialty. The encounter between a physician and a patient is mediated by character as much as by society, though somewhere back in the traditions of sociological reasoning about the medical profession, the study of professional character was subordinated to more ambitious attempts to analyze the nature and function of all professions as corporate enterprises. Whether or not public and academic discourses on physicians will ever again be encouraging of their personal vocation, rather than critical or even condemning of their current place in the "health care delivery system," will depend on whether or not those doctors influential enough to speak out to a broad audience about their work can do so in ways that will help their profession regain what it has lost in terms of public trust.

Medicine has always been in a constant negotiation with the public that depends upon it, sometimes adulates it, and sometimes holds it in contempt. The delicate fabric of trust between this profession and the public depends not simply on the effectiveness of medical treatments but also on the effectiveness of physicians in conveying that they are doing the best they know how to do for everyone who comes under their care. Here, of course, the transformations in the structure of delivery have combined with public uncertainties about the personal commitments of physicians to create extraordinary challenges to our understanding of how physicians and patients understand one another.

With this book I have not undertaken to write another social history of medicine, but I am obviously indebted to this important tradition of accounting for historical and organizational change. However, in the end I believe that in order to understand a crucial dimension of the profession—the nature and scope of the physician's moral authority—it is necessary to address the intellectual and religious traditions out of which the physician's distinctive twentieth-century reputation as trustworthy arose. Because for decades the academic emphasis has been on the management and economic reform of medicine, I risk challenging some in my own discipline who believe that all professions are rapidly and dangerously accommodating themselves to the demands and constraints of business. I have little argument with them about the existence of such accommodation in general, but I am less persuaded that physicians in particular are on the verge of completely abandoning their historic vocation. Patients, thus far, will not let them.

Throughout the world of pagans and Christians, Hippocrates represented the autonomy of medicine as a sphere of life. With his system and many of its practices discarded, he has yet not ceased to do so.

—Owsei Temkin, *Hippocrates in a World of Pagans and Christians*

To assert the autonomy of medicine as a sphere of life is to acknowledge the millennia of efforts on the part of physicians to delineate and come to terms with their special responsibilities in human affairs. Today many questioners, both within and from outside the profession, address what are routinely described by the mass media in the United States as the most pressing and crucial dilemmas confronting modern medicine and modern society. Among these, abortion, euthanasia, and organ transplantation rank very high in public and professional visibility. Less is heard about what medicine represents as a sphere of life and a culture of practices, organized and directed by physicians themselves, which encompass ideas about calling and character, competence and ethics.[1]

At the same time, recent attempts to balance the often severe criticisms of the "health care system" with an uplifting catalogue of the virtues of the "health care provider" illustrate the competing rhetorics that have increasingly dominated public discourse about health and well-being for the past several decades. The nature of this discourse has allowed for multiple conversations about who occupies the central position of informed critic of medicine, and about the past deficiencies and future challenges of medicine as a profession. To date, sociological and anthropological studies of system and provider have produced relatively few ethnographies—that is, descriptive works—of medical practice as compared to a vast range of quantitative social-scientific research, but these ethnographies present a much more complex view of what might constitute a contemporary definition of medical "virtue" than do the ever-growing number of normative analyses made by medical ethicists.[2]

Other sociologists have written about medicine in terms of both deterministic theories of professional dominance and idealistic theories about professional virtue. With this book I am seeking to return attention to the making of the physician in a characterological sense—which involves tensions about the enduring basis of trust between patients and health care professionals in the context of a changing backdrop of increasingly institutional systems for providing that care. Several decades ago, many of the complaints about medicine—especially during the years in which the professional dominance model seemed fresh in its approach to understanding medical self-confidence—were rooted in the political conviction that medical consumers suffered a false consciousness about their health and well-being. It was said that by giving themselves over too easily to the dictates of medical authority, patients rendered themselves incapable of recognizing and asserting their own interests. This sociological critique was directed against the bourgeois character of patients, especially women, as much as it was aimed at giving patients more control over their own treatment. Lost in the argument was any sustained examination of what social standing doctors possessed or what cultural values they might be said to embody.

For more than a century—from the 1860s to the 1970s—the American medical profession relied on a combination of commitment to rigorous training in medical science and a dedication to professional ethics that made it a revered and respected vocation. But how was this combined commitment and dedication understood by others? In the first half of this book, I will examine a connection between the rise of trust in physicians and the role played by Protestant and Catholic clergymen and thinkers in the second half of the nineteenth and first half of the twentieth centuries. These members of the religious community defined and bolstered the moral authority of modern medical professionals, whose responsibility to patients was grounded in the willingness of patients to trust their individual doctors. Protestant clergymen, in particular, helped to shape that trust by insisting that the physician was and would be a person of integrity and high moral character, while the Catholic perspective focused on specific moral dilemmas that physicians faced in everyday practice, thus adding an important dimension to judging medical decision-making in terms of morality and ethics as well as by purely technical standards.

In the second half of the book, I will present an account of how doctors, who were once publicly perceived in this country as healers engaged in a sacred vocation, began to lose their moral authority as they increasingly became more valued for their technical competence than for their noble character. Doctors themselves were not entirely responsible for this turn of events, as I will illustrate by examining how social critics—long after the clergy of previous decades had lost their own central presence in the culture—contributed to a loss of public trust more generally in all professions. In medicine in particular, an acknowledgment of the changing nature of the problems that patients in ever larger numbers will come to face is also important to understanding why physicians must now negotiate between a vast world of knowledge (both certain and uncertain) about the possibilities offered by science in the arena of health care and the worries, beliefs, and concerns of their patients. In this book I hypothesize that the layperson's ability to trust in doctors will face even greater challenges in the future, as medical professionals grapple with the dilemmas associated with an increasing capacity to extend life indefinitely.

Over the past few decades, the now largely historical image of each and every physician always being "on call" has been replaced on the one side by eighty-hour work weeks for those in medical training, and on the other by the nearly insurmountable barriers established by those dictates of group practice that tend to separate patients from their personal physicians. However, these kinds of changes do not diminish in the slightest the anxieties that patients express about what they expect from their physicians. Today the perceived character of the practitioner—as concerned or indifferent—remains at the center of the dynamics of trust.

I offer here some historical insights and an apologetic for the figure and persona of the physician, a person who may wonder what the legacy of respect and veneration for doctoring was all about now that it may seem to be compromised. The asymmetry of the doctor-patient relationship is not an illusion, nor does our need to trust in others represent a blindness to the dynamics of power. But what I see as a decline in the public's trust in the moral authority of the physician over the past few decades is an illustration of a much broader decline in the public's trust in the superiority of the judgment and competence of "experts" in all fields. Why this is the case with regard to the medical profession in particular is an important question to address. The physicians of tomorrow are always born of today's expectations about their character and conduct. Trusting doctors is about the hopes and despairs of everyone, doctors and patients alike, as they come to terms with new realities in the context of the profound, age-old inevitabilities of sickness and death.

PART ONE

Religious Foundations of Trust in Medicine

That is what people are like in my district. Always expecting the impossible from the doctor. They have lost their ancient beliefs; the parson sits at home and unravels his vestments, one after another; but the doctor is supposed to be omnipotent with his merciful surgeon's hand. Well, as it pleases them; I have not thrust my services on them; if they misuse me for sacred ends, I let that happen to me too.

—Kafka, "A Country Doctor," 1918

CHAPTER 1

Protestantism, Piety, and Professionalism

Whether trusted or not, doctors have used the Hippocratic oath for two thousand years as the equivalent of a social contract between the medical profession and the public, administered in modern times at graduation from medical school. Even though the legacy of that contract may now seem to raise more questions than it answers about the physician's duties, the original oath has been described as "the Medical Decalogue [equivalent to the Ten Commandments], universally accepted as such."[1]

That original, as translated by Ludwig Edelstein in his book *The Hippocratic Oath: Text, Translation, and Interpretation* (1943), reads as follows:

> I swear by Apollo Physician and Asclepius and Hygieia and Panaceia and all the gods and goddesses, making them my witnesses, that I will fulfill according to my ability and judgment this oath and this covenant:
>
>> To hold him who has taught me this art as equal to my parents and to live my life in partnership with him, and if he is in need of money to give him a share of mine, and to regard his offspring as equal to my brothers in male lineage and to teach them this art—if they desire to learn it—without fee and covenant; to give a share of precepts and oral instruction and all the other learning to my sons and to the sons of him who has instructed me and to pupils who have signed the covenant and have taken an oath according to the medical law, but no one else.
>>
>> I will apply dietetic measures for the benefit of the sick according to my ability and judgment; I will keep them from harm and injustice.
>>
>> I will neither give a deadly drug to anybody who asked for it, nor will I make a suggestion to this effect. Similarly I will not give to a woman an abortive remedy. In purity and holiness I will guard my life and my art.

I will not use the knife, not even on sufferers from stone, but will withdraw in favor of such men as are engaged in this work.

Whatever houses I may visit, I will come for the benefit of the sick, remaining free of all intentional injustice, of all mischief and in particular of sexual relations with both female and male persons, be they free or slaves.

What I may see or hear in the course of the treatment or even outside of the treatment in regard to the life of men, which on no account one must spread abroad, I will keep to myself, holding such things shameful to be spoken about.

If I fulfill this oath and do not violate it, may it be granted to me to enjoy life and art, being honored with fame among all men for all time to come; if I transgress it and swear falsely, may the opposite of all this be my lot.[2]

A more contemporary adaptation was written in 1964 by Louis Lasagna (1923–2003), who was for many years the academic dean of Tufts University Medical School. As an introduction to the central concerns of this book, it is worth comparing the two.

I swear to fulfill, to the best of my ability and judgment, this covenant:

I will respect the hard-won scientific gains of those physicians in whose steps I walk, and gladly share such knowledge as is mine with those who are to follow.

I will apply, for the benefit of the sick, all measures [that] are required, avoiding those twin traps of overtreatment and therapeutic nihilism.

I will remember that there is art to medicine as well as science, and that warmth, sympathy, and understanding may outweigh the surgeon's knife or the chemist's drug.

I will not be ashamed to say "I know not," nor will I fail to call in my colleagues when the skills of another are needed for a patient's recovery.

I will respect the privacy of my patients, for their problems are not disclosed to me that the world may know. Most especially must I tread with care in matters of life and death. If it is given me to save a life, all thanks. But it may also be within my power to take a life; this awesome responsibility must be faced with great humbleness and awareness of my own frailty. Above all, I must not play at God.

I will remember that I do not treat a fever chart, a cancerous growth, but a sick human being, whose illness may affect the person's family and economic stability. My responsibility includes these related problems, if I am to care adequately for the sick.

I will prevent disease whenever I can, for prevention is preferable to cure.

I will remember that I remain a member of society, with special obligations to all my fellow human beings, those sound of mind and body as well as the infirm.

If I do not violate this oath, may I enjoy life and art, respected while I live and remembered with affection thereafter. May I always act so as to preserve the finest traditions of my calling and may I long experience the joy of healing those who seek my help.[3]

Lasagna's updated pledge is a recasting to accommodate to more modern times: the Greek gods are no longer invoked, the language no longer refers to male family lineages or "pupils who have taken an oath" only, and the dismissal of "the knife" has been changed to acknowledge that surgery is often a key component of medical treatment.

Today, however, even relatively contemporary formulations like Lasagna's or an earlier one adopted in Geneva in 1948 by the Second General Assembly of the World Medical Association might seem dated. In fact, according to a recent graduate of Harvard Medical School, her class wrote its own, even newer pledge. Much has changed with regard to the moral and ethical challenges today's doctors face—and with regard to the implications of those challenges for the bond of trust between physician and patient. What has not changed is that within the profession of medicine the tradition of making a solemn commitment to adhere to certain standards of character and morality endures. And even in times that present them with many new dilemmas, fledgling doctors still vow to uphold those parts of the ancient oath that are seen as timeless. Respect for one's teachers; cooperation with one's colleagues; and above all, the protection of patients' interests, including a promise of confidentiality—these assurances are deeply embedded in the institutional foundations of what it means to be and act as a physician.

These foundations do not, for our purposes here, determine what a physician actually does; rather they represent a key to understanding the historical belief in the United States that doctors are worthy of our trust. The Hippocratic oath was the first rhetorical foundation of that trust, the pagan halo under which all subsequent collective efforts to stipulate the physician's duties emerged.[4] And the sacred nature of that pledge, in all its contemporary variants and in the broadest sense of the word "sacred," still resonates in American society—despite an erosion of personal and public trust in doctors in recent decades—because of the historical connections between religious beliefs, religious establishments, and the medical profession.

The Protestant Vision of Medicine as a Sacred Vocation

During the nineteenth century, formal codes of guidance for physicians in the United States were the direct inheritance of the work of three British physicians, John Gregory (1724–1773), Thomas Percival (1740–1804), and Michael Ryan (1800–1841).[5] In particular, Percival's *Medical Ethics, or a Code of Institutes and Precepts, Adapted to the Professional Conduct of Physicians and Surgeons* (1803) was the principal source for the "Boston Medical Police," a code of conduct promulgated by members of the Boston Medical Association in 1808. Medical societies in eleven other states adopted some version of this code in subsequent years, and on May 6, 1847, the American Medical Association approved the first national code of medical ethics at a gathering of physicians in Philadelphia.

Echoing the Hippocratic oath, these various codifications of expectations about medical conduct included specific directives about the duties of physicians to their patients (and vice versa), the obligations of physicians to one another, and the obligations of the profession to the public (and vice versa). The principle of reciprocity between physician and patient and between profession and public, as the late historian of medical ethics Chester Burns noted, was exemplified in the work of one American physician, Worthington Hooker, who published the only full-length study of medical ethics to be brought out in the nineteenth century. In writing about Hooker and his time, Burns concluded,

> No American claimed that codes guaranteed medical righteousness. Codes simply provided physicians with some knowledge of the difference between right and wrong professional conduct. Without some ideals and some means of institutionalizing them, there would be little chance to alter professional evils anywhere.[6]

As the medical profession continued to evolve in this country, "righteousness" was indeed an issue, and the question of whether the meaning of this word relates to religion, to morality and character, or to strictly secular standards of conduct is central to the broader question of trust. Historians of nineteenth-century medicine in the United States have long taken for granted its white, Protestant character, so much so that one key to understanding the nature of the public's almost universal trust in medicine, beginning in the middle of the nineteenth century and lasting until the middle of the twentieth, was the near uniformity of its practitioners not only in terms of their race, class, and gender, but also in terms of the kinds of cultural expectations that pertained to how they should act with respect to society, colleagues, and their patients.

In his book *The Therapeutic Perspective: Medical Practice, Knowledge, and Identity in America, 1820–1885*, John Harley Warner writes,

> In a commencement address to Cincinnati medical students in 1877 on "the dignity and sanctity of the medical profession," the speaker asserted that "its chief excellence is not that it is scientific, but that it is redemptive."[7]

To understand and explain illness were important parts of the physician's task, but they did not constitute the whole of it. The physician was more than a natural scientist; he was also a healer. Warner goes on to argue that the commencement speaker, Nathaniel West, was dissenting from the "still novel view that professional identity in medicine should be defined chiefly by science," and in an article titled "Science, Healing and the Physician's Identity," he interprets the "redemptive" dimension of medicine as being the humane impulse to act, whether or not the action taken had been scientifically proven to be therapeutically efficacious.[8] It is significant, however, that the speaker Warner chose to quote on this point was not a physician, although his talk was entitled "The Medical Science and Profession," but rather a Presbyterian minister.[9]

The Reverend Nathaniel West Jr. (1824–1906) graduated from the University of Michigan and the Western Theological Seminary, and served in pulpits in Pittsburgh, Cincinnati, Brooklyn, and St. Paul.[10] In the clerical tradition of working through the relation of revealed truth to practical conduct, West followed the general practice of many other ministers who used the occasion of a commencement speech to put forth their own views about what was at stake in the fledgling physician's obligations to patients and profession.

Quoting Ovid, "Non est in Medico semper releveter ut aeger" (The cure of the patient is not always in the physician's power), West remarked,

> If any one, therefore, will seek the true occasion of the rise of the medical profession, he will find no sufficient explanation of this in science itself, but in an historic fact antecedent to all science, the

first violation of moral laws imposed upon man by his Creator. It involves questions which do not belong to medical science, as such, but to a totally different department of investigation—none the less important on this account, but all the more worthy of moral consideration, as throwing a peculiar sacredness around the profession itself.[11]

The "peculiar sacredness" West attributed to medicine was his way of acknowledging that, far from being hostile to science, the theological beliefs of enlightened Protestants encouraged an examination and justification of how the clerical and medical professions were engaged in a common pursuit of both physical and spiritual well-being.

West insisted that his remarks should not be interpreted as sanctioning all practices alleged to be medical. Charlatans were present in both the medical and clerical professions, he noted. He did not describe in any detail who, in his opinion, walked on the right side and who did not, but he did convey an overall view to his audience similar to that expressed several years earlier by Oliver Wendell Holmes Sr., who concluded in 1869 that although improvements had occurred in the relations between clergymen and physicians, "Whether the world at large will ever be cured of trusting to specifics as a substitute for observing the laws of health, and to mechanical or intellectual formulae as a substitute for character, may admit of question. Quackery and idolatry are all but immortal."[12]

It seems clear that even while admonishing students about the limits and temptations of their vocation, West hoped to join the "scientific" with the "redemptive" in order to secure both a scientific basis for medicine and a theological guide for physicianhood. His long encomium to medicine was not nostalgic but rather intended to reinforce the idea that the new methods of scientific investigation were confirming of, rather than destructive to, Christian truths:

> The skillful anatomist will cut away a whole hemisphere of the brain, slice by slice, and find the Apostle's Creed or the Ten Commandments, faith in God and hope of immortality, with all the mental faculties, just as strong as before the chloroform and knife began their work. The living spirit is the same, its creed the same. Its ethereal essence survives the knife, the martyr's flame, the tomb![13]

In an age of rapid change and development, conflict among physicians about the therapeutic efficacy of differing approaches to disease and treatment did influence clergymen's opinions of the medical profession.[14] But their central concern was contained in the advice they gave to physicians about their moral responsibilities, advice that was intended, at least in part, to define new strategies for professing and promoting Christian faith and values in an era rapidly substituting scientific agnosticism for divine revelation. And in the end, modern codes of medical professionalism owe as much to this professing as to any advances in therapeutic technique.[15]

How ministers communicated the importance of specifically Protestant Christian piety in this context can be seen in a literature of preaching that was directed at medical students and, presumably, their teachers. Both Nathaniel West and Charles Quintard (whose pronouncements we will quote later) were among those ministers who used the occasion of a commencement ceremony to outline Christian ideals as they pertained to medical practice. It is difficult to reconstruct completely who was asked to deliver such addresses, and the vast majority of them, in any case, were not published.[16] But extant versions of speeches, sermons, and eulogies, a list of which is contained in appendix 1, provide ample illustrations of how Protestant clergymen approached the vocation of medicine during the greater part of the nineteenth century.[17] (Clergy asked to deliver commencement addresses to medical students during the second half of the century were overwhelmingly Protestant and male, although Lucretia Mott [1793–1880], the Quaker abolitionist and participant at Seneca Falls, made a speech to medical students in 1849 in Philadelphia,[18] and rabbis delivered several addresses that survive. Catholic priests, however, were virtually invisible in such quasi-public ceremonies.)[19]

Luckily enough for researchers, the preservation of some of the speeches and sermons delivered to medical students in one context or another was assured by an academic custom commonly employed throughout the nineteenth century. Graduating students would request in writing a copy of the graduation speaker's address for the purposes of publication and dissemination to a wider audience. The custom was routine in some places, for example, at the National Medical College or Medical Department of Columbian College, founded in 1822, which is today the George Washington University School of Medicine. At George Washington, only members of the medical faculty were called upon to deliver the address, and the same is generally true for older university medical schools established in the eighteenth century, such as Yale and the University of Pennsylvania.[20] In Philadelphia, a leading center for medical education throughout the nineteenth century, medical schools did not routinely invite clergy to speak to medical students at graduation, although they were regularly asked to open and close such occasions with prayer. But commencement speakers at newer, less tradition-bound institutions—like Tulane University, the University of Arkansas, the University of Maryland, Wayne State University, and the University of Michigan—included a variety of people other than physicians, such as clergymen, senators, governors, lawyers, writers, and university and college presidents.[21] In addition, a handful of surviving published talks by clergymen to medical students in other contexts suggests that both groups often sought one another out in other ways.[22] (See appendix 2.)

A very instructive example, which I will focus on in some detail, is the sermon that the Reverend Henry Augustus Boardman (1808–1880), who led the Tenth Presbyterian Church of Philadelphia for more than forty years, delivered to invited medical students from the University of Pennsylvania and the Jefferson Medical College in 1844, at a special evening gathering at his church on Sunday, November 24. Two days later he received letters from representatives of each school, requesting that he make his sermon available for publication. In all, thirty-two students and faculty members signed the request, indicating that they were speaking for a larger audience in attendance that evening as well.[23]

Boardman began his sermon by quoting from the New Testament book of Colossians 4:14, which refers to "Luke, the beloved physician." He was careful to observe that the term "physician" did not mean the same thing in Luke's time as it did in his own. Striking a theme that would remain central to the Protestant clergy's anxieties about their own duties regarding the well-being of their flocks, he concluded about medicine that "there is no science, theology excepted, which opens a nobler field of inquiry to the human intellect—none which is more intimately associated with our earthly happiness—none which is more entitled to the respect and veneration of society."[24]

The training of physicians demanded "eminent qualifications, both of head and heart," Boardman insisted, but one of these qualifications was "inculcated in the class-room only in an incidental way"—and that was the necessity of cultivating "personal religion." The phrase "personal religion" was not meant to affirm a "bare intellectual assent to the truths of Christianity" nor "a rigid conformity to all the peculiarities of any particular denomination of Christians." It was meant to be "synonymous with true piety," consisting, "in general, in the renewing and sanctifying of the heart by the Holy Spirit, a cordial reliance upon the merits of Jesus Christ as the only ground of acceptance with God, and an habitual desire and aim to lead a holy life, and walk according to the pure morality of the Scriptures."[25]

The ingredients of "true piety," Boardman maintained, were available to all who were willing to subscribe to them, but he went on to outline seven reasons why physicians, in particular, might be vulnerable to both a lack of personal religion and to what he termed infidelity.

One concern of Boardman's was that because of the demands of the profession, a physician might have insufficient time or motivation to examine the subject of religion, or to attend Sabbath worship. He also expressed concern that science itself might "inspire men with inflated views of the sufficiency of human reason on *all* subjects; and thus, from questioning the necessity, they may easily come to deny the fact of a Divine revelation," comparing "the habit of reasoning from induction and analogy which belongs to every scientific physician" with "the argument from miracles which constitutes so material a portion of the external evidences of Christianity." He also concluded that physicians were more likely than others to see too much of the world of human suffering, and that this might erode their religious faith. "It may be worthy of consideration," he stated, "whether familiarity with such spectacles has not sometimes assisted in fortifying them against the requisitions of Christianity, and even [hastened] them into infidelity."[26]

The admonition that the scientific imagination could have a corrosive effect upon the moral character of the physician had to be carefully made to an audience of physicians in an era when science was subjecting traditional beliefs of all kinds to empirical inquiry. In this context, Boardman was careful not to attack science as such but only the indifference to spiritual needs that could arise from too great an absorption in the strictly medical. He then proceeded to examine specific attributes of character that were essential to the right conduct of the Christian physician, and the dangers to that character.

The first was that "physicians are exposed to peculiar *trials of temper*, as well from the unprofessional conduct of their brethren, as from the inconsiderateness, caprice and resentment of their patients." Although personal religion "cannot secure them an exemption from these vexations ... the temper fostered by religion—the meek, patient, forgiving, benevolent, ingenuous temper everywhere inculcated in the Bible, not simply as a graceful appendage of Christianity, but as one of its essential elements—is the best safeguard a physician can have against the wrongs we have been contemplating, and his best antidote to them when they *are* inflicted":

> A man with this temper will be uniformly just to his brethren and his patients. He will be slow to give, and equally slow to take, offense. He will be free from envy and suspicion, and will put the best construction upon all doubtful passages. He will be as jealous of his professional as of his popular, reputation. . . . Where he has perpetuated a wrong, he will not be ashamed, on discovering it, to acknowledge the offense, and make every reparation in his power. . . . All this, and much more than this, a physician will do, not because his interest will be promoted by it, nor simply because it is his duty to do it, but also because it is the very course to which his feelings prompt him, and which he finds his happiness in pursuing.[27]

In these characterizations of the ideal doctor, the qualities of action on the part of the physician were seen as not merely technical or formulaic; rather the Reverend Boardman described the discovery of personal happiness in the intensification of professional obligations inspired by religious commitments. The fulfillment of duty for duty's sake was not sufficient:

> The life of a fellow-being, and the earthly happiness of a family, may be suspended upon their decision of a question so nicely balanced that they [physicians] shrink from deciding it either way. The load of anxiety they sometimes feel in these circumstances must well nigh crush them to earth. The image of their patient follows them like their shadow; it puts them upon a reexamination of the authorities in their libraries; it throws a gloom over their fire-side enjoyments; it sits beside their couch at night; it makes them feel, for the time, that all the emolument and honors of the profession are no equivalent for its trials.[28]

To place squarely upon the physician all of the anxieties about the medical fate of the patient exaggerates the day-to-day reality in which most doctors, then and now, find themselves. The key to this aspect of Boardman's characterization turns on the degree of self-imposed pressure to redirect the "load of anxiety" into a constructive engagement with patients and their families, while at the same time his reference to "the emolument and honors of the profession" signals changes in the status of the profession within society.

The Tension between the Vision of a Calling and the Rise of Professionalism

The professionalization of medicine in the United States during the second half of the nineteenth century has been the subject of numerous histories.[29] Scholarly efforts to describe the conditions of medical practice during this time have yielded a remarkable consensus about how scientific discoveries transformed the powers of physicians to heal. The improving economic fortunes of the profession have also been well documented and debated since the turn of the twentieth century.[30] Gradually, as scientific research was pursued in newly organized programs of undergraduate and professional education, the physician became the most popular symbol of professional authority.

At the dawn of this new era, the Reverend Charles T. Quintard (1824–1898), second Episcopal bishop of Tennessee, who practiced and taught as a physician before entering the ministry, had this to say about the tension between character and medical skill within the profession itself:

> I have thus glanced at some of the moral characteristics of the true Physician, and have alluded, incidentally, to his mental qualifications.

These last, however, are sometimes, and I may say often found disconnected from the former. Brilliancy of intellect and profundity of learning, do not pre-suppose either benevolence of disposition, or purity of heart. . . . Good men are not all physicians, nor are all physicians good men. I may esteem and honor a man for his purity, but I cannot esteem a physician who trusts alone to kindness of disposition for the performance of his duties and responsibilities.[31]

Quintard, like many other ministers, was not indifferent to the powerful claims of an emerging scientific medicine. He was especially aware of the new as well as the enduring meanings of physicianhood. At this point, it is worth noting, the basis of the profession's increasing cultural authority derived from the proximity of the established, but declining, public influence of the clergyman alongside the growing public visibility of the doctor.

An illustration of the latter can be found in the self-congratulatory depiction of the final dinner of the sixth annual meeting of the American Medical Association in 1853 in New York City. "No assemblage in America," wrote a correspondent to the *Ohio Medical and Surgical Journal*, "perhaps in the world, ever met combining so much moral worth, self-denial in the cause of humanity, disinterested exertion for the advancement of science and a more thorough identity of educated alliance to our free institutions than this did." Toasts offered at the occasion included "Divinity, Law, Medicine—Three graces, all of which combined, support each other." Responding to this toast, the Reverend Samuel Osgood remarked that divinity and medicine were "interpreters of the same heavenly mercy," and he "gave the following sentiment, after speaking of medicine as nature evangelized":

> Medicine and Divinity—The two stood together in the beginning, when science was darkened by superstition; they shall stand nearer together at the end, when science and faith shall be recognized as different, but harmonious, aspects of the same divine wisdom and goodness.[32]

The ritual comparison of each of the learned professions (law, divinity, and medicine) to one another was often made on formal occasions that celebrated professional authority, and the Reverend Osgood's remarks would appear to secure the pious end of that comparative spectrum. But such comparisons were also the source of revealing humor, if not impiety. Delivering the valedictory address to the University of the State of New York Medical Department in 1860, Dr. Seth L. Chase observed,

> The physician's duties [are] more arduous than those of other professions. The clergyman prescribes once a week to his patients *en masse*, each one of them selecting the medicine best adapted to his

neighbor's case. (Laughter.) The lawyer can with impunity allow the scales of justice to continue vibrating for an indefinite time. On the contrary, the physician must go when and where he is called, leaving the quiet fireside, the interesting book, pleasing society, his bed, everything, to answer the call for aid against the destroyer.[33]

Compare Dr. Chase's observations to those of Dr. Troyen A. Brennan in 1991:

> To allay his [a patient's] fears, Dr. A. drove over to the hospital, excusing herself from a dinner party. . . . This kind of visit is one of the most gratifying aspects of medical practice. But it is not really part of relations between citizens in the liberal state. Dr. A. could have called the house officer physicians and ensured that the blood counts were to be checked. That would have been adequate. Yet it would not have fulfilled the sense of duty and affection Dr. A. and other doctors have for their patients. . . . While I would hardly call a simple visit like this one a virtuous or altruistic act, it does represent a morality in which more than a simple "contract" between two autonomous people is expected.[34]

The contrasting assumptions that underlie these two quotes captures the very different expectations about the calling or vocation of medicine in 1860 as compared to 1991, and in so doing raise the question about how the expectations about doctors' duties in 1860 became the cultural expectations of both patients and physicians for more than a century. A second question is how the "sense of duty and affection" relates today to what is "adequate," and what both have to do with trusting doctors.

Meanwhile, returning again to the nineteenth century, no well-educated Protestant minister in the United States could ignore the public consequences of the physician's emerging powers. The gradual disestablishment of Protestant authority in America led those in religious offices to accommodate themselves to new leadership in the medical community that sought to organize and direct an overtly professional system of higher education.[35] Daniel Coit Gilman (1831–1908), first president of Johns Hopkins University, had considered the ministry but resisted because he sought, finally, to impose a duty on society rather than on individuals. Contemplating a vocation in 1854, at the age of twenty-two, Gilman wrote:

> I told him [Noah Porter, who later became president of Yale University] that if I should become a minister I should want to preach about every day affairs—not in the style of H.W.B. [Henry Ward Beecher] if I could get above it, but in a more dignified manner— and that instead of dwelling long and regularly upon such points as

original sin and the doctrine of election, I should urge the practical application of the Bible to common events and daily habits.[36]

Gilman recognized early on that the future of medical education required organizational changes that no church-affiliated leader or church movement could be relied upon to help effect, and within decades Johns Hopkins University Medical School had become the exemplar of contemporary medical education and research as the new discoveries of science enhanced its prestige in ways that religious elites could no longer emulate in the older, more established schools, all of which rapidly followed the lead set by Hopkins during the first quarter of the twentieth century.[37]

In an important defense of the professional order fostered by elite physicians during the second half of the nineteenth century, Barbara Gutmann Rosenkrantz dismisses as "a post-Flexnerian myth" the argument that professional authority was achieved exclusively by "wringing out the medical economy through reducing the number of poorly trained doctors."[38] The old ethics, she contends, embodied in the AMA's code until its substantial revision in 1903, were neither antiscientific nor antiprofessional; rather they were rooted in specific qualities of professional tolerance that were being transformed by the demands of a new professional order that included considerations of "standing in medical school, hospital staff membership, and participation in specialists' societies," and which replaced "the outworn armatures of latitudinarian collegiality."[39]

Rosenkrantz has described the prebureaucratic features of medicine as its practitioners began their adaptation to the new rules of scientific meritocracy at the end of the nineteenth century. Who, in fact, was qualified to enter medical school, to practice, and to consult, were all questions that new forms of accountability would settle, at least in principle. But at the time, for the elder statesmen of the profession, "a professional ethos in which accountability to science replaced relations with colleagues and patients was a crack in the wall of tradition that had supported the reputation and authority of medicine in the past." Trust in physicians was still affirmed first in their social relations with peers and patients. Rosenkrantz sees the emergence of a new professional identity as not simply "a transformation of vocation authorized by the growth of scientific knowledge," but also as the transformation of the "reputation and authority of medicine."[40]

The idea of a "transformation of vocation" requires further elaboration, insofar as the collegial culture of physicians—a key element of the legacy of the Hippocratic oath—is viewed from their standpoint alone. As important as the medical profession's internal disputes about new theories and treatments may have been to physicians themselves, notice was also taken by others. Humorous aphorisms, composed by outsiders to medicine over millennia, were again quoted to confirm the fact that little real progress had occurred in the physician's understanding of disease and its treatment—a point that harkened back to an earlier vein of popular distrust of physicians. As the transformation of vocation under the new dispensations of science proceeded, the threatened ethos of physicianhood as defined in part by gentlemanly and collegial authority was rescued once again with the ever persistent tradition of personal authority whose origins we can trace in this country to the endorsement and beliefs of Protestant ministers.[41]

In this context, I would argue that what remains of the moral authority of the doctor today resides in what is abstractly called the "physician-patient interaction." In his sermon of 1844, Boardman referred to the Puritan divine Richard Baxter, who "remarked [that] what belongs to the pastor *ex officio*, belongs to the physician *ex charitate*." Unlike the pastor, the physician "has access to individuals whom no clergyman can reach," and

> the same counsels uttered by him would be more likely to produce a good impression than if they came from the lips of a clergyman, because, in the latter case, they might be heard as the promptings of professional duty, while in the other, not only would they be ascribed to a generous and disinterestedness kindness, but they would derive additional weight from the presumption, on the part of the patient, that they proceeded from one who understood his physical condition.

Boardman concluded that the physician "has an ascendancy" over the patient "which no other person can have—that his imagination (to borrow the expressive language of a learned and venerable professor in one of our medical schools) has 'conferred on him the attributes of a *tutelary divinity*.'"[42]

Acting in the capacity of a "tutelary divinity" was, in Boardman's view, the physician's most important role: "There can be no doubt," he stated, "that the sick sometimes suffer intensely from *suppressed anxiety* in relation to their spiritual state. . . . A few kind words of spiritual counsel, kindly offered, have, in some instances of this sort, done much to tranquilize the system, where the best pharmaceutical agents have failed." Here, early on, we can sense the tension between the commitment of doctors to religiously based moral precepts and the emergence of new ways of evaluating their conduct. Boardman acknowledged that "different cases require different treatment," but maintained that "the responsibility of physicians is not restricted to their merely technical duties."[43]

The practice of inviting medical students into Philadelphia churches continued with a sermon preached by Joel Parker (1799–1873) in the Clinton Street Presbyterian Church in 1848. The Reverend Parker spent most of his career in New York City and was an early president of Union Theological Seminary. Parker began his sermon by quoting Luke 4:23, "Physician, heal thyself," noting that this was one of several places where Christ compared "the functions of the spiritual teacher to those of the healing art." Parker's comparisons were clearly sociological: "Neither Clergyman nor the Physician, have anything to do directly with the estates, the social position, or the political relations of their fellow citizens."[44] The pastor's and the physician's influence alike were directed toward persons as individuals; thus, the pastor or the doctor "cannot exercise the influence of a good man without *being* a good man. He cannot banish bad moral influences, without being himself personally averse to them."[45] But Parker also cited a symptom of the changing balance in terms of public regard for ministers and doctors, one that points to the tension between the professions, when he observed:

> It is not uncommon for Physicians to resist the visits of clergyman till the last hope from medical remedies is extinct. That there are cases which demand such a procedure, no thoughtful person can doubt. But when it is made a rule to pursue this course, it creates an impression in the community of such a character, that the moment the clergyman is sent for, the sustaining influence of hope is suddenly taken away, and you might as well sound his funeral knell in the ear of the patient, as to propose a visit from the minister of the gospel.

Parker also commented that "corrupted forms of Christianity [thus referring to Roman Catholicism] . . . pronounce incantations over the dying, and anoint the extremities with oil, and exorcise evil spirits by shreds of unclassical Latin."[46] His view of the physician's responsibilities required that the doctor maintain a more than strictly medical relationship with the patient, but also that the clergyman be available to assist at other times than during the final hours of life. The Catholic approach did not preclude such a relationship between a doctor, his patient, and a member of the clergy, but Parker and other Protestants saw "spiritual counsel" as distinct from and superior to ritual practices.

Despite the scorn expressed by Parker about "corrupted forms of Christianity," he acknowledged that Protestant ministers were also sometimes a source of anxiety from the perspective of doctors and patients. Physicians "are afraid that he [the clergyman] will present religion in its gloomy aspects and agitate the patient with oppressive fears or fill his mind with hot and injurious excitement," he noted, and he expressed the hope that doctors would not ignore the useful function of the clergy because the zeal of a few might disturb their patients.[47]

The clergyman's interventions were complicated by this issue, but the physician's interventions, particularly on matters of personal conduct, required careful guidance as well:

> Men will apply to you to heal diseases occasioned by intemperance, or other vicious indulgences. A sound ethical code undoubtedly requires it of you, not to injure the reputation of those who entrust you with a knowledge of their faults. When you know their secret sins, however, and when you are careful not to use that knowledge to their disadvantage, you have the finest opportunity to employ the power of reproof successfully. You can prescribe virtue as a remedy.[48]

The idea of "virtue as a remedy" falls squarely between a religious hope and a medical responsibility, especially in those matters pertaining to the conduct of a patient that might have adverse effects on health. The responsibility to reprove a patient about failure with regard to the virtue of temperance, for example, was something a physician could consider valid both religiously and medically. The key to understanding the specifically Protestant dispensation on how a physician was to think about this responsibility is contained in the word "prescribe."

What seems clear in retrospect, after more than a hundred years of the institutional displacement of religious authority in the United States, is the inevitability with which physicians, in particular, were regarded as the successors to ministers in matters of individual moral guidance, at least insofar as the behaviors so guided had medical implications. Not every physician viewed this part of the medical practitioner's role in specifically Christian terms, but even as its influence waned, the Protestant establishment's insistence that the physician must first be a believing Christian, and thus a righteous person, gave added public credibility to the rising status of the physician's office, that is, his position of authority in society.

In other words, in Parker's system of values, the personal *was* the official, and his caricature of Catholic ritual was a rebuttal to anyone who argued that person and office could be separated. Martin Luther had noted that any office might inspire respect even if those who held it were not pious, but Parker's view of society insists that the inspiration of public confidence in any such offices or authorities rests on the spiritual condition of those who occupy them. Returning to this theme again and again, he concluded,

> You cannot win for yourself the esteem, the heart-felt confidence that is cheerfully awarded, by almost every one to a pious physician, without being a good man; without fearing God and keeping his commandments. You may think you are doing it by substituting

a spiritual finesse for piety. . . . Yet, if you be not a true Christian, men will penetrate your sinister management.[49]

"Physician, heal thyself" thus became, in Parker's vision, an opportunity to offer a renewal of confidence in the office of the medical doctor against the ever-lurking prospects of "sinister management" that might develop if the physician lost sight of the sick-chamber as a sanctuary:

> We turn again to the solemn scene, and listen to the sobs of the widow and the orphan, and there stands the physician, a cold skeptic, or an indifferent man of the world. How shall he administer spiritual comfort? He cannot do it. He is himself bereaved. In his patient, he has lost a friend. He has need to heal himself.[50]

Parker knew that he was instructing by analogy. "Gentleman," he told the medical students in his audience, "you may think that I am endeavoring to impose upon you responsibilities which belong only to my own profession. . . . Our duties arise from our relations and our opportunities for doing good."[51] This slightly ambivalent attempt to encourage unity of purpose by appealing to the complementarity of roles of religion and medicine was also evident in many other clerical addresses on the physician's moral authority. (A brief aside: The origins of today's new arenas of specialization in the administration of what nineteenth-century Protestant ministers spoke of as "spiritual comfort" may be attributed to the public's wide exposure to diverse religious ideas and psychological theories in more recent decades. And later attempts—by social scientists, for example—to disestablish further the special status of physicians must first be understood in light of this historical background of the efforts of Protestant ministers to transfer something of their own authority to their professional peers in medicine.)[52]

In the same year that Joel Parker delivered his sermon, the Reverend Joseph Frederick Berg (1812–1871) of the Reformed Church, spoke to medical students from another school, Pennsylvania College, in much the same vein. Berg emphasized especially the healing powers of Jesus: "He gives but one prescription, and that is *faith*. All who trust him are healed."[53] And he did not shy away from insisting "that whatever may be said respecting the propriety of the Christian minister's being qualified to practice the healing art, there can be no doubt that every physician should be fully prepared to preach the gospel."[54] "The physician cannot work miracles, neither can we," he stated, and then he asked, "But can we not console them?" The Protestant vernacular, which was used in discussing how divine revelation related to everyday matters, touched often upon the matter of consolation, carefully avoiding any special claim by the minister to provide such, but insisting that the physician, like the minister, should recognize the necessity and the challenges of doing so: "And that may be in our profession as decidedly malpractice as it is in yours, to administer a sedative when the system needs a most powerful stimulant."[55]

Another important element of the Protestant contribution to the enduring values first espoused by the medical profession in the nineteenth century is exemplified in the sermons of Elias Root Beadle (1812–1879), pastor of the Second Presbyterian Church in Philadelphia, who preached twice to medical students from Jefferson Medical College and the University of Pennsylvania, in 1865 and 1874. Although Beadle drew many of the same conclusions about faith, moral character, and the vocation of medicine that his fellow Philadelphia clergymen had endorsed, he was more direct about the hierarchy of callings:

> I greet you here, and hail you only to give you words of cheer. I respect your choice. I disparage no other profession. My presence here to-night, is evidence that there is one which I prefer before it. I wish you had done the same; but I leave that with God and you. I honor all professions and all lawful callings.[56]

And, while still using the vocabulary of faith, he put a new kind of moral pressure upon the emerging profession, insisting, for example, that doctors minister to the poor: "Though they cannot recompense thee; but, '*thou shalt be recompensed at the resurrection of the just.*'"[57]

Beadle spoke about the physician's obligation to what would later be termed public health in both his sermons. In 1865 he observed,

> And the question is fairly pressed upon you at this moment, whether you cannot arrest the physical degeneracy, so apparent in our time, and restore human life to its normal conditions. Whether by insisting upon a better mode of life, more nutritious food, purer social enjoyments, higher mental culture; by retarding the speed and lessening the pressure of all commercial and business life, you may not again enlarge its boundary and change the whole face of human society.[58]

By 1874, as the United States became more and more industrialized and both migration to the cities and immigration increased, Beadle's perception of the effects of urban crowding on public health had become more sophisticated and more specific:

> As population has largely increased, and necessities of civilization compelled men to herd in cities, to crowd manufactures, to gather in large armies, to live in unhealthy localties [sic] and labor under influences adverse to health, many questions will arise which the

wise and thoughtful physician can alone properly deal with and answer. Clear and decisive sanitary knowledge must be reached and disseminated. Causes which impair public health and shorten human life must be sought out and removed. City life, prison life, different forms of labor and all forms of exposure, must be studied and the essential conditions of health, ascertained and made known.... The command to "Heal the Sick" [Matt. 10:8] covers much ground. It is both to work cure and remove cause.[59]

Combining a deeply religious and thus conservative view of the ideal character of the doctor with a progressive outlook about the most significant health problems of his time, Beadle balanced an evangelical approach to public health with the classic mission of saving souls.

In no other hands are such sacred trusts deposited as in yours. You are the confidant of families. You carry the strange and often sad secret of human hearts. You are admitted to privacies which are denied to all others.... It is here, in the very citadel of all sacred relations and social excellence that your integrity will be tried and your character as men and physicians put to the severest test.[60]

By admonishing his listeners about the "sacred" character of the "strange and often sad secret of human hearts," Beadle was also endorsing the authority of physicians to minister in special ways when clergy could not.

In the end, what resonates above all in the speeches given by Protestant clergymen to physicians throughout the nineteenth century is the deeply held conviction that the vocation of medicine added up to more than the sum of training and ability. Preaching to the medical students of Jefferson Medical College in 1863, the Reverend Stephen Townsend, M.D., concluded,

To follow a calling involving such duties and responsibilities, something more than an intimate acquaintance with anatomy, physiology, chemistry, therapeutics and the principles and practice of medicine, surgery and obstetrics is required. You must be filled with an exalted sense of the onerous duty, the moral and religious obligations, and the profound responsibility which are inseparably connected with your mission; and you must come to the work, moreover, with an earnest, sincere and truthful desire to advance the interests of medicine, and thereby the prosperity of men, as far as in you lies the power.[61]

It is this now seemingly ineffable and indefinable "something more" that shines, like a halo, above those callings in which success demands both personal presence and personal understanding, in a word, trust.

CHAPTER 2

The Influence of Catholic Perspectives

Unlike the Protestant heritage that coincided so effectively with emerging ideals about professional authority in the United States—and played a large part in defining those ideals—another religious tradition, sometimes entangled in public disagreements with the dominant culture, offered its own, more deliberate approaches to complex matters involving religious teachings and medical ethics. As a sociologist, I would argue that Catholic clergy and physicians represent an important case of professional exceptionalism in the history of American medicine.[1] And to this day, by virtue of religious belief rather than professional training, Catholic physicians and Catholic hospitals think and act differently with respect to key medical matters, especially such matters as contraception, end-of-life care, and abortion.[2]

In this chapter I will focus on one aspect of the last of these issues for discussion—the nineteenth-century debate about by what means, and to what end, a physician might be allowed intervene in cases where a threat to both a mother and her unborn fetus was either determined in advance or evident in crisis during childbirth.

The Tradition of Pastoral Medicine

Because, as historian Burton Bledstein and others have argued, Protestant ideas about "vocation" have been so dominant in defining the culture of professionalism in American life,[3] less attention has been paid to the importance and influence of Catholic thought in medicine in particular. But that influence has been there throughout our history as a nation, and it pertains not only to the religious foundations of our trust in doctors but also to current debates about medical ethics.

In a historically significant summation of the Protestant perspective on character and duty, published in 1919 and entitled "Vocation in Medicine and Nursing," William Osler, an exemplar of Protestant medical professionalism, described the "four great features" of the medical guild: its noble ancestry, its solidarity, its progressive character, its singular beneficence.[4]

At the time, Catholic thought did not dissent from the vision of the medical profession celebrated by Osler, but it had evolved separately over many centuries and represented a specific and different tradition of reasoning regarding the moral dimensions of the choices doctors make in treating their patients.

The dominant Protestant culture of nineteenth-century America endorsed scientific professionalism over and against both medical and religious forms of sectarianism but continued to advance the view of medicine as a vocation or calling. In Catholicism, however, a calling still referred first and foremost to a life served in the church;[5] put sociologically, part of the suspicion directed toward Catholics in this country during the nineteenth century arose from the Protestant belief that service to an overarching institution and its traditions was less inspired than service based upon individual conscience.[6] Yet as Protestant reliance on the dictates of individual conscience began to reflect a less and less cohesive public consensus about such matters as abortion, the Catholic tradition of moral reasoning about medically complex cases—what came to be called pastoral medicine—offered frameworks to both the medical profession and the public about how to deliberate upon and resolve the issues they raised.

Medical ethicist David F. Kelly has described three "cognate predisciplines" to twentieth-century medical ethics: (1) medical jurisprudence;[7] (2) "medical etiquette" as derived from codes of ethics;[8] and (3) pastoral medicine. The field of pastoral medicine attends to the relationship between theology and medicine, and is part of the larger tradition of casuistry as guided by what was seen as natural law.

Casuistry is a specialized term that originally referred to the application by theologians of general principles of morality to specific cases—especially those in which a person might face conflicts of conscience or duty—in order to determine what should be done and how responsibility should be defined. It is worth noting that from the eighteenth century on, for English speakers the word carried slightly sinister connotations which implied that the complexities of the reasoning involved might be used to permit an evasion rather than an adherence to the call of duty or conscience—and that these connotations may have been connected to anti-Catholic sentiments. Nevertheless, as a part of this tradition as it was originally understood, the field of pastoral medicine initially provided medical information for the rural pastor "in caring physically for people lacking proper medical care" as well as "moral treatises from moral theology intended to inform medical personnel of their ethical responsibilities,"[9] and it has addressed a multitude of specific and hypothetical cases over many centuries.

Kelly cites the seventeenth-century figure Paolo Zacchia, personal physician to Pope Innocent X for eleven years (1644–55), as the "first of the real forefathers of pastoral medicine." According to Kelly, Zacchia's "most important contribution to the development of medical ethics was his opinion that the ensoulment of a fetus takes place at fertilization."[10] Anticipating the growing power of science on medical thinking about many matters, Zacchia's three-volume Latin treatise, *Quaestiones medico-legales*, reviewed a broad range of problems that could be said to be medical in their implications, including "fetal development, pregnancy testing, multiple births, causes of fetal death ... mental illness, poisons ... sexual impotence, sterility, dissimulation of illness and epidemics, miracles, virginity, and rape, fasting and Lent, wounds, mutilation and castration."[11] (And this was only the first volume.)

The two further volumes of Zacchia's treatise examined "the physician's liability before the law for his mistakes, torture and legal penalties for criminals, and the order of rank between doctors and lawyers ... [as well as] monsters, the obligation of hearing Mass and reciting the Office during illness ... stigmata ... pestilence, tobacco, coffee, liquor." The treatise concluded with a compilation of, as Kelly puts it, "canonical precedents in the medical-theological and medical-ethical area."[12]

Kelly's extensive review of the Catholic perspective also includes a discussion of the work of the seventeenth-century Belgian theologian Michael Boudweyns, who is credited with being the first writer to focus on the moral dilemmas that could arise in medical practice in particular. In his 450-page work *Ventilabrum medico-theologicum* (1666), Boudweyns posed questions addressed to the physician, under seventy-four topics, that foreshadow many of the issues doctors still face today, especially those related to what is now known as "reproductive medicine." These questions included the following:

> May he impede the production of sperm, or destroy the genitals? May he suggest masturbation in order to regain health? May he, for someone's health, break the hymen? May he advise his patient to marry for health? May he impede conception? May he procure an abortion? ... May the impotent marry and what advice should be given to them? ... Are married people allowed to have intercourse at any time and in any manner, when health is not at issue? May pregnant women or nursing women fast, and are they obliged to? ... Is a mother obliged to nurse her child herself?[13]

Seventeenth-century questions should not be anachronistically assigned twenty-first-century implications, yet the persistence with which such questions were raised—especially, but not only—in the Catholic tradition is striking, given the consistent absence of similar perplexities and analyses among Protestant clergymen. (Orthodox Jewish interpretations of biblical and Talmudic sources can be viewed as a parallel source of discussion,[14] but since during the time period in question they were not widely influential, they lie outside our purview for now.)

Balancing Lives: Direct or Indirect Abortion versus Cesarean Section

Historian James Mohr attributes to nineteenth-century Protestantism a "blackout" on the subject of abortion, and it does appear that during that time Protestant clergymen did not pronounce on the subject in a way that is comparable to the Catholic pastoral tradition.[15] But to attribute such "silence" only to ambivalence or indifference on the part of Protestant ministers may misconstrue the role that American Protestantism played in shaping the public character of medical professionalism, especially with regard to this issue. The focus on "medical ethics" and "medical etiquette" by the leadership of the American Medical Association from its inception in 1847 was in every vital respect Protestant in tone and character, as these elite ranks were in the vast majority Protestant men, but the medical literature on abortion written by these physicians did not endorse the procedure; rather they were intent on retaining control over any variants of it, against other medical entrepreneurs to be sure, but also in response to their own culture, in which the performance of abortion was understood as at least problematic and most likely sinful, depending on the circumstances under which it occurred.

In fact, American Protestant physicians had succeeded in securing their professional authority in part by campaigning to outlaw abortion except in rare cases and only if performed by licensed physicians. The discussion of circumstances under which abortion and other medical procedures might be permitted was therefore not an exclusively Catholic preoccupation by any means. The debate about abortion in American society was first taken up by doctors whose Protestant moral bearings were informed by religious convictions that had much in common with Catholic moral reasoning. ("Criminal abortion" was a term widely used for the performance of any procedure that resulted in the termination of a pregnancy except under dire and specifically medical circumstances.) But in the end, distinctively Catholic perspectives on the choices doctors must make in the course of medical practice provided an initial and enduring framework in which debate about what is morally permissible and what is not continues to take place to this day.

Until the nineteenth century, the deliberations that arose out of the Catholic casuistic tradition of pastoral medicine were conducted almost exclusively in Latin. The emergence of a literature in languages other than Latin (primarily German) began in the early nineteenth century, coinciding with the ever larger role that physicians rather than priests then played in decisions about medical cases that had fallen for hundreds of years in Europe under the canonical authority of the Catholic Church.

The first publication in America of an English translation of a Latin work on Catholic pastoral medicine appeared in 1878; the original had been written by Carl Franz Nicolaus Capellmann (1841–1898), a German Catholic physician.[16] Published in New York and Cincinnati by Friedrich Pustet, printer to the Holy Apostolic See and the Sacred Congregation of Rites, Capellmann's *Pastoral Medicine* was translated by a Pennsylvania parish priest, William Dassel, who in his preface remarked straightforwardly about the book's intended audience:

> As this work is addressed *exclusively* to priests and physicians, I have endeavored, with the author, to lessen the disgust necessarily provoked by unavoidable details, by putting them into a Latin disguise, when that could be done without any risk of misunderstanding.
>
> Nevertheless, I reiterate, most earnestly and solemnly, that the work is intended *wholly*, *exclusively*, and *entirely*, for the *professional* use of priest or physician, and that it is altogether unfit for the perusal of the lay or general reader; as indeed must all works be, treating of similar subjects.[17]

Dassel's intention to cite the authority of Capellmann's deliberations as well as to promote the responsibilities of a select audience—namely clergymen and physicians—for whom such deliberations were intended, required a careful reticence, exemplified in the selective use of Latin phrases even in the English translation. (This tendency persisted, no matter what the personal cultural background of the physician might be. Long after the disappearance of Latin substitutions for what were once construed as indelicacies in English, such reticence would be interpreted, especially in sociological criticism, as an element of "professional dominance"—that is, an assertion of special knowledge not accessible to, and thus not appropriate for, the "lay or general reader.") And Dassel certainly did not intend his translation to imitate any strategies of reformation that might undermine the church's authority to pronounce on the moral matters of medical practice. As Capellmann, the original author, noted,

> In whatever is written in this work, it has been my intention to be in complete accord with the doctrines of the Holy Roman Catholic Church. Should anything have been inadvertently advanced ever so little at variance with them, I recall and disavow it, by anticipation, unconditionally.[18]

Among Capellmann's most pressing concerns was the approach taken by medicine toward the unborn child. In addressing the interruption of

pregnancy, he asserted what has become a fundamental, if not *the* fundamental, tenet of contemporary right-to-life doctrine:

> We must maintain that the human embryo is endowed with the
> rational soul at the very instant of conception, and that the impreg-
> nated human foetus is an individual human being. Each individual
> human being, and consequently the impregnated human foetus,
> has the right to live.[19]

In this context, the concept of a "rational soul" that was embodied at "the
very instant of conception" was intended to counter long-standing claims,
inherited from Aristotle and others, that presented other opinions about
when the human soul came into existence.

Capellmann's logic proceeded, then, with clarity. The "right to live"
cannot be disputed except under two circumstances: "1) The individual is
deprived of it by acting against divine and human laws, or by trespassing on
all natural and social order; or unless, 2) By any unlawful attack on the body
or life of another, this other is justified, in self-defence, to harm the unlawful
assailant, even to the depriving him of his life in order to preserve his own."
In both circumstances, the fetus cannot forfeit its right to live because, in
the first instance, it is unable to act and thus cannot be condemned for any
action, and in the second instance it cannot be considered an "unjust aggressor," thus ruling out the claim of self-defense.[20]

At this point, Capellmann acknowledged the progress of medical science,
and in so doing he subtly reframed important issues for future debate. His
outlook, while informed by church teachings, explicitly acknowledged that
new developments in medical practice would have profound implications
for how those teachings would be applied. In his treatise, while keeping close
to a faith-based system of values, he gave voice to an understanding of fetal
development that derived principally from medical rather than theological
considerations. He argued, for instance, that while abortion may never be
used *directly* to save the life of the mother, a medical treatment other than
abortion that is deemed necessary to save her life but which might at the
same time cause abortion might sometimes be permitted;[21] in other words, if
an abortion is not the intent, the physician may proceed with his treatments
of the pregnant woman, so long as "every precaution [is] taken to avoid the
forbidden effect."[22] And in his view, one particular medical condition did
allow for interpreting an otherwise "direct" operation as an "indirect" one.
It was not as if this condition was new in the medical sense; rather, the medical understanding of its cause had improved. Abortion would be permitted

> only in the single case where the uterus, with the foetus, is locked
> in the upper strait, as may happen through, retroversion, sinking

and prolapsus of the pregnant womb. If all other known means of turning or replacing the uterus fail, I believe it is to be *allowable* to induce abortion indirectly, by procuring the discharge of waters, or by the perforation of the foetal membranes. (Emphasis added)

In this medical emergency, Capellmann noted, when the "mother's life is in an immediate danger" and there "is no other means of saving the mother,"[23] abortion of the fetus might be induced, but the use of the term "allowable" was immediately qualified in a footnote:

I have learned that some theologians do not approve of indirect abortion even in this case. I see no reason to recede from my opinion, until my reasonings are refuted and until I am convinced that there is wanting one of the conditions which make, according to the above, the operation allowable.[24]

It could be argued that the great achievement of obstetric medicine throughout the course of the twentieth century was its continuous progress in eliminating strictly medical indications for the interruption of pregnancy,[25] and it seems clear that decades earlier Capellmann was already trying to anticipate what future developments might mean in terms of the doctor's dilemma with regard to any procedure that would have that result, and also that he recognized that the obstetric medicine of his own day could and would likely change in the future. In the end, however, remaining close to the teachings he had inherited from the church, he argued that if medicine could find another way to save the life of an endangered mother without sacrificing the life of the unborn child, then the proscription against abortion would be valid without exception.

But what if medical progress created a further dilemma, one in which the safety of a particular abortion procedure became the justification for its use? The case in point, debated among physicians in the United States throughout the second half of the nineteenth century, addressed the relative safety for the mother of craniotomy (the destruction of the fetus in utero) and Cesarean section during the later stages of pregnancy. In 1882, Capellmann had acknowledged that the practice of perforating the uterus to accomplish delivery was known to the ancients.[26] In an earlier work devoted to the comparative risks of craniotomy (certain death for the child but the possibility of survival for the mother) and Cesarean section (possible survival for the child but probable death for the mother), Capellmann did not deny the place of casuistic reasoning in defining the status of the unborn, but he held out the medical-scientific perspective, underwritten by the use of comparative statistics, as essential to understanding how knowledge of the outcome of many cases could aid in reasoning about what would be permissible in any individual one.[27]

Until improvements in surgical technique and anesthetics were achieved, Cesarean section was regarded as always fatal to the mother. But as medical techniques evolved, Capellmann was among those who enlisted the aid of statistics to demonstrate that, at the very least, "the death-rate ensuing from the Cesarean operation is certainly decreasing, owing to improved surgery and treatment";[28] and that in cases where the lives of both mother and child were in danger, despite a growing use of craniotomy requiring the certain destruction of the fetus, the statistics favoring the relative safety for both of Cesarean section "should suffice to make us reject any such operations [e.g., craniotomy], even from a simply utilitarian standpoint."[29]

Capellmann's observations about Cesarean section in particular provide insight about the long-standing public fears toward the prospect of pain and death then still associated with it. Medical historian Martin Pernick, in documenting the huge changes that the new science of anesthesia brought to medicine during the course of the nineteenth century, has confirmed the difficulty leading physicians faced in changing opinions about the procedure while trying to appease the fears (both professional and public) associated with its use.[30] In this changing medical environment, Capellmann commented that Cesarean section

> is not so much to be dreaded as non-professionals imagine it to be, especially when the patient is placed under the influence of an anesthetic. Sometimes, even now, this operation is performed without an anesthetic. I had several times occasion to observe that an average amount of moral courage does enable the patient to endure its pain even without chloroform.[31]

An "average amount of moral courage" notwithstanding, the fusion of a religiously derived commitment to saving life with statistically derived evidence about the utility of Cesarean section gave ample strength to Capellmann's conviction about the superiority of one much-debated procedure over the other. (The medical utility of Cesarean section has been more or less self-evident for over a hundred years; so much so that at the beginning of the twenty-first century the scales have tipped in the other direction, arguing against any unnecessary resort to the procedure. But this only confirms how medically safe it has become for both mother and child, even as innovations in the monitoring of "normal" deliveries have improved their outcomes as well.)

Capellmann concluded his discussion of Cesarean section with a remarkable reminder of how closely the physician and priest were bound by religious precepts about the sanctity of life. Physicians throughout the nineteenth century were regularly advised by clergy—both Catholic and Protestant—about the ways in which they were obliged, as Christians, to attend to the spiritual needs of their patients. Within the Catholic tradition, this advice was also pressed forcefully in the other direction, that is, in terms of the priest's obligation to be familiar with certain medical procedures in order to fulfill his religious duties. The concern for the baptism of a living child led Capellmann to propose that after the fourth month of pregnancy it was appropriate to perform a Cesarean section in the event of the death of the mother, although he cautioned that on occasion it might not be easy to "ascertain conclusive signs of death, especially if they were sudden or quick. But to ascertain these signs belongs to the province of the physician, who may . . . perform the operation with as much caution as if he were performing it on a living woman, in the event she may still be alive."[32]

"But," Capellmann asked, "what shall be done in the event of a physician not being at hand? Should not the priest, who, in cases of serious illness is almost invariably summoned, perform the operation?" This question puts issues about the medical versus the theological as they affected people's everyday lives into stark relief. As to attending birth, Capellmann encouraged the rural priest in particular to "go through a course of midwifery" in order to be able to help not only spiritually but also physically in difficult situations. And, although its assumptions may surprise us, his answer about whether priests should perform Cesarean sections graphically summarized the ever clearer boundaries between physicians and clergymen:

> But to perform this operation is not only indecorous, but even dangerous, on the part of non-professionals. Apart from the difficulty of proving death certain, the operation requires a detailed knowledge of the parts and great technical ability, which non-professionals cannot have, even should they know by heart an exact description of the operation. To perform the Cesarean operation on the warm, new corpse is exciting even to professionals; especially as there is generally no assistance from a brother-physician, and no time to be lost in procuring such. The alarm caused by the occurrence, the anxious apprehension lest the supposed corpse should move, the copious gushing of the warm blood, . . . all these circumstances allow only professionals to maintain a mental equilibrium, because they are well informed, and accustomed to bloody operations.[33]

This snapshot of the circumstances in which physicians routinely found themselves as compared to what would have been extraordinary circumstances for "non-professionals" adumbrates a theory of professional responsibility (and accountability) that would be made more explicit throughout the twentieth century, especially in sociological descriptions of modern medicine. What was "exciting even to professionals"—by which Capellmann meant challenging and nerve-wracking—added greater weight to the view that professionalism was something more than simply a trained response to emergency situations. The skills associated with such surgical performances to this day require more than a recipe knowledge of what to do, as Capellmann fully appreciated.

The Catholic case for choosing Cesarean section over craniotomy in cases where if nothing was done the likely outcome would be the death of both mother and child was based on specific appeals to the sanctity of the unborn life; and it preceded the medical-scientific consensus that eventually endorsed Cesarean section on the grounds of safety to both mother and child—a consensus that was not rapidly achieved. But on this topic the character of American medical professionalism (read here as Protestant authority) coincided with the appearance in English of Catholic accounts of the European debates about the *medical* superiority of one procedure over another.

Protestant-Catholic Connections

Dr. Samuel Clagett Busey (1828–1901) was among the most outspoken physicians of his time dedicated to improvements in obstetrical care. With respect to Cesarean section, he led the way in establishing medically what those writing in the Catholic pastoral tradition had concluded theologically and morally.[34] He was president four times (1877, 1894–96) of the Medical Society of the District of Columbia, first president of the Washington Obstetrical and Gynecological Society (1883), and, though a Protestant, a continuing member of the faculty of the medical department of the University of Georgetown—a Catholic university founded in 1789. (Georgetown's medical department—now its medical school—was established in 1851 with a commitment to the Jesuit ideal of *cura personalis*, "the care of the whole person.") In offering his reminiscences of a life in medicine, Busey observed,

> I have uniformly contended for the honor and dignity of the medical profession, which I have believed could be more effectively maintained by the dicta of a high *esprit de corps* than by the penal provisions of a code of ethics but rarely enforced; that the highest standard of medical education was demanded by every consideration of professional duty and obligation, and that the profession should assert its prerogatives of right and power, in that legislators and all others in authority should come to know that science must dominate public opinion in all matters pertaining to preventive and remedial medicine.[35]

In the Protestant tradition, Busey summarized the aspirations of a profession in which science and the physician's conscience, rather than a code of ethics or political opinion, would assure its public reputation. "Duty and ob-ligation" signified internalized understandings of individual responsibility, in contrast to bureaucratic mandates intended to assure such responsibility by a professional code. A code of ethics, regardless of its implications for the organization and practice of medicine, did not actually impose duty and obligation on practitioners; rather, formal deliberations to establish such a code reflected uncertainties within the profession about how to achieve "honor and dignity" without further intensifying public scrutiny and moni-toring of physicians' actions.

But despite his vigorous defense of the primacy of science and indi-vidual conscience, Busey also endorsed a religiously based perspective. In a commencement address delivered in 1877 to the graduating students of the Medical Department at Georgetown, he offered his reflections on the "true" physician:

> Ghouls, harpies, and vampires may wear his title and usurp his place even as the false prophet "steals the livery of heaven to serve the devil in"; but they feast upon the credulity of the ignorant only. They are never found in the haunts of poverty, speaking words of comfort and administering to the bodily needs of those stricken with disease. The nobility of our profession recognizes no national-ity, no creed, no condition of life. It is founded on the broad basis of Christian philanthropy.[36]

By "broad basis," Busey meant to convey a very different kind of certainty about the physician's authority than was contained in either an official medi-cal society professional code or any specific approach to medical treatment.

It is reasonable to propose that at this historical moment a parallel existed between medical-scientific debates over how to evaluate the effec-tiveness of various treatments and procedures and the religious ferment in America over the nature of temporal authority and its public representa-tions. Describing the clergy's role in shaping public opinion in America, the historian John R. Bodo has argued that the turn against lingering ele-ments of a Puritan theocracy in the early nineteenth century had produced Unitarianism and other movements that placed an enduring emphasis on individualism, whether set against any "God-given pattern for the national life" or in the forms of Theodore Parker's "crusading humanitarianism" or Ralph Waldo Emerson's "aloof transcendentalism."[37]

The antitheocratic ideals of Parker, Emerson, and others were sometimes allied with and sometimes pitted against various efforts led primarily by Prot-estant clergymen to reform the nation. In the case of the movement to abol-ish slavery, they found themselves united, but in the case of alcohol, despite one theocratic moment, namely the era of Prohibition, the antitheocratic temperament prevailed.[38] Protestant individualists advocated a belief in human nature that saw it as at least potentially perfectible by the assurance of liberty and the strict exercise of conscience. Yet as the hopes of some for a religiously based state diminished, numerous "benevolent" or voluntary associations carried forward theocratic designs by other means. Even as Alexis de Tocqueville was praising the American patchwork quilt of voluntary associations, others were more skeptical about the ambitions of certain associations. If no particular religious tradition could shape a national morality, then the various surrogates to such traditions, in the form of domestic and international missionary movements, were not likely to do so either. Theocratic and antitheocratic movements have nevertheless defined the course of American struggles to incorporate into law and morals some notion of the limits to individual liberty, a matter unsettled to the present day.

It is in this context that the appearance of a specifically Catholic vision of morality in the realm of medicine should be considered. During the first half of the nineteenth century, American physicians did not speak with one voice about morality as it affected their profession, except on a very abstract plane, and we might see this as a legacy not only of Protestant religious pluralism, but also of Jacksonian democratic individualism, both of which allowed for a broad definition of who could be called and practice as a doctor.[39] Only toward the end of the nineteenth century were codes of professionalism devised and effectively incorporated into medical education in America, and then only as a result of decisive developments in medical understanding, both scientific and clinical. Meanwhile, Catholic moralists did not seek to challenge the scientific bases of medicine but rather to influence its clinical practices and outcomes. In so doing, these moralists, first from abroad, found unusual allies, and Samuel Busey was among them.

Busey described his Protestant faith as descending from his mother (his father having died when he was a young boy), who "was a consistent, but somewhat austere communicant of the Presbyterian denomination, and attended service on alternate Sundays, ... and on intervening Sundays attended the Concord Methodist Church."[40] He did not dwell on religious subjects in particular but noted further that his mother was "careful to inculcate the highest qualities of good morals, probity, and frugality, but was, perhaps, more especially concerned in regard to our education."[41] The effects of this upbringing were not inconsequential for Busey's tendency to formulate subtle but incisive moral distinctions about many matters.

In recalling his father's pursuit of sport, Busey observed,

> Fox-hunting was, in those days as it is now, a gentleman's amusement, if chasing an innocent animal to his lair or to death, by a kennel of bawling and devouring dogs, that the first at the finish might,

followed by the yelping hounds, bear the brush, in triumph back to a sumptuous, if not a riotous, feast, is a rational enjoyment for cultivated gentlemen. . . . The simple but graphic story of my father's devotion to the sport that owes its pleasures to the pain of the dumb animals excited in me a lively and lasting prejudice against gaming the animal for the trophies of death and tail tufts.[42]

This sensitivity regarding moral matters was conveyed in another way when as an adult Busey briefly entered the fray over the religious affiliation of John Charles Frémont, the explorer and mapmaker who ran as the Republican presidential candidate against James Buchanan in 1856. During the 1850s, before slavery became the preeminent public issue, disputes over the presence of Catholicism in American life flared, especially when anti-Catholicism was politically useful.

In a pamphlet published in 1856 and entitled *The Romish Intrigue: Frémont a Catholic!!* a long series of letters was reprinted, attesting to the fact that its subject was indeed a Catholic. Rather than engaging in the debate over who was a true American or whether Frémont had at any time in his life been Catholic, Busey complained,

The mere fact of his denying his religion should be sufficient to open the eyes of all honest men. He who would deny his religious faith for votes, is unworthy the support of honest men. I hold that it is a much greater crime to deny one's religion than to be the believer in any creed, however untenable that creed may be.[43]

However obliquely he may have endorsed religious pluralism with this statement, Busey's criticism signaled a devotion to what he saw as truth that led him to become specifically associated with Catholic teaching on the surgery of craniotomy.

In 1883, and then again in 1889, Busey addressed the issue directly. As the first president of the Washington Obstetrical and Gynecological Society, he devoted the entirety of his 1883 annual address to "the great importance of the subject and the increasing interest which it is now exciting, hoping that with the re-examination now in progress there will result a modification of the extreme views which have been held by a large majority of the ablest and most renowned obstetricians of the past, and perhaps, of those living of equal ability."[44] By virtue of its ancient practice, used during the times of Hippocrates and Celsus, the operation of craniotomy had achieved a visibility and medical venerability that was not easily challenged; and in times of difficult labor, recourse to various surgical interventions, including forceps, had been widely established as permissible. (Of course, Capellmann's work on *Pastoral Medicine*, already available in English several years before [1878], provided both theological and medical arguments against craniotomy, but Busey made no mention of this work.)

Objecting to the hastiness with which resort to this procedure took place, Busey noted "a case where a living child was born while a messenger had gone for the instruments of death, and more than once the shocking illustration of bungling haste has been exhibited in the cries of a mangled infant."[45] In contrast, Cesarean section, especially with the advent of antisepsis, was praised for its results, although it had been so rarely used during the first half of the nineteenth century that Busey recorded in a footnote the following curiosity (which might be seen as foreshadowing our contemporary fascination with "test-tube" babies and cloning):

> Several of the subjects of Cesarean delivery have reached advanced life in the United States, the oldest known being sixty-eight and seventy-four respectively. Several of the children have been heads of families, and one in this city [Philadelphia] is now forty-eight years old, and has given birth to eight children, three of whom have grown up.[46]

The necessity to recite anecdotally the survivability of those born by Cesarean section indicated how uncertain the profession—and public—still was about the use of this operation.

Weighing the arguments about various strategies of intervention in difficult labors, Busey appealed not to the sanctity of life but to utilitarianism as his rationale for why craniotomy should be abandoned:

> [Craniotomy] subordinates the life of the fetus and the larger number of lives to the possible enhancement of the chances of life to the mothers, and relegates the resources of obstetric science, which offer in the aggregate largely more favorable results, to the category of methods of dire necessity and almost hopeless resort. It is not, then, the greatest good to the greatest number, but the offer of possibly improved prospects to the chosen few. Is that the humanity which the science of medicine should espouse and proclaim to the world as an illustration of its beneficence?[47]

Carl Capellmann had also raised the "utilitarian standpoint" in his argument against craniotomy, but with a different sensibility about where a utilitarian defense stood in the hierarchy of moral considerations. Capellmann championed the "relative safety" of Cesarean section, whereas Busey saw it as a new example of the "beneficence" of medicine. This is a seemingly small difference, but it underscores the importance both gave to the moral dimensions of medical decisions, and therefore to how the public and individual patients might understand them.

The Protestant character of Busey's reflections is worth remarking. Medical progress, like science, was a species of permanent reformation, a renunciation of past beliefs and practices in favor of better ones. The image of utilitarian beneficence, founded upon a deep belief in the autonomy of the individual, led him to conclude,

> The relative value of two lives cannot be the only arbiter, for every life is of equal value to every holder. It is true that the fetus has not gained an independent existence. It is, nevertheless, true also that in these cases it is the life of a woman who cannot give birth to a living child *per vias naturales*. And such incapacity is the one and only claim of right to destroy the fetus. Can such a right rest exclusively upon such a basis, when it is established that other procedures offer almost, if not quite, equal chances of the mother's recovery, and rescue the larger number of children imperiled?[48]

Busey's logic was ostensibly devoid of appeal to religious belief, and in this sense, it embodied an ideal of vocation that was Protestant in character but professional in outlook. Indeed, he drew the line himself by declaring, "I have endeavored to consider the question in its scientific aspect, and entirely free from the influence of ecclesiastical doctrines."[49] It was medical rather than doctrinal piety that led him to his conclusions, he maintained. But his views on the merits of craniotomy versus Cesarean section, as it happened, coincided with Catholic values.

Of course, Busey's association with a Catholic institution of higher learning was not unrelated to his interests, but he went out of his way to emphasize a Protestant temperament about Catholic subjects. Georgetown University's relation to its Medical Department assumed no supervisory authority of its operation; the department did not rely on financial assistance from the university for many years; and its faculty members were not selected or retained for their doctrinal loyalties. As Joseph T. Durkin, S.J., notes in his history of the university, "the unselfishness and loyalty to Georgetown by her non-Jesuit faculty members of all departments is . . . one of the most shining features of the University's story."[50]

It is all the more interesting, therefore, to discover that Busey's high reputation among Catholic educators extended beyond Georgetown. In his memoirs he reprinted a Latin citation that accompanied the conferring of an honorary degree of doctor of law from St. Mary's Seminary in January 1888. The Latin text specifically praised his work on craniotomy, and in a brief letter in English, Alphonse Magnien, S.S., D.D., who led St. Mary's, wrote,

> Your well-known merit, your science and zeal in the promotion of good morals and the sound principles of Divine and natural law

in your profession as a medical doctor, have won for you the esteem and even admiration of many, and principally of the Catholic clergy, whose high mission you so well understand, and have constantly seconded with much success.[51]

Busey wrote back to Magnien, reiterating his commitment to the disinterested search for truth, coincident as that search may have been with Catholic goals.

> The high distinction comes to me, as stated in the diploma, for the maintenance of convictions which were the result of considerations entirely free from ecclesiastical influence. . . . The convictions referred to relate to the obligations of physicians to save life, and the belief that science and religion are not antagonistic. My abhorrence of the operation of craniotomy induced me to review this subject in its scientific aspect, and, when the conclusion which you so heartily approve had been reached, duty compelled me to promulgate it.[52]

The Protestant physician of late nineteenth-century America was not beholden to external authority or imposed values but rather to duty—that form of motivation inspired in the face of incontrovertible facts. Only after reviewing "this subject in its scientific aspect" was Busey finally compelled to condemn it. He thus reversed the stream of authority in which the value of life itself would dictate the facts determining how life was treated. Instead, Busey's assumption was that a determination of the facts themselves would lead to the values to be embraced.

But what "induced" Busey to conduct his review in the first place? His "abhorrence" was the underlying inducement to investigate the possible disutility of craniotomy in scientific terms. Catholic pastoral considerations were not above citing such disutility, but their focus on the issue of the fetus's right to life was one part of a much larger ecclesiastically induced endeavor to illuminate moral truths in all forms of human activity. The embrace of Busey by those less specialized than he was, then, amounted to an expedient form of deference to his more scientifically based point of view in the service of a unity of purpose that brought Catholics and Protestants together as Christians first. The extent to which this unity was tentative has much to do, finally, with the weakness of abhorrence as a form of moral authority, which left medical statistics, and such doctrines as "relative safety," as the only surviving forms of casuistry in Protestant, and thus professional, approaches to contentious moral matters.

Having been honored under Catholic auspices in early 1888, Samuel Busey set out one last time to summarize his views of craniotomy in the sixth annual "Address of the President" before the Washington Obstetrical and

Gynecological Society on October 19 of the same year. At the age of sixty, he had already witnessed a vast transformation in the progress of medical science. But in the relatively short five years since he had first publicly addressed the issue, in 1883, Busey could take some delight in remarking to his colleagues, "You will pardon my expression of the pleasure it gives me to recur to this subject, not, as then, a postulant, canvassing the issue of justifiability, but now, as a predicant, asserting the wrong of craniotomy upon the living fetus."[53]

In distinguishing craniotomy from criminal abortion, Busey was careful to argue that he had no wish to be associated with those who would welcome enactment of laws against it, any more than he would be with those who would diminish the role of professional conscience in determining its use in obstetric practice:

> I will not characterize craniotomy upon the living fetus as a crime in the ordinary acceptation of the word—that is, a deliberate, willful, and malicious malefaction. Nor would I invoke the enactment of penal laws upon the subject. [Here Busey cites a medical authority calling for such laws.] Nor do I assume censorship of professional conscience. Neither do I maintain that one who may differ with me is necessarily wrong. I concede to every qualified obstetrician the right of private judgment, and recognize the moral responsibility of every one for his own acts. Nevertheless, I would seek to cultivate and disseminate a higher and broader conception of moral duty than that which reposes in conscientious security upon the assumed right to kill an unborn child "in the interest of the life of another, responsible for its existence," when there is sufficient evidence to justify other procedures "equally in the interest of both mother and child."[54]

This kind of cautious and well-considered avowal of professional conscience and autonomy echoed throughout the professional societies of physicians for decades. It was the avowal of professional authority informed by an earnestness about "a higher and broader conception of moral duty" that transcended both temporal laws (and their absence) and casuistic reasoning that operated outside the bounds of clinical realities.

Indeed, within medicine those clinical realities had changed profoundly in many realms of practice, and perhaps nowhere as rapidly as in the arena of childbirth:

> The present has surpassed any previous century in scientific discovery and advancement. In no department of science has this advance been more marked than in medicine; in no branch of medicine

more than obstetrics, and in none of the subdivisions of obstetrics more than in the saving of maternal and infantile life.[55]

Chastising those well-established colleagues who still found reason to resort to craniotomy, Busey insisted that they were simply and tragically behind the times and that Cesarean section was something that eventually "every country practitioner ought to be able and always prepared to do."[56]

At the same time, he dismissed those arguments that condemned the use of craniotomy on the basis of what had been, at least of late, Catholic grounds for moral reasoning: "The argument that craniotomy upon the living and viable fetus is the indirect killing of an unjust aggressor is a trivial sophism." Referring to the "intuitive obstetric practice of primitive peoples," Busey also condemned the belief that the causes of difficulty in pregnancy were attributable to faults in the child and mother, but he noted that "the savage inhumanity of such a doctrine evinces a broader sense of justice than is exhibited by the craniotomists of today, in that it recognized the culpability of the mother to be equal with that of the child."[57] As for any "rights" that pertained to the use of one procedure over another, Busey admitted that "those dying after craniotomy might have been saved by section, and *vice versa.*"[58]

It was the prospect of saving the lives of both the child and the mother that could now be promised by Cesarean section. However, if the right to destroy the child was paramount in choosing the method used to resolve a threat to both lives, then, as Busey recognized presciently, an altogether different future loomed than the one for which he hoped:

> If a pregnant woman possesses the natural and inalienable right to terminate the life of her child at term, she cannot be denied the right to terminate it at any period of gestation, and criminal abortion would then become an accomplishment of the highest significance. The early destruction of embryonic life would be the simplest and surest escape from the perils of utero-gestation and parturition; would effectually withdraw from further scientific pursuit the advances in obstetrics which seek the elimination of craniotomy; more certainly extinguish the instincts and attribute of maternity; nullify the laws of reproduction; and reduce woman to a level more degrading than any to which the most barbaric of primitive people consigned her.[59]

Busey's sentiment about "the instincts" of maternity could not resolve the dilemmas created by the simultaneous demands for better and healthier lives on the one hand, and greater control over life—whose control?—on the other. To imagine, as he did, however opposed he was to it, a mother's "natural and inalienable right to terminate the life of her child at term," Busey anticipated the contemporary debates about "partial-birth" abortion, though the logic of abortion freedom started in his mind from "term" back to conception, rather than, as has come to be the case, from conception to term. In this sense, the twentieth-century logic about abortion depended first upon the nineteenth-century achievement of a new possibility in obstetric practice, namely, the use of medical procedures to end rather than save lives.

Contemporary debates about abortion in general—including the procedure called dilatation and evacuation, usually performed earlier in a pregnancy and not necessarily for strictly medical reasons—must be seen in the light of Busey's crusade against craniotomy.[60] Although the high hopes of nineteenth-century physicians about setting firm ethical boundaries around abortion within the practice of obstetrics were grounded in a moral consensus that no longer operates at the beginning of this, the twenty-first century, they still have great influence on how doctors, patients, and politicians approach the issue.

Convergences and Divergences

Between Capellmann's and Busey's time and our own, the Leviathan of the state, especially in its fascist and totalitarian forms, has played a role in determining what the medical profession's greater control over life might mean. Yet the sensibilities their writings reflect have remained influential even in the face of the social forces and changes that have uniquely defined the present era. Beneath the veil of either individual or professional autonomy, some form of deliberation obviously still occurs about what decisions patients and physicians alike (and together) may make and why.

The legacy of Busey's arguments against the practice of craniotomy displays the distinctly Catholic and Protestant variations on the theme of moral authority. The Catholic approach derived from the long tradition of pronouncements sanctioned by the church and focused on the adjudication of particular kinds of moral dilemmas. The Protestant approach, in effect, consecrated the authority of the practitioner to determine what was in the best interests of the patient and of life generally without direct appeal to outside authorities other than science. The two approaches were sometimes aligned, sometimes in conflict. It can be argued that as arguments for a woman's "natural and inalienable rights" regarding the control of birth gained acceptance within the medical profession and in public discourse throughout the twentieth century, the influence of Catholic doctrine and ideas about natural law were diminished.

Nevertheless, the Catholic perspective has, despite all appearances to the contrary, been victorious in form, if not strictly in content. Busey's approach represented a Protestant dispensation that, in deferring to mutable facts, did not anticipate that the rights of all concerned (e.g., doctors and patients) could become decisive over and against any "science" pertaining to unborn life. In the meantime, the authority of the physician in its ministerial inheritance was challenged by the very process of fact-finding that had served so well for a time in assuring that Christian-informed values would form the foundation of the profession's refusal to countenance abortion, or any other surgery threatening to unborn life, except in dire emergency.

Catholic pastoral medicine met Protestant science at a moment when the moral alignments between the two faiths had yet to fracture sufficiently to make medical practice per se, rather than medical morality, the subject of both public and expert scrutiny. But writing in 1905, more than a quarter-century after the appearance of Capellmann's work in English, the Reverend Andrew Klarmann, offering what he described as his "rigid opposition to traditional methods of pastoral medicine," concluded that it "has been held in such scant esteem, by the medical profession, at least, that succeeding authors contented themselves with copying each other."[61] Klarmann's work nevertheless addressed anew many of the problems that had received so much attention in the tradition of pastoral medicine, including abortion, ectopic conceptions, embryotomy, and vasectomy. The question of who had the authority to speak on such matters was nearly as important as what was spoken.

The Catholic case for medical morality was complicated from the outset by how the lines of authority were established. Protestant clergymen remained conspicuously silent about such matters, leaving the Protestant stamp of authority only on the medical profession itself. This stamp of authority is what was eventually called "professional autonomy," insofar as medical decision-making came to be seen as the exclusive purview of physicians. Meanwhile, pastoral medicine, to the extent that its questions were subsumed beneath pastoral theology and a Catholic view of natural law more generally, found popular expression in such periodicals as the *Homiletic Monthly* (and later the *Homiletic and Pastoral Review*) and the *Ecclesiastical Review*. Two such popularizers were Father John Ambrose McHugh (1880–1950), and Father Stanislaus Woywod (1880–1941), who compiled a collection (eventually in five volumes) of "Cases of Conscience." Although intended primarily for priests, their publication marked a popular codification of sorts about those kinds of cases that were of interest to a broader lay Catholic audience, including Catholic doctors.[62]

In the first of Woywod's volumes, published in 1906 and revised in 1924 in light of changes in canon law, seventy-four cases were presented, including "Mixed Marriage before a Protestant Minister," "Hysterical Scrupulousness of a Nun," "Forbidden Books," and "Confession by Telephone?" The cases that implicated medical knowledge or the physician in some direct way included "Sudden Sick Calls" and "The Medical Secret." In the former case, the question taken up was about how to determine the moment of death, since the performance of the last sacraments (including extreme unction, a sacrament specifically for the critically ill) was supposed to be done before death occurred. The author concluded, with reference to "Dr. Capellmann," that it was less urgent to determine for sure that someone was dead than to assume that they might not be, thus allowing for rites of absolution to be performed. The lesson was clear: "The priest, on being called to the sick, should not delay in hastening to them."[63]

The case of the medical secret was more complex and bore directly upon the issue of what patients might expect of their physicians. The early twentieth century marked a heightened public awareness of the communicability of disease, and in particular, of syphilis in marriage. Was the physician obligated to disclose his knowledge of a male patient's medical condition if this would, for example, affect the decision of a woman to marry him? Extraordinary discretion was given to the physician to find a way not to have to break his confidence and disclose the secret he was privy to, but "neither justice toward the patient nor the interests of the social order require of a physician that he keep inviolate the secret of a patient who is determined to commit a crime, the cause of which crime or the incentive to it is contained in the secret."[64] The physician was expected to acknowledge a higher law than his professional duty to protect his patient's confidentiality, or even the necessity to protect himself from legal liability. Rather than enumerate all the possible cases in which such acknowledgment would be required, Woywod encouraged the physician to recognize when such moments of truth might be upon him. Here was another convergence of sorts between Catholic assessments of troublesome cases and Protestant trust in professional character.

It was this convergence that would shape much of the American public understanding of physicians' responsibility until the last quarter of the twentieth century. In medicine as in theology, the complexity of a case required regular and certain measures of both moral and clinical assessment. The divergence between an official religious position on medical practices and the determination of how those practices are chosen or advocated by physicians themselves has been alternately described as part of the process of secularization (from the religious side) or professionalization (from the medical side). These two processes appeared to be in flight from religious authority, however it was established. Yet, however attenuated, the religious bases underlying the question of a physician's authority and public trust in that authority persist to this day.

CHAPTER 3

The Scientific Challenge to Faith

As we have documented, in nineteenth-century America comparisons of the three learned professions often included specific judgments about those who practiced them, judgments that focused on questions of character, and thus of trust. In an introductory address to the opening session of the Kentucky School of Medicine in 1858, Dr. George Wood Bayless (1816–1873) described the contrasting types—those who were worthy of public trust and those who were not—found within the professions of medicine, law, and the ministry:

> Medicine has her votaries, who love her science and are proud of her noble benevolence; and she has her charlatans, who would "sell her birth-right for a mess of pottage."
>
> Law has her lofty jurists, who find the highest pleasure in the pure waters of ethics, and who would scorn to compromise their noble calling for mere gain; and she has also her miserable crew of pettifoggers, who would torture *truth* to give it the appearance of falsehood, cloth *right* in the shocking habiliments of injustice, and rob *innocence* of bread and fair fame, all for a bribe.
>
> The Ministry has her grave theologians and pure minded divines, who have an eye single to the sacred character of their work, and it can boast its long list of martyrs, who have died for principle; but she sometimes finds in her ranks, men who will huckster their hypocritical cant for the highest price the market will afford.[1]

Even while warning that not all professional practitioners were honest, Bayless implied that most were, and he rested his remarks on the assumption that medicine, law, and religion were of equal stature in society. At the same time, however, the comments of others comparing the professions were beginning to reflect a general shift in relative cultural authority among them. In 1852, for example, the Reverend Edwin Hubbell Chapin (1814–1880) had this to say about the tireless work of the physician: "No profession is more arduous. Not only does it make laborious days, but encroaches upon the limits of needful sleep, admits no qualifications of personal ease, no excuses of climate, no consideration of weariness and hazard, at hours when the tired lawyer may lay down his case, and the toilsome pastor resign himself and his flock to the sleepless watch of the Great Shepherd."[2]

Thirty years later, the weekly Philadelphia *Medical Register* editorialized on "The Relation of the Medical and Clerical Professions," repeating observations that had already been made decades earlier by numerous Philadelphia clergymen about the physician's responsibilities to patients, but including a statement that presaged the changing relationship between doctors and pastors: "All clergymen will find their usefulness abridged who forget their intimate relation to the medical profession."[3]

By the middle to late nineteenth century, then, to answer the call in medicine had begun to mean, in the eyes of many, to fulfill a duty distinct from those of the other learned professions.[4] Preaching came in many varieties to suit many tastes and beliefs, and Dickens's *Bleak House* was the popular symbol of the slow progress of justice, but with its new commitment to scientific progress and a new emphasis on the character of the physician, the medical profession, sometimes distrusted over the centuries, was now bolstered by an increasing acceptance of a worldview that challenged the assumptions of tradition and faith.

The Dialogue between Religion and Science

Dr. Oliver Wendell Holmes Sr. depicted the cultural tensions between the declining authority of the clergy and the rising power of the medical profession in his novel *Elsie Venner*, published in 1861. Holmes spent his life challenging the complacency of his fellow doctors, calling upon them to recognize their limits as agents of cure. At the same time, until his death in 1894, he expressed little sympathy for the orthodox clergy of which his own father had been a moderate representative. His urging on of his colleagues, combined with a loss of feeling for organized religion, led him to examine, with the leisure of Boston Brahmin self-confidence, vexing questions about the dynamics of professional authority in America.

Holmes's novel recounts the illness and death of Elsie Venner in a small New England village. During the last months of her pregnancy, Elsie's mother is bitten by a rattlesnake, a creature conveniently abundant in the mountains nearby. This unfortunate event results in a number of curious features in the child, including a peculiar birthmark, diamond-shaped eyes, and hypnotic powers not unlike those of a snake. Elsie falls in love with a well-born medical student from Boston who has been forced to teach literature at her school to obtain the funds to continue his studies. Her death, in Holmes's account, is the result of unrequited love—and the fact that snakes do not live as long as humans do.

Although Holmes is not regarded as an important writer of fiction, and *Elsie Venner* was described by a friend as a "medicated novel,"[5] his point of view is revealing. In depicting the relations between the country doctor who attends to Elsie and the local parson who is incapable of providing an explanation for her lapse into madness, Holmes describes a larger contest between medical and theological authority with regard to understanding and ameliorating human pain and illness. The doctor is clearly the hero of the novel. He represents an acquired wisdom of medical insight and sympathy that directly confronts the clergy's religious interpretation of human actions and events.

At one moment in a conversation between the doctor and the parson, the doctor remarks, "Our libraries are crammed with books written by spiritual hypochondriacs who inspected all their moral secretions a dozen times a day. They are full of interest, but they should be transferred from the shelf of the theologian to that of the medical man who makes a study of insanity."[6] Appearing after widespread challenges to the theology of predestination, Holmes's "spiritual hypochondriacs" were pious, typically female wanderers in a post-Calvinist and increasingly physician-led world. (In a sense, Holmes could be said to have anticipated Freud's contempt for the misuse in America of his psychoanalytic approach to well-being as versions of his therapy were increasingly coming to serve a world in which spiritual hypochondria was a major industry for less and less talented practitioners in all of its many forms, including ostensibly religious ones.)[7] In Holmes's view, and that of many other champions of science, it would be the doctor, not the clergyman, who would be responsible for all authoritative diagnoses of individuals, mental as well as physical.[8]

What Holmes was describing was a process of gradual change in every small town in America, as the tools for handling the complexities of human anxiety and despair were gradually being transferred from clergymen to doctors. In this context, the status of the medical profession was immeasurably improved by its appearing to have something more substantial to offer than the consolations of faith or the promises of an afterlife, yet in seeking some aspect of the truth about oneself from the physician rather than the pastor, patient-parishioners experienced fresh uncertainty about just how much the physician could really deliver. The brightest religious minds recognized this and attempted to forge new alliances between the two professions.

The Theory of Evolution versus Biblical Literalism

Even as American ministers and doctors sought in particular ways to define the medical and public situations in which each one's special training was relevant, the battle over the theological and cosmological implications of evolutionary theory—most famously put forth in Charles Darwin's *On the Origin of Species by Means of Natural Selection*, published in 1859—was raging and had put every aspect of religious proclamation under scrutiny by the advocates of science. In England, John Tyndall (1820–1893), one of the great Victorian polemicists for science, championed the clarifying powers of the scientific attitude over and against the various unchallenged orthodoxies of religious faith. Tyndall, an Irish Protestant, took his place among the ranks of "agnostics" and "freethinkers" whose objections to religious authority were intellectual as well as institutional. By questioning the intellectual substance of religious authority, he offended the Victorian propriety of religious belief. The idea that the scientific imagination appeared to have no limits deeply troubled religious people of many different faith traditions,[9] and Tyndall appreciated the implications of his skepticism toward certain aspects of religious authority, whose public spokesmen became increasingly defensive in habit and tone.[10]

In his presidential address to the British Association for the Advancement of Science in Belfast in 1874, Tyndall offered some of his most controversial and enduring observations about the rise of science and the displacement of theology:

> The impregnable position of science may be described in a few words. We claim, and we shall wrest, from theology the entire domain of cosmological theory. All schemes and systems which thus infringe upon the domain of science must *in so far as they do this*, submit to its control, and relinquish all thought of controlling it.[11]

The religious responses to Tyndall's Belfast Address, as it came to be known, were nearly unanimous in their condemnation of his misuse of office and, in his own words (in a counterresponse titled "Apology for the Belfast Address"), "making an unjustifiable raid into the domain of theology."[12] In his "Apology" Tyndall dismissed those who said that he was necessarily endorsing atheism in his criticisms of certain claims of religion, but maintained that he was determined nevertheless to defend the freedom of scientific inquiry:

> And looking at what I must regard as the extravagances of the religious world; at the very inadequate and foolish notions concerning this universe which are entertained by the majority of our authorized religious teachers; at the waste of energy on the part of good men over things unworthy, if I may say it without discourtesy, of the attention of enlightened heathens; the fight about the fripperies of Ritualism, and the verbal quibbles of the Athanasian Creed;

the forcing on the public view of Pontigny Pilgrimages; the dating of historic epochs from the definition of the Immaculate Conception; the proclamation of the Divine Glories of the Sacred Heart—standing in the midst of these chimeras, which astound all thinking men, it did not appear to me extravagant to claim the public tolerance for an hour and a half, for the statement of more reasonable views—views more in accordance with the verities which science has brought to light, and which many weary souls would, I thought, welcome with gratification and relief.[13]

Tyndall's plea for the "verities" of science against "these chimeras, which astound all thinking men," invoked the broader calls for religious toleration in England and America, while at the same time it pandered to conventional hostilities toward Catholicism. His and others' disagreements with England's clergy have been further summarized by the historian Frank M. Turner: "The intellectual authority frequently ascribed to the clergy, the Bible, and theological concepts such as divine providence exerted a pernicious influence on the practical affairs of everyday life. Traditional religious authority provided the justification for sabbatarianism, restrictive marriage laws, prayers to change the weather and to prevent disease, religiously dominated education, and other social practices that inhibited the discovery, diffusion, and application of scientific truth."[14]

Any hold that Anglican clergymen had on the "practical affairs of everyday life" was weakened further by Tyndall's effective strategy of playing off religiously absolutist claims (e.g., miracles, Ultramontanism) against socially conventional forms of establishment religion that had become the substance of Protestant civil society. The intellectual warfare between science and religion—exemplified in John W. Draper's *History of the Conflict between Religion and Science* (1874) and Andrew Dickson White's *A History of the Warfare of Science with Theology in Christendom* (1896)—was portrayed as a battle between worldviews that, once settled, would transform the intellectual and practical organization of higher education throughout the world.

The theory of evolution was not only a challenge to individual religious belief, it was also a challenge to Anglican control of and influence upon major social institutions, institutions that were supposed to function for the edification and uplifting of all people, whether or not they were Christian. In a reminiscence of Thomas Henry Huxley (1825–1895), one of the most persuasive proponents of Darwin's basic thesis, Wilfrid Ward gave personal force to the cultural stakes of this conflict:

I felt my impression of Carlyle's dogged unsympathetic persistency, in measuring everything by his own ideas, sensibly deepened by a story which Huxley told me of their mutual relations. Carlyle and he were for long good friends, but had a serious difference on the evolution question in the early stages of the controversy. Their personal intercourse ceased in consequence. After an interval of many years Huxley happened to see the Scotchman crossing the street in London, and thinking that bygones might be bygones, went up to him and spoke to him. Carlyle did not at first recognize Huxley, but when he succeeded in identifying him, he at once said, with his Scotch twang, as though he were continuing the last conversation of years ago, "You're Huxley, are you? You're the man that's trying to persuade us all that we're the children of apes; while *I* am saying that the great thing we've really got to do is to make ourselves as much unlike apes as possible."[15]

In recent decades, historians have offered a revisionist claim about the "battle" image. Some have argued for a less traumatic shift of power from religion to science, particularly in the context of the development of higher education and the disputes about evolution.[16]

Yet, in that very context, Tyndall's and others' public challenges to religion's role in everyday life did open a second front in the larger struggle between religion and science. In the American case, pushing westward geographically and downward in the social class system, the struggle that had been effectively settled in the administrative and faculty offices of universities by the end of the nineteenth century continued to break out periodically elsewhere throughout the twentieth century, and once again in the twenty-first. Although the Scopes trial in Tennessee in 1925 and the many subsequent court battles over the teaching of "creationism" in the public schools have not seriously threatened the material or organizational interests of universities, they have been characterized as worrisome by a host of critics,[17] and the fight for the hearts and minds of elementary school students has lately been termed part of the "culture wars." In contrast to the nineteenth-century intellectual struggle between science and religion, these conflicts of beliefs and values have amounted to disputes over the social and cultural consequences of a welfare state that is also a secular state.[18]

The conflicts created within the secular state, for example, about how the law is supposed to pertain to the everyday life of Americans—especially in the realm of medicine—has had less to do with science as a social institution than with political beliefs about where the line should be drawn between the protection of public assertions of religious dogma in society and the individual rights of citizens. While "scientific truth" appears to stand against the religious "superstitions" of the past, today it also appears peculiarly defenseless in the face of the "right" of citizens to "believe" that the world is flat or was created literally as the Bible describes. Much is at stake for the practical conduct of life, especially in terms of what various institutions are obliged to teach, or may not teach, to future generations. The debate over the origin of species may have been more or less settled by the beginning of the twentieth century, but the same can hardly be said about the question of the nature of society.[19]

John Tyndall challenged many ideas and practices that he believed were inadequately defended by religious authority. Historian Stephen S. Kim has argued that it was not Tyndall's goal to disestablish the clergy's authority over spiritual matters, but rather to counter its broader claims about religious revelation versus natural knowledge. In this revision Tyndall is depicted as a promoter of secularism over and against religious orthodoxy, leading Kim to conclude that "Tyndall's agnosticism was a sincere appeal to let religion mind its own turf (feeling) and science its (intellect)."[20] This now conventional account of the force of secularization in the West still has its polemical uses. The secular, it is argued, is that which diminishes the influence of authority based on criteria other than reason. Tyndall did not seek to reconcile religion and science as much as intellectually sanitize the boundaries between them, so as to further the impression of peaceful cohabitation. By consigning feeling to religion alone, critics like Tyndall dismissed any of the intellectual countermovements *against* science as isolated and irrational attempts to undermine it by principles other than free thought. Yet Tyndall's idealism betrayed a lack of consideration of the enduring nature of human institutions, including religious ones. He sought a purely intellectual religion as much as an intellectual science, leaving the messy details about how to run such institutions to others.

The Prayer-Gauge Debate

Unlike papal infallibility or the miraculous healing powers of relics, prayer as a petition for divine acknowledgment can hardly be described as narrowly sectarian. And insofar as prayer was confined to individual and private worship, it was not a subject of public controversy during the nineteenth century.[21] The clergy in England had established over several centuries special days for prayers and fasting, which in the nineteenth century included specific petitions for the cessation of excessive rain, for the end of a cholera outbreak and one of the cattle plagues, and for the recovery of good health of members of the royal family. Frank Turner cites four separate occasions, in 1853, 1860, 1865, and 1871, which brought the clergy in direct conflict with various and new authorities—for example, government, public health, scientific, medical—all of which championed the advances of science over the use of prayer to effect a particular result.

In 1853, for instance, a request to appoint a national fast day to combat cholera was rejected by government officials because they believed they understood well enough the causes of the outbreaks to address them effectively. In defending the actions of the government not to sanction the clergy's efforts, Charles Kingsley, a liberal clergyman and advocate of public health measures, rejected the simple-minded attempts to attribute the disease to "Maynooth, the Crystal Palace, the Jerusalem bishopric, the neglect of the Church fasts, the neglect of the worship of the Virgin, the increase of the worship of the Virgin, Free-trade, Protection, any and every cause but that palpable one of which the poor unwashed gas-poisoned hearers were but too well aware."[22] The steady improvement of knowledge about disease in particular turned such attributions into careless and irrational forms of explanation. But a deeper impulse was also at work, one that apparently survives no matter how powerful the case for scientifically based causal explanations and strategies might be. The impulse to make correlations between one phenomenon and another, between one sphere of life and another, is rooted in the process of making things meaningful and establishing the kinds of explanations that may put certain questions to rest, if only temporarily.

Although during this period the English clergy may have been hoping to reassert their authority over matters of national concern, another intriguing aspect of these calls for national prayer was the assertion by some pastors that the wet weather was a punishment for sin. One minister attributed excessive rainfall to the passage of the Divorce Act of 1857 and to other specific events in the nation's recent history.[23] The correlation of human actions (e.g., sin) with unwanted natural occurrences (e.g., excessive rain) was followed by the correlation of human actions (e.g., prayer) with supernatural intercession and absolution. A belief in the palpable and intercessory qualities of the divine was not only a demonstration of the appeal of individual will, as in the case of prayer, but also a strategy to move large numbers of people to see their common bonds in the face of hostile circumstances. This collective aspect of the rituals of prayer and fasting had a long history in Britain and other European nations.

In 1860, a call for prayers for better weather (to counter wet weather, which was detrimental to farming) was met in some quarters with the same skepticism as Charles Kingsley had expressed, and with the outbreak of cattle plague in 1865, the sides were clearly drawn between attempts by governmental and scientific authorities to address the disease (by slaughtering the affected livestock) and by the clergy's call for national, collective prayer. The archbishop of Canterbury "issued a special prayer for use in schools, households, and families."[24] Reaction in the public press was by now predictable, with a broad separation between those, on the side of science, who saw nothing constructive in such calls and those, on the side of religion, who still correlated disease and disaster with the moral decline of the nation. The defenders of a scientific approach to these problems could not claim that they knew what to do to prevent bad weather, but with regard to the cattle plague, as had been the case with cholera,[25] even without a complete understanding of all of the reasons for the outbreaks, science's effective efforts at halting the spread of disease were evidence that some aspect of causality had been determined.

A decade before his Belfast Address, John Tyndall had figured in these emerging public controversies over the utility of prayer in such national circumstances. In late 1865, in the *Fortnightly Review*, he criticized prayers being offered to end the plague.[26] In response, Arthur Penrhyn Stanley, dean of Westminster Abbey, wrote to Tyndall, asking him to propose a form of prayer "in which the heart might express itself without putting the intellect to shame."[27] Faced with having to conduct a service to pray for an end to the cattle plague at the request of the bishop of London, Dean Stanley assured Tyndall that he would not mention to anyone that he had written to him. Tyndall's response was blunt: "I hope and think—and pardon me for thus hoping and thinking—that you will *not* pray as others will for the staying of this plague, but will ask on the contrary for strength of heart and clearness of mind to meet it manfully and fight against it intelligently."[28]

At this point in the history of the West, the use of prayer to influence a particular circumstance appears to have been controversial in part because it exposed a certain lack of knowledge about causality itself. The tension persists today between determining and treating disease at the deepest level of causality or preventing it long before the need to treat it arises. Much of the controversy in England was, as Frank Turner has persuasively argued, between established religious authority and fledgling scientific authority, but it was also about the nature of human understanding of the meaning of the events themselves. One legacy of the disputes in England is that debates over the "efficacy" of prayer presage the ways in which public policy about health is presently debated under what remains the enduring human condition of uncertainty.

In 1871, when Edward, the Prince of Wales, contracted typhoid, special prayers were offered on his behalf. Within several days, his condition improved, and by mid-February the nation was in a state of euphoria over his recovery. This was taken as evidence by some clergymen of the real efficacy of prayer, while the doctors who had attended the prince were hardly acknowledged in the popular press, and much of the publicity about his recovery itself focused on the role that the public and the clergy had played in petitioning for divine intercession. British medical journals, on the other hand, bristled at this affront to the important role that medicine—and, increasingly, public health measures—played in the treatment and prevention of the disease. Frank Turner concludes, "The physicians and their allies in other scientific professions saw their hopes for new public recognition and social prestige dashed and the triumph of their skill and methods turned into a fete for the monarchy, the church, the politicians, and the physical efficacy of the prayers for the sick in the Book of Common Prayer."[29]

The illness of Prince Edward and the chagrin of the British medical establishment set the stage for what became known as the prayer-gauge debate.[30] Unlike the previously recounted episodes, American interest was also stimulated in what would be the last public controversy on the matter. The ensuing debates touched upon important questions about the nature of causality and probability, concepts that were associated with science and medicine alike. And the newly emerging intellectual attacks on religion put pressure on all figures in authority to justify that authority on the basis of skill and competence. The public's sense of the trustworthiness of physicians was to undergo a transformation that would create a new balance between trust in doctors and expectations about the outcome of medical treatment.

The specific controversy began in the pages of the British periodical *Contemporary Review* in July 1872. Again John Tyndall figured prominently by introducing a proposal to determine the efficacy of prayer for healing the sick. The proposal itself was unsigned and presented as a letter to Tyndall. Scholars now believe it to have been written by Sir Henry Thompson, a prominent London surgeon, and for the purposes of this narrative we will assume that is the case.[31] In his presentation of the proposal, Tyndall noted that "the writer seeks to confer quantitative precision on the action of the supernatural in Nature." The question for all to consider was whether it was possible to propose some way of measuring such an effect. The proposal itself assumed a matter-of-fact tone, described by Tyndall as "conciliatory," and the author proceeded to list four classes of "legitimate objects of supplication" contained in the Book of Common Prayer.[32] Although Dissenters did not use it as their prayer book, Thompson noted that they did embrace much of its content, if not its form. In this sense, not unlike many other nineteenth-century critics of religion, he did not distinguish among faith traditions but treated them as functionally equivalent. In so carefully stipulating the many "legitimate" uses of prayer, Thompson, with Tyndall's endorsement, offered a comprehensive view of the use and misuse of particular religious practices.

Thompson then asked which types of supplication might be amenable to testing and found that "there appears to be one source from a study of which the absolute calculable value of prayer (I speak with the utmost reverence) can almost certainly be ascertained. I mean its influence in affecting the course of a malady, or in averting the fatal termination."[33] He described two types of prayers that were made on behalf of the sick, those offered weekly as general prayers for all who were ill and those offered specifically for individuals who enjoyed "one of the advantages of rank and gentle birth in England," that is, "special prayers . . . made for such, every week at least, in most churches throughout the country."[34] Special prayers were intended to concentrate many minds on the recovery of one person in particular and thus imitated more direct therapeutic intervention, while general prayers were made for the population of ill persons at any given moment in time. In this latter respect, general prayers were as much in keeping with strategies of prevention as with those of intervention.[35]

In this way Thompson was able to argue for a clinical approach toward prayer, an approach that was already being used by physicians and researchers in their work to ascertain the effectiveness of medical treatments: "A new remedy has been proposed, or is said on high authority to be efficacious; and as authority does not suffice in medicine, further than to recommend a given course, and never to prescribe it, the remedy is carefully tested."[36] Long before debates about the efficacy of "alternative" or "integrative" medicine, Thompson called for an epidemiology of prayer by insisting that scientific method could be applied to domains as yet untested by science. But he was also endeavoring to alter common assumptions about the function of religion generally. The prayer-gauge test would follow the same methods as those used for determining the efficacy of medical treatments, using a case-control design in which patients with a diagnosed illness would be divided into two groups, one treated by whatever measures had been used before and the other treated with the new remedy, in this instance, prayer.

The essence of Thompson's proposal was to ask that special prayers be offered for patients on a single ward or in one hospital, "under the care of first-rate physicians and surgeons, containing certain numbers of patients afflicted with those diseases which have been best studied, and of which the mortality-rates are best known." Such prayers would be offered for a period of three to five years; "at the end of that time, the mortality-rates should be compared with the past rates, and also with that of other leading hospitals similarly well managed during the same period."[37] This prospective study of prayer was simple and elegant in its design, requiring little expense and, the author slyly remarked, providing "an occasion of demonstrating to the faithless an imperishable record of the real power of prayer."[38] Thompson's feigned ingenuousness was intended to be disarming, but it elicited pointed responses in Britain's leading periodicals.

The earliest reply appeared in *The Spectator* in the form of an editorial that took immediate exception to "this elaborate sarcasm" and "unworthy piece of literary irony," and chided Tyndall for associating his name with it.[39] The editorial writer argued against the characterization that special prayers in particular were made only for members of the British aristocracy: "In most churches, one hears prayers for the sick poor every Sunday; while the

reserve of the rich usually prevents their asking the prayers of the congregation, even where they are not skeptical as to the value."[40] (These competing
images of whose access to the benefits of prayer was greater have been recycled into debates over the inequalities in access to medical care. Whether
conceptualized as involving "time with the physician," "expensive tests," or
"magic bullets," contemporary controversies over access to medical care and
treatment are anticipated in these earlier arguments about who in the larger
society did or did not benefit from the uses of prayer.)

The Spectator's editorial writer approached the problem of measuring
prayer by denying its external possibility: "But we should be much surprised
to learn that any man who had really given up his mind to thoughts of this
kind at all had ever regarded his prayer as a sort of petty dictation to God,
the effect of which might be measured, like a constituent's pressure on his
representative in parliament, by the influence it exerted on the issue." Dis-
closing what he believed to be the true purpose of prayer, he concluded,
"You pray, if you pray in the spirit of Christ at all, not for a specific external
end, but because it is a deep relief to pour out your heart to God in the
frankest way possible to limited human nature, and in the hope that if your
wish is not granted, your *want* may be."

The contrast here could not be more striking. On the one hand, a test of
prayer was proposed to determine its alleged external influence upon others
and the world generally. On the other, prayer is envisioned as "a deep relief,"
in other words, as a source for relieving the anxiety that was provoked by a
concern for oneself or others. In this second formulation, the anxiety of not
knowing what might happen next—"limited human nature"—is the central
motivation for any faith at all: "What your prayer really consists of is the confession of the blank you fear for yourself, and still more, perhaps, for others;
of your dread of losing the moral help and sympathy so essential to you; of
the yearning that this trouble may not come on those whom it threatens."[41]

This was not a selfish anxiety but one that animated the deepest sense
of concern about the control of one's life individually and in relation to
others—for example, the concern about the health of one's children, spouse,
or a close friend. It was all the more important, therefore, to make clear what
might be called the authenticity of the prayerful request itself: "How should
we think of any one who prayed—i.e., who ought to be pouring out the
deepest longings of his soul—for the restoration of certain persons of health,
only to make a delicate experiment on the relation between the spiritual and
physical forces of the universe? Does it follow, because, in some sense, God
answers true prayer, he would answer the demand for a scientifically scaled
prayer-gauge?"[42] According to the writer of the editorial in The Spectator,
instead of being a test proposed to assist the recovery of dearly beloved persons, the prayer-gauge proposal was aimed at "the scientific determination

of our moral command of the fountains of divine mercy"—in other words, prayer offered in this context would be inauthentic and an affront to, and test of, God.

The problem, then, was not one of research design or even noble scientific intention but of fundamental disagreements about the nature of faith. From a sociological point of view, we might say that whereas several hundred years earlier wealth had already been thoroughly "rationalized"—that is, integrated into Protestant theology as a sign of being "chosen," as Max Weber put it in his seminal book *The Protestant Ethic and the Spirit of Capitalism*— at the end of the nineteenth century any such rationalization of health was only beginning, and the "determinants" of health, from an epidemiological (scientific) standpoint, were only beginning to be understood. The prayer-gauge proposal was obviously insincere on some level, but it pointed the way toward an expanded approach for exploring both the causes of illness and the effectiveness of treatments. Prayer was "the simplest expression of [peoples'] anxieties,"[43] but might it not also be the "cure" for them?

In mounting a defense of what was being dismissed by many as a crude assault on the dignity of the Anglican Church and its doctrines, Francis Galton (1822–1911) entered the fray. Already having established himself as the preeminent Victorian observer of sundry phenomena in his work *Hereditary Genius: An Inquiry into its Laws and Consequences* in 1869, Galton was well prepared to offer comments obliquely supporting the concept of a prayer-gauge test.[44] First he used the words of ministers against them by quoting from various books in which prayer was defined and by citing many examples of the use of prayer for temporal advantage in all religions. He then addressed the relative advantages of conducting a study of "large classes of cases . . . guided by broad averages" over and against examining "isolated instances." This approach to statistical significance added another layer upon the previously proposed investigation of the use of special prayers over general prayers. Instead of focusing a congregation's efforts on, say, one hospital ward over several years, and then comparing the morbidity and mortality rates of that ward with those of wards that had not received special prayers, Galton moved closer to a modern experimental design: "We must gather cases for statistical comparison, in which the same object is keenly pursued by two classes—similar in their physical, but opposite in their spiritual state; the one class being prayerful, the other materialistic."[45]

Galton's professed interest was in results: "We simply look to the main issue—do sick persons who pray, or are prayed for, recover, on the average, more rapidly than others?" Yet rather than pursuing this particular line of inquiry, Galton introduced his own "data" on the effects of prayer. Whether inadvertently or not, Galton included another category of the possible influence of prayer on health when he mentioned sick persons who pray, in effect, for their own recovery. He pointed out further that "in all countries and in all creeds, the priests urge the patient to pray for his own recovery . . . but," he acknowledged, "I have been able to discover hardly any instance in which a medical man of any repute has attributed recovery to the influence of prayer."[46]

Putting forth his own evidence about prayer's efficacy in the form of information that he had gathered for other purposes, Galton looked at the mortality rates of men in different occupations, including members of royal houses. He argued that prayers offered on their behalf or made by them for themselves resulted in no difference whatsoever in how long they lived. In presenting data in this way, he claimed to isolate prayer as the singularly and causally ineffective element in the determination of whether clergymen lived longer than physicians or whether royalty lived longer than the rest of the population, and concluded that physicians outlived clergymen and that royalty were outlived by those they ruled. The search for conclusive data, apart from polemically useful inferences drawn from them, is itself a constant challenge to the authority of beliefs and assumptions at any given moment in time. (A half century later, actuarial claims about mortality rates between clergymen and physicians in Wales were exactly reversed,[47] but this only reinforced the necessity of constant monitoring of trends over time, which, in addition to studies of effective treatments, is the hallmark of modern scientific medicine.)

Galton was not satisfied with depicting the higher mortality rates of clergymen in England, despite their prayerful lives, over and against other professions. He also pointed out that missionaries were especially vulnerable to shortened lives and were not "supernaturally endowed with health." In other words, religious piety was no prophylactic against the strenuous conditions of missionary work, although it is interesting to note that Galton did not propose examining the mortality rates of those who were not ministers who may also have worked in charitable missions around the world,[48] and that he also pointed out that insurance companies did not calculate any special "immunity from danger" to missionary ships as distinct from commercial vessels.[49]

At the same time that Galton was calling into question the influence of any specifically religious practices upon health, the medical literature of the time did acknowledge, if not even promote, other investigations into such effects. In 1874, for instance, the British Medical Journal noted an international call for scholarly papers on the healthfulness of the Sabbath:

The Swiss Society for the Sanctification of the Sabbath offers 1,200 francs (£ 41), in one prize or in accessits, for the best essay or essays on the hygienic importance of rest on Sunday, especially for those engaged in laborious occupations. The following points must be discussed, in as popular form as possible:—1. The favorable effects of such rest on the individual at different ages, and its influence on families and on nations; 2. The diseases which continuous labor provokes or aggravates in those whose occupations deprive them of weekly rest—for example, those employed in works that require constant attendance, workmen in certain manufactories, railway, telegraph, and post-office employees, etc.; 3. The practical application of the facts ascertained.[50]

The implications for health of various religious activities were part of a larger interest that had developed among Western societies with professional classes who supported the recording of census figures not only in the interest of promoting democratic government but also for understanding the health of their populations. The British case, however, perhaps revealed a distinctive form of class and cultural conflict about whose voice would prevail in national debates over the various meanings of health. Tyndall and Galton received much attention for their pronouncements and proposals about the efficacy of prayer, but the gradual growth of a medical interest in other religious activities proceeded alongside these more publicly visible controversies. (Fasting for religious purposes, for example, was given a thorough examination by "A Committee of Clergy" in 1897, long after the prayer-gauge debate had subsided. In the case of fasting, the purpose was not to debunk its intrinsic worth, as was the case with petitionary prayer, but rather to determine if there should be exemptions made to the requirement to fast on the basis of health.[51] The door to twentieth-century medical hegemony was thus opened by those endorsing the superior, and measurable, interests of health as it could and eventually would be described epidemiologically.)

Meanwhile, in the ensuing debates about prayer, Galton's statistical approach, in particular, foreshadowed important disagreements that would emerge more forcefully in the twentieth century about the use and value of such statistical (or epidemiological) data in determining the efficacy of various medical treatments and preventive measures. One of Galton's challenges to prayer's efficacy was to appeal to the vast amounts of accumulated data about mortality rates in order to ask strictly empirical questions about cause and effect, and his data indicated no correlation between prayer and the length of life.

Most initial objections to this statistical approach were more bellicose than reasoned, but in 1877, John Hewitt Jellett (1817–1888), rather than dismissing entirely this approach to evaluating the influence of religious practices on medical outcomes, attempted to find a middle ground. Jellett, who had formerly been president of the Royal Irish Academy, set forth his reasoning in what became known as the Donnellan Lectures, later published as *The Efficacy of Prayer*.[52]

Jellett pointed out, to begin with, that Thompson's proposed experiment to measure the effects of prayer on the sick had never been actually tried. Supposing, he went on, that it had been tried and that "no difference between the respective percentages of recovery could be detected. What does the principle of the method of differences require us to infer from this? The general inefficacy of prayer? Certainly not; but the inefficacy of prayer *under the conditions of the experiment*."[53] But what if the differences were measured by observation instead of experimentation—that is, what of the claim that the effects of prayer were beneficial might be confirmed in other ways? Referring to the many kinds of statistical data then emerging about prayer and mortality, Jellett conceded that "the method of differences, and statistics as its proper auxiliary, are applicable to every case in which an asserted cause and an asserted effect are both within the cognizance of man." And further, that

> this condition is fulfilled in the present case. The effect, namely the longevity of a certain class, is altogether within human cognizance; and although the same cannot be said of each individual unit in the complex cause—for we cannot look into each man's heart and decide whether his prayer be real or merely formal—yet we are justified in assuming that, among so great a number of prayers, many are genuine. The use, therefore which this argument proposes to make of statistics and of the method of differences appears to me to be quite legitimate.[54]

Jellett's concession was strategically important for a defense of the possible role of religion in human health. He recognized the emerging and eventually ubiquitous power of statistical reasoning, meeting Galton's rejection of the beneficial effects of prayer on the longevity of royalty, for example, with this insight about the nature of scientific skepticism:

> Suppose it to have been proved, by an examination of the statistics of the case, that Kings do on the average live longer than other men. Suppose now that some advocate of the doctrine of the efficacy of prayer were to adduce this fact as evidence in support of the doctrine for which he contended—what reply would be made to him? It would be said, this is not a legitimate application of the method of differences; for Kings differ from ordinary men in other respects besides the fact that more prayers are offered up for them. It may be that they are more carefully reared in their youth. It may be that they live easier lives than other men—in a word, the effect which you attribute to prayer may be due to a quite different cause. Even if

no such cause can be pointed out, the phenomenon is too complex to justify you in assuming that no such cause exists. This objection seems to be reasonable.[55]

Jellett's arguments, couched in part in what would become the language of epidemiology, were indicative of the rapidly changing mood among the religiously faithful who sought better accommodation with the shifting balance between the authority of revelation and the powers of science. This balance favored the powers of observation, leading Jellett to conclude that "the statistical argument is theoretically applicable to every case in which the relation of cause and effect, or of condition and result, is supposed to exist between two phenomena which are, more or less completely, within the range of human knowledge."[56] That everything could, theoretically, be correlated with everything else, but for the lack of human and material resources required to carry out such an endeavor, was a compelling way to announce the seemingly endless project of science, whether natural or social. The positivism of Auguste Comte, which by the 1870s had its own adherents in England,[57] had yet to shed its own religious ambitions, but Jellett already identified the principal modus operandi of future scientific positivism, with its ambition to correlate everything with everything else.

Jellett's insight was also more instructive than the polemical insistence of Tyndall, Galton, and others that religion and science had to retain sanitary borders between faith and reason. What was at stake, finally, in such a theoretical possibility was the unleashing of fresh anxieties about what could be known. These anxieties would sweep across the twentieth century, less noticed and remarked upon than the suffering created by politics and war during the first half of the twentieth century, but emerging in the United States in fuller force with rising prosperity and relative peace in the second half.

Jellett's disagreements with Galton over what statistics proved were also raised in connection with the nature of physicians' beliefs about healing. Galton had asserted that physicians did not believe in the efficacy of prayer, and in any event, they did not recommend to the friends and families of patients that they pray for their recovery. Jellett countered:

Physicians do not habitually urge the practice of *every* thing which they regard as important to the recovery of their patients. There is nothing, for example, more important than kindness and love on the part of the friends who surround the sick man's bed. Yet I do not suppose that physicians habitually urge upon them the medical importance of kindness: and the reason of this silence is not, certainly, that they regard kindness as *un*important, but that they assume as a matter of course, unless they have proof of the contrary, that the friends of the sufferer *will* be kind to him.

So, too, in the case of prayer. That a person who has faith, even a weak faith in its efficacy, will pray for one he loves when attacked by a dangerous illness, is as certain as that one of affectionate disposition will be kind to him. The physician who himself believes in the efficacy of prayer knows this perfectly. He knows that it is quite as superfluous to exhort a person, who has even a small measure of this faith, to pray for a suffering friend as it would be to exhort one of a loving disposition to be kind to him. Even a clergyman would probably consider any very strenuous exhortation to the practice of this duty unnecessary. He knows that at such a moment submission, not prayer, is the really difficult task.[58]

Jellett's proposed agreement between clergyman and physician about the superfluity of "strenuous exhortation" to pray for a suffering friend, while at the same time he acknowledged the importance of "kindness and love," was part of the consensus of a civil society in which a general, though vague, correspondence existed between particular religious beliefs and general expectations about how to live. It was precisely this consensus that Galton and others sought to undermine, however respectfully. Jellett was the better ethnographer, but Galton's was the more accurate vision of the future.

The American Reaction to the Prayer-Gauge Debate

John Tyndall made one visit to the United States, beginning in October 1872—a few months after the appearance of the prayer-gauge proposal in *The Contemporary Review*—and culminating in a farewell banquet in his honor at Delmonico's restaurant in New York City before his return to England on February 5, 1873. In the same month Tyndall arrived, one of the first responses to the proposal from American shores appeared in *The Contemporary Review*, written by James McCosh, who had been president of Princeton College (later University) since 1868. (A year earlier, in 1871, McCosh had delivered lectures at the Union Theological Seminary on "Christianity and Positivism" in which he pursued a theological reconciliation with the theories of Darwin in the hope of advancing the causes of both religion and science.)[59]

McCosh's reaction to the idea that the physical efficacy of prayer could be measured was not only unsympathetic but also important for the effort to establish a demilitarized zone between religion and science even as the musings of scientists encroached further and further into the religious domain: "I believe that the time has come when the intelligent public must intimate pretty decisively that those who have excelled in physical experiments are not, *therefore*, fitted to discuss philosophical or religious questions." And McCosh specifically admonished John Tyndall: "Prof. Tyndall has faith in the ordinances of nature; and he, and those who read his works, have profited by it. I have no evidence that he has studied so carefully the method of earning fruit in the kingdom of grace as in the kingdom of nature. But of this I am sure, that with a like faith in God, in his providence and word, as he has in science, he will reap a yet greater and more enduring reward."[60]

Other criticisms were made by Mark Hopkins (1802–1887), president of Williams College, and Hugh Miller Thompson (1830–1902), an Episcopal priest. Both Hopkins and Miller scoffed at the idea of a prayer test, Hopkins noting that "but for the endorsement of Prof. Tyndall, the proposal of such a test would probably have been attributed to a wag with a long face, and have excited no serious notice."[61] Miller concluded that "all we know is that prayer is a factor of human life itself, as eating, drinking, thinking, reading, and working are factors of human life, and a universal factor, from which no man can be excluded, from whose effects you can shut in no man."[62] (Tyndall himself was not entirely unsympathetic toward those who expressed discomfort about his views, writing in a letter that "there have been people praying for me, and writing to me about my soul and its future prospects, at such a rate. Some of the letters so full of indescribable sweetness, that it is a pain to give such people pain by differing from them.")[63]

By the time Tyndall had returned to England and delivered his Belfast Address as the new president of the British Association for the Advancement of Science in 1874, the debate over science and faith had become a familiar one in America. In September of that same year, Edwin Lawrence Godkin, editor of *The Nation* published an editorial, "Tyndall and the Theologians," in which he formulated a clear set of distinctions between the functions of religion and science, much like James McCosh had done the previous year. Tyndall and Huxley, he wrote, did not "occupy the position of religious prophets or fathers. They preside over no church or other organization. They have no power or authority to draft any creed or articles which will bind anybody else, or which would have any claims on anybody's reverence or adhesion. No person, in short, is authorized to bring science into an alliance with religion or anything else."[64] Godkin was less impressed with Tyndall's challenges to religious ideas, noting that "these speculations are very old, and have, after all, only a remote connection with human affairs." Godkin was more concerned about the sociological significance of the popularization of science:

> We may fear the growth of something in the nature of a scientific priesthood, who, tempted by the great facilities for addressing the public which our age affords, and to which nearly every other

profession has fallen a victim, will no longer confine themselves to their laboratories and museums and scientific journals, but serve as "ministers of nature" before great crowds of persons for the most part of small knowledge and limited capacity, on whom their hints, suggestions, and denunciations will have a dangerously stimulating effect, particularly as the contempt of scientific men for what is called "literature"—that is, the recorded experience of the human race and the recorded expression of human feelings—grows every year stronger, and exerts more and more influence on the masses.[65]

In Godkin's view, there was no "authority" of science, except to discredit already existing authority, which he defined as "the recorded experience of the human race and the recorded expression of human feelings"; the noble ideal that scientists would "confine themselves to their laboratories and museums and scientific journals" competed with the all-too-human desire to seek public approbation for scientific ideas about many matters, including ostensibly religious ones.

Two months later, in another piece in *The Nation*, Godkin noted that the responses to Tyndall's latest address had sought ways to reconcile science and religion. Unfortunately, in his opinion, while a consensus about the nature of science might exist, less agreement was evident about how to define religion. Reconciliation was thus a feeble attempt at bringing otherwise separate spheres together again, and Godkin rejected the effort.[66] A response criticizing Godkin's earlier editorial "Tyndall and the Theologians," entitled "What is the Business of Scientific Men," appeared in the same periodical a month later, at the end of 1874. The author of the letter insisted that "the influence of the conclusions of science on theological thought is certainly not unimportant" and went on to argue that the development of theology and philosophy without taking into account the findings of natural science would turn the former into superstition and the latter into scholasticism.[67]

At this point, William James joined the debate, praising Godkin and chiding the "fearful" figure he called Scientist for encouraging the immodest ambitions of those who "cut loose from the old traditions of taking things piecemeal and contentedly ignoring much, and commit themselves to vast theories which, whether true or false, stand at least as much unverified today, in the strict scientific sense of the word verification, as any of the theosophies of the past." James concluded, "In 'science,' as a whole, no man is expert, no man an authority; in other words, there is no such thing as an abstract 'Scientist'—fearful word!"[68]

That "fearful word" was characterized as such because in this new climate no concept of the ineffable in any religious tradition was immune to scientific skepticism. In response, Rabbi Frederick de Sola Mendes

(1850–1927) wrote in 1874, after Tyndall's visit to the United States, "And further, that school is false that teaches the falsehood of the inconceivable, the inconceivable *is* sometimes true."[69] The defense of religion, which a generation earlier had rarely united Protestants, Catholics, and Jews, was galvanized by people who understood that once *all* aspects of religion were subject to the accusation of superstition, it was only a matter of time before *all* explanations would be judged exclusively as either scientifically proven or "unscientific." No such either/or was acceptable to William James, but he, like so many others, was hard-pressed to do much about it other than bemoan scientific grandstanding and its corrosive effects on the larger public.

A quarter century later, in delivering the Gifford Lectures at Edinburgh in 1901–2, subsequently published as *The Varieties of Religious Experience*, James revisited the controversy that brought scientists and clergymen into open conflict—not about Darwinism, but about prayer:

> We have heard much talk of late against prayer, especially against prayers for better weather and for the recovery of sick people. As regards prayer for the sick, if any medical fact can be considered to stand firm, it is that in certain environments prayer may contribute to recovery, and should be encouraged as a therapeutic measure. Being a normal factor of moral health in the person, its omission would be deleterious.[70]

James obviously elided the question of whether there were differences in praying for oneself and praying for others, but it mattered less in the therapeutic realm than in the scientific one. In the therapeutic realm, the idea of "moral health" encompassed a much broader range of possible measures than those that could be tested and confirmed scientifically. What James achieved in a few short sentences was a disengagement from the intellectual challenges that scientists a quarter century before had raised against organized religion: outside the laboratory and in the world of human encounters, questions about cause and effect were less easy to disentangle, and so the answers were more varied and personal.

Anxiety, Authority, and Trust

In the end, the reception of the prayer-gauge debate in America, if it could be said to have been different from that in Britain, was less about whose institutional authority was being challenged and more about the nature of authority itself, that is, about the diverse functions of belief in a society steeped in practical problems and proposals for their solution. American physicians, in particular, did not necessarily see the scientific worldview as an ideological point of departure for discussing the deficiencies of other worldviews. On the contrary, even as the physician avoided the pitfalls of being too closely associated with "men of the cloth"—indeed, men in black—he acquired, however deservedly or undeservedly, the trusting persona of the ministering angel by taking on a part of the minister's role. And although the practice of doctors wearing white coats had to do with sanitary concerns, it also provided, more profoundly, a vision of light against the darkness of being ill and dying unaided. In the main, however, in America prayer was not seen as a threat to scientific work or to medical practice; it was another element acknowledged in the vocation of medicine, something possibly greater and more enduring than whatever may have been inside the doctor's (black) bag at any given moment in time.[71]

Nevertheless, the legacy of the prayer-gauge debates that began in the last quarter of the nineteenth century continues to influence contemporary ideas about the connections between religion and medicine. From the side of science and statistics, the problems that come with constructing a study of the power of prayer to affect healing and health, not to mention defining and measuring such effects, have been raised consistently in every decade during the past fifty years.[72] From the side of religion and alternative medicine, the pursuit of evidence about the need for a greater integration between the increasing technical powers of medical science and broader ideas about the definition and maintenance of human health has led to substantial investment in research and reports.[73]

Yet anxiety about illness and death, whether mediated by a trustworthy doctor or a respected member of the clergy, has not disappeared. The principal lesson of the nineteenth-century controversies presented here is that beneath the well-established contours of reassurance assumed by the complementary roles of physicians and clergymen, a craving persists for some type of certainty about one's fate in life. The British publicists for a strictly scientific worldview, such as Tyndall, Huxley, Galton, and others, had proposed a new, scientific approach to studying the nature of cause and effect in all realms of human life. But despite its ascendancy over the next century, this approach has not resulted in absolute certainty, even with regard to medicine. Why do some drugs work better for some people than others? What are the dangers of this or that "style" of living? Why are some people healthier than others? These are some of the questions about health and well-being that still loom large in the field of medicine. The anxiety that accompanies them, whether personal or collective, is timeless, and it continues to have implications for trusting doctors.

CHAPTER 4

Public Health, Public Trust, and
the Professionalization of Medicine

LOU GEHRIG: Give it to me straight, Doc. Am I through
    with baseball?
DOC: I'm afraid so.
GEHRIG: Is it three strikes, Doc?
DOC: You want it straight?
GEHRIG: Sure I do, straight.
DOC: It's three strikes.
GEHRIG: Doc, I've learned one thing. All the arguing in the world
    can't change the decision of the umpire.
—*The Pride of the Yankees, 1942*

As American medicine matured and the authority of the physician rose, public health movements—now ubiquitous in American life—and the export of both medical expertise and Christian ideals to nations around the world paralleled the growth of medical research and hospitals in this country. In a sense, both of these efforts—internal and external—were, broadly conceived, missionary movements, and originally their religious and medical aspects were often linked. As they diverged, efforts at Christian proselytizing have retained the label "missionary," while efforts to improve the health of nations on principles derived from "sanitary science," as public health was first called, have been more consequential to the politics and culture of American life over time.[1]

Medicine as a Mission

Signaling the beginnings of a shift from an emphasis on trust in the individual physician to the responsibilities of the profession as a whole, the physician Daniel J. Macgowan, in an address entitled "The Claims of the Missionary Enterprise on the Medical Profession," delivered to the Temperance Society of the College of Physicians and Surgeons of the University of the State of New York in 1842, implied that duty was greatest where the greatest good could be accomplished. Macgowan also drew a distinction between the missions of the clergyman and the physician:

> The facilities afforded the physician for commending Christianity to the degraded and benighted heathen, are so great that it would seem his imperative duty,—if not going himself to the rescue,—to co-operate in every possible manner with those who *have* gone forth. There are none of us who are not indebted to that gospel, and in the order and freedom it has established amongst us, and in the science it has cherished, and the arts it has aided to cultivate. The physician has access to communities and families in heathen lands as a missionary laborer, where the evangelist is not permitted to enter. He has it in his power at once, to give to the distrustful heathen palpable demonstration of the benevolence of his errand. This he can do with comparatively an imperfect knowledge of the sufferer's language. The minister of the gospel, on the other hand, can do nothing of his appropriate work without the language.[2]

During the nineteenth century, in missionary work abroad, the minister of the gospel was already at a comparative disadvantage to the physician, whose skills could fuse two kinds of healing, one physical and the other spiritual. That a necessary division of labor was required to demonstrate the "benevolence of his errand" was sustained more easily abroad, where the varieties of paganism were all equally subject to the spiritual healing of Christianity as well as the physical healing of the physician.[3]

The worldwide influence of medical missions was in full force by the second half of the nineteenth century. In Great Britain, W. Burns Thompson, M.D., published the *Medical Missionary Journal*, and historians of missions, such as James S. Dennis, described the considerable growth in the number of physicians from Europe and the United States who had elected to practice abroad.[4] At the same time, the success of these endeavors was often measured and argued by reference to the different strategies undertaken by Protestants and Catholics in their efforts to evangelize and "civilize" the world.[5] In the midst of these controversies, which were exacerbated by national loyalties and colonial realities, the medical doctor struggled to rise above the fray insofar as he could be represented as exemplifying more broadly humanitarian motives.[6]

Expanding upon previous pronouncements about the moral obligations of doctors at the Centennial Celebration of 1876 in Philadelphia, J. G. Kerr,

M.D., reported to the International Medical Congress that "every physician is called to administer to the poor and destitute, with no hope of reward but the consciousness of having used his skill for the relief of those who were in need."[7] He portrayed this purity of heart in his account of various leaders in medical missions:

> While the work of the medical men, of whom I shall speak, has been, in most cases, in connection with the missionary societies of various denominations and different countries, still the medical work possesses an importance independent of its connection with these societies, and many persons, with no sympathy for their special object, having witnessed the working of missionary hospitals, have most warmly approved of them, and contributed liberally for their support.[8]

Support for medical work associated with or sponsored by religious groups thus transcended the evangelical goals of the mission movements themselves. Most of these missionaries, medical ones included, worked tirelessly and often in life-threatening circumstances far from the public eye,[9] although several were accorded recognition in the popular press as well as in religious circles. As the medical and religious goals of these movements began to diverge, however, the work and charismatic personality of Albert Schweitzer (1875–1965)—whose dedication as a medical missionary brought him worldwide celebrity status during the first half of the twentieth century (and a Nobel Peace Prize in 1952)—attracted a great deal of media attention and had a significant influence in shaping new ideals within the medical profession about the promotion of health and well-being at home as well as abroad.[10]

The Changing Relationship between Physicians and the Clergy

The missionary impulse that extended abroad was adapted at home to the conditions of an ostensibly Christian country in which the varieties of Protestantism were defined by doctrinal and ethnic differences, and this diversity was one factor in eventually reducing the direct influence of organized religion upon medicine in America. But during the last quarter of the nineteenth century, when ministers still served as trusted bridges between the new powers of medicine and public skepticism about them, the clergy helped to foster a new vision of medicine as a whole. Forty years of commencement addresses between 1860 and 1899 at Long Island College Hospital (LICH), which was the first hospital-based medical school in the United States, and which is now the State University of New York Health Science Center at Brooklyn College of Medicine, provides many examples that can help us trace the new relationship between Protestant clergy and the medical profession (for a full list of dates and speakers, see appendix 3).[11]

In contrast to the more familiar comments about the character of the physician by clergymen to the medical students of Philadelphia, the variety of speakers called upon to exhort the graduates of LICH reflected as much the cosmopolitan interests of New York City and ongoing changes in the organization of hospitals and medical education as it did any concerns about the medical practitioner's individual moral authority.[12] And these ministers' labors to keep the importance of religion relevant to medical practice reveal strategies that were intended to inspire both individual souls *and* social institutions toward the further improvement of human health as well as a trust in the moral ideals behind this effort.

It should be noted here that nineteenth-century observers of the commencement ceremonies of the day were not necessarily reverential. Mark Twain's Pudd'nhead maxim captures the essence of some of their comments: "To be good is noble; but to show others how to be good is nobler and no trouble." In the course of complaining about overcrowding (what he called "the bread-and-butter question") and other issues affecting the medical profession in 1876, Dr. George F. Shrady, M.D., editor of *The Medical Record* (of New York), offered his opinion of the function of the commencement address:

> But the commencement orator, allowing for the sake of the argument that the ranks are crowded, still maintains that above the common struggling mass of ordinary intellects there are vacancies of position which every conscientious worker may help to fill, and still there will be room. This is to be understood as that higher realm of thought in which their teachers dwell, and in which there is none of that base rivalry for preferment, and none of that meanness of purpose which characterize the lower stratum of professional society. While we forgive the innocence of such an assumption, we are discourteous enough to deny the fact. If some of these young men should ever dare, unsupported by some college ring, by social influence, or political patronage, to apply for a hospital appointment or professorship, they may be somewhat astonished at the amount of jostling, elbowing and toe-treading there is in the upper and roomier realms of professional distinction. Talk of the dignity of their profession![13]

Eleven years later, Shrady turned again to the topic, no longer pausing to acknowledge that he was being "discourteous" but still obliquely implying that the lofty sentiments expressed might be overblown:

> This is the season when the history of medicine is reviewed from the earliest time to the present day by eloquent commencement-orators.

It is a period when thousands are refreshed with the story that medicine is the noblest and grandest of professions, and when the young medical graduate is surprised by being told that he is just on the threshold of a new career in which he is destined to hush the groans of millions with the joy of health.[14]

At around the same time, *The Nation's* editor, E. L. Godkin, in an essay entitled "Commencement Admonition," concluded,

Authority has with the last hundred or even fifty years undergone a serious loss of power, and this loss of power has shown itself nowhere more markedly than in the work of education. It has indeed almost completely changed the relation of parents and children, and teachers and scholars, so that it is now almost as necessary to prove the reasonableness and utility of any course of action which is required of boys as of mature men. Persuasion has, in other words, taken the place of command, and there is nobody left whose dictum owes much of its weight to his years of his office.[15]

Besides making an early, progressive case for a different form of education, Godkin confirmed what many in positions of religious authority already felt: their sermons from the pulpit could no longer be counted upon as being seen to instruct youth effectively, and in any case, the reach across from sanctuary to the larger society was no longer easily accomplished.

Increasingly, until the present era of celebrity and sound-bites, the commencement ceremony was anachronistic, drawing from an allegedly authoritative past at a time when veneration of professional authority was more a matter of tradition than an occasion for public inspiration or entertainment. Both Shrady's and Godkin's assessments are sufficient caution about what the public effects may have been of ministers talking to graduating medical students. An empirical review of what they actually said is thus all the more useful for determining whether they were arbiters of a glorified past of "command" or the harbingers of some new dispensation whose origin can be traced specifically to more liberal pronouncements about medicine and health.[16] This is all the more important in helping to show how, as the clergy's public authority was in decline, many ministers recognized that doctors were beginning to assume the mantle of public trust.

The roster of personages who delivered commencement addresses to graduating medical students in New York provides a snapshot of an important and influential era in the history of the Protestant clergy in America. Approximately half of those invited to speak during this period were ministers. And in numerous instances their reputations preceded them. They came from all the denominational ranks of Protestantism, and they were regarded as civic leaders both in Brooklyn and beyond.

During the first five years, only members of the medical faculty addressed the graduating students.[17] The first minister asked to deliver the main address was the Reverend Richard Salter Storrs (1821–1900), in 1866, who had led the Congregationalist Church of the Pilgrims in Brooklyn for more than fifty years. His influence in Brooklyn during the second half of the nineteenth century was rivaled only by that of Henry Ward Beecher (1813–1887), who delivered an address to the graduates of LICH in 1881.[18] Besides his reputation in Brooklyn, Storrs's presence at LICH in 1866 and again in 1873 was indicative of his work on two important fronts in what formed the religious impulse toward twentieth-century progressivism. Along with Beecher and others, he helped to organize the Sanitary Fair in Brooklyn in 1864.[19] (The United States Sanitary Commission, which provided medical care to injured and dying Union soldiers, was assisted by many fund-raising efforts on the part of municipalities throughout the northern states.) Storrs, like his father before him, was also a leader in the national conversation on missions both at home and abroad.[20]

This was the era during which the emerging powers of medicine were joined with the waning authority of religion in the pursuit of medical missionary work. Among Long Island College Hospital's earliest graduates were sons of a famous medical missionary, John Scudder. Both of Scudder's sons, John Scudder and Jared Waterbury Scudder, pursued missionary work in India.[21] The Reverend Henry Martyn Scudder, D.D., M.D. (1822–1895) spoke to the graduates of LICH about the poor quality of medicine in India.[22] The call of the missionary doctor was to alter centuries of accrued ignorance, and Scudder hoped that students would be thankful that "you, as medical students, have been trained in the enjoyment of advantages which civilization and science have bestowed upon you."[23] At the same time, the medical press occasionally observed that encouraging some physicians to practice abroad might alleviate the perceived overcrowding in the profession.

In 1867, the Reverend Abram Newkirk Littlejohn (1824–1901), who a year later would become the Episcopal bishop of Long Island, delivered the address to the medical graduates. Littlejohn developed three themes—on vocation, service, and the new threat of materialism to medical practice—all of which were reminiscent of the earlier concerns of the Philadelphia clergymen, but he admonished the students without invoking Christian themes specifically, and he was more deferential to the physician's specific knowledge and competence:

> Some crafts and callings are prized because the technical skill required to enter them renders them exclusive and select; others,

because protected more or less from the popular gaze by a veil of mystery, and others, because they are lucrative in fame and money. The medical vocation may profit somewhat from each of these sources, but its real dignity, its intrinsic worth rests on a foundation independent of them all. It is lifted high among the professions and clothed with attributes which challenge the esteem of mankind, because it affords one of the noblest possible exhibitions of learning and educated talent brought in practical sympathy with human suffering and formally bound to the alleviation of ills which are the universal inheritance of our nature.[24]

By describing the inner "calling" of medicine, its "intrinsic worth," Littlejohn noticed also the universal application of medical skill:

When I think of all this, and the thousand memories it awakens in the cells of prisons, the wards of hospitals, the bloody furrows of battle, the garrets and cellars of the poor, the ceiled mansions of the rich, along highways and upon the paths of the sea, over which hover the white wing of commerce, sure I am that the common suffrage of the race has not been just in its awards to this profession, or suitably grateful for the inestimable service it has rendered.

While Littlejohn lamented ingratitude on the part of many of those served by medicine, he also warned his audience about the consequences of neglecting the spiritual aspect of life itself:

Physiology has of late been bending itself to the task of giving us a chemistry of humanity. It has thrown this complete nature of man into the retort, and reported that an exhaustive analysis discovers only so much dirty water and fetid oil—so many ounces of scientific dust. It has been handling him not so much as a human being with a spirit inside (whose destiny we have told how to read), as a plaster statue of nucleated cells whose life is manifested in growth and decay, or as a mass of organized compost capable of distillation into gases or resolution into acids and alkalis—the whole to vanish sooner or later in hollowness and oblivion.

The concern that scientific progress would overshadow the spiritual aspects of human life was not new, of course, having already been voiced by other clergymen in the course of their addresses to physicians. But the development of a "chemistry of humanity" was now inevitable, and Littlejohn was among those ministers who continued to address the spiritual condition of the practitioner himself and beseech new doctors not to "permit the art of healing, scarcely less than divine, to be dragged in the mire of such blank materialism."[25]

The Reverend Littlejohn's dilemma was over what the consequences would be if ideas other than those inspired by revelation were to gain sway over human affairs.[26] As he stood before an audience on whom the grip of religious authority generally was weakening, he was careful to conclude,

> Preserve all the franchises of free thought, but maintain also the rights, obligations and beliefs of faith which is only the projection of reason in the realm of the unknown; study the body in its vital connections with the soul; recognize with candor and in the interests of scientific truth that there is something there which no physiologies or chemistries or anatomies will ever fire on the point of the fallible analysis. Behold God as the sovereign principle of all in the flesh and the spirit of humanity.[27]

As science was rapidly becoming the new source of revelations by means of reason instead of faith, and skepticism about religious dogma grew, the ministers who delivered such addresses to medical students were compelled to reframe the expectations they had about the "fit" between religion and medicine.

The difficulties of establishing guidelines for the minister on how to counsel individual souls was not unlike the physician's dilemma in treating difficult patients. Spiritual hypochondria was a constant distraction:

> No soul should be encouraged to rely upon the *extraordinary* while the *ordinary* has not been exhausted, to come to the minister to quiet his conscience, when he has not done what he could, previously, to do so himself, or to open his grief when he has only vague notions of what his grief is, and leans upon the priest to tell him what it is. So, with over-scrupulous persons, and persons given to doubt and despondency on very slight grounds; if treated too seriously, made too much of, allowed to tell their special trouble too often, they soon sink into the tone of feeling exhibited by beggars who parade their nakedness or deformity to excite the charity of the passer-by.[28]

Littlejohn appreciated the dilemma of a religious authority that was either too remote or too forgiving. Like the physician in the medical precinct, the pastor could not afford either to be indifferent to pain or to indulge it unnecessarily.

As for the specific responsibilities of the minister, Littlejohn reiterated a distinction that has long illuminated the nature of authority:

> There are two kinds of authority, the disregard of either of which will impair his influence and hinder his work. There is moral authority, the essence of which is love, and the outward form of which is character shaped by love. This is the highest sort of power which one soul

can wield over another. Stubborn wills and alienated hearts and soiled consciences bow down to this when they would do so to nothing else. But besides, there is the authority of a Divine Commission of a Sacred Office, in virtue of which the priest is required to exhort the people "to obey them which have the rule over them." The two authorities blended together so that we cannot precisely discern where the one begins and the other ends, make the perfect guide of souls. Some are indifferent to the authority of office, but none will be indifferent to the authority arising from moral elevation, loving sympathy, and an evident desire to lighten the burdens of the wary and heavy laden. Where the former will not serve us, the latter must be our resource.[29]

The divine commission of a sacred office carried the minister only so far. It was his outward *status*. But Littlejohn emphasized the corresponding development of inward commitment within that status, and he put the matter as clearly for the clergymen as it would be for anyone in any professional office:

The fervid tongue in the pulpit somehow dwindles away into cold silence in the chamber of sickness and in the house of the mourner. How sadly, sometimes, able and godly men disappoint themselves and others in their private ministrations amid scenes of trial and grief, where sermons about Christ the Consoler must give place to counsels fresh from the heart of Christ and bound upon the aching, lacerated soul as the skillful surgeon puts the lint into the gaping wound or the bandage on the broken limb. . . . We were ordained to console as well as to preach.[30]

The analogy to medicine was more than a convenient means by which to distinguish between competence and caring. As we have already seen in numerous ways, the medical doctor was subject to precisely the same kind of problem, except that the doctor was judged first on competence and then on character, whereas the minister could not be deemed competent without already possessing a caring character. The casuistry of spiritual caring in pursuit of the cure of souls required a genuine and cultivated sympathy within the minister.[31] But this was not the same as possessing scientific knowledge and medical skills. As the balance of authority between the two professions was shifting, the remarks of the Protestant clergy reflected that shift and the growing public confidence in the revelations of science.

New Definitions of Medicine as a "Calling"

A decade later after Littlejohn's address, in 1878, Octavius Brooks Frothingham (1822–1895), who disdained the title "Reverend" and who was among the most famous Unitarian ministers of his time, reiterated the problem of being *both* doctor and minister when he told LICH students about a physician friend in Boston who had recently died:

> He studied medicine with enormous industry, with a patience that was exemplary, and became one of the most thoroughly qualified physicians in the City of Boston. Not a brilliant man at all. Never made a discovery. Always walked in the beaten track. Never knew anything that a great many other physicians did not know. Failed to know things that physicians of his time absolutely knew. But there was always this singular combination in the man of moral feeling, keen sensibility, acute and large human sympathy with medical skill . . . he succeeded in combining the two professions with such perfect aptness that he never could tell where the one began and the other ended. When he came into the sick room he was just as much a priest as he was a physician. His voice, his manner, his interest in things, his soothing tone and bearing, all had an effect upon the nerves and the physical condition, so that his patient was prepared to be cured—not to be killed. [Laughter and applause.][32]

Nothing in Frothingham's remarks contradicted his long-standing devotion to Auguste Comte's later doctrine of the Religion of Humanity. The physician was to be the exemplar of a new professional ideal. The clergymen might "walk through his routine," but the physician "must be the master of all the science that his age could master." The rising expectations about doctors' abilities were enormous. "The aim of the physician [is] to make life long and happy," Frothingham commented, but he also acknowledged, referring to a British study of physicians who had failed in their profession, that the challenges doctors faced were great: "Was it any wonder that men left, neglected, abandoned, swore off from a calling that meant to all but the most brilliant and the most fortunate of small support limited popularity?"[33] By the time he finished his address, the image of the Boston physician whose adequate abilities had been offset by his priestly character was tempered by a more bitter truth that physicians would invariably be blamed for their mistakes regardless of the public's growing idealization of their vocation.

Frothingham also reminded his audience that they were duty-bound to treat all patients according to their infirmities and not their stations in life, as did the Reverend William A. Snively (1833–1901), a year later, in 1879:

> To the true physician, devoted to his calling, these varieties of human condition are but faint and temporary distinctions. Absorbed in

the philanthropic errand of his life, sickness levels all ranks, and through the varied exterior he sees but one fact of suffering humanity, which it is his mission and task to relieve.[34]

Gradually, the Protestant ministers who engaged their audiences with lofty rhetoric about the vocation and mission of medicine imposed less and less in the way of specifically Christian doctrine in their strong endorsements of the physician's calling. The absence of references to Jesus Christ, for example, was a concession to the scientific orientation of the audience addressed, but it also reflected clerical anxiety about challenges to religious traditionalism. Another minister asserted that "humanitarianism is coming home to roost,"[35] reminding students that a true vocation was above the mere pursuit of monetary rewards, not only progressive but also uplifting for those doctors who might continue to struggle in their occupation for many years to come. One kind of home mission, then, was to minister to patients without judging them, at least according to their means. As another clergyman stated to an audience of LICH graduates in 1892, "The grandest and best men of your profession today have learned how to reach the heart and conscience and will of those with whom they are dealing and have learned that this is the greatest aim of their profession."[36]

These addresses to medical students also touched upon the topic of the impaired physician. The Reverend James M. Buckley (1836–1920), a Methodist, told the LICH graduating class in 1880, "I have, in a ministry of twenty-two years, seen a score of brilliant doctors going to ruin by drink.... A drunken doctor is worse than a drunken minister, for a drunken minister is an awful warning and his bad sermons do not kill people." He also warned against physicians becoming callous.[37] Similarly, in 1898 the Reverend Thomas B. McLeod concluded,

> I want to say plainly the man who has no respect for a man as a man, who has no reverence for woman, who cannot meet and match delicacy with delicacy, sorrow with sorrow, prayer with prayer, and enter the sanctuary of suffering with unshod feet, clean hands and a clean heart, that man is not fit to be a physician and should seek occupation in a slaughter house.[38]

Other ministers denounced therapies other than those being taught by "regular" physicians:

> The faith cure is a fraud. [Applause.] It commits suicide by its own name. [Applause.] Faith without works is dead. [Applause.] We have no right to ask God to help us if we do not do all we can to help ourselves at the same time.[39]

Two of the most well-known and flamboyant ministers in America also delivered addresses at Long Island College Hospital: Henry Ward Beecher in 1881 and Thomas De Witt Talmage in 1888. Beecher's reputation brought him numerous invitations to deliver such addresses, and in one worth examining here, which he had delivered earlier, in 1872, to the graduates at Columbia University's College of Physicians and Surgeons, he formulated a thesis about the doctor's mission that exemplified the rise of the new concept of public health as a realm of medicine and the new challenges that doctors would face as patients lived ever longer and healthier lives:

> Take my own profession. . . . There was a time when it was hardly right for a man to be born without the priest to sanction it; and all through life, at every turn, he must call in the priestly aid and counsel. Now, men not only are born, but they marry and die without our help; they have appropriated to themselves a thousand offices that were once our sacred and exclusive privilege. But we have gained far more than we have lost; have been deprived of those manifold duties which were hindrances, only to give us freedom for broader and higher growth; and I rejoice in it. So in medicine. The intelligent mother is now your rival. The laity know more than the wisest of you did two or three centuries ago. Yet the field of your own work is not narrowed, but marvelously enlarged; and it is destined to be extended more and more with the advance of science and its popular recognition. . . .
>
> You are no longer to be simply ministers of healing to the sick; a large part of your future duty is to be toward the well. The community looks to you to develop and enforce the whole science of private and public hygiene; it looks to you, moreover, for instruction in mental and moral philosophy.[40]

In his comments about the future responsibilities of physicians, however, Beecher did foresee how the physician's broadening mandate to "minister" would incorporate all aspects of the science of medicine. Not all physicians were enthusiastic about such an expansion of authority, but Beecher signaled a decisive way in which the conscience of the nation could be stimulated by this new mission of medicine. And in the end, public trust in the profession of medicine would depend on how this mission was defined and by whom.

At the same time, Beecher insisted that the social problems of the day required medical attention:

> A part of [God's] revelation is in our own physical constitution; and in the progress of truth we are to learn what is the connection between bodily conditions and moral states. I say, as the result of

long observation and experience, that, very largely, the causes of wrongdoing are morbid conditions of body and unfavorable circumstances. . . . I aver, then, that a sick man can hardly be a moral man; can hardly conduct himself as a free moral agent, when every nerve and fiber of his body is crowding temptation upon him. There is sin enough in one single organ, the liver, to call it the devil's den. You are to interpret for us this connection between physical and moral disease; to help us clear the way for larger conceptions life and duty. . . .

To whom shall we look for the diffusion of knowledge on these subjects among the people, if not to you?[41]

Although it had been inarguable for millennia that alcoholism has profound effects on an individual's health, the theory that it also has an organic basis would be pursued off and on throughout most of the twentieth century. Beecher still saw this issue and others in moral terms and public health measures as a link between the ends of medicine and the end of sin as it related to the ills that plagued society in general. By so doing, he added further encouragement to the ideal of making all human problems amenable to medical solutions:

It devolves, then, upon the physicians of this age to make themselves felt as a power in public as well as in private. In every effort to elevate the standard of personal purity; in every discussion of the best means of preventing crime; in every attempt to gain a sounder philosophy of education, and to apply it in the direction of public institutions, or in the training of individual children—the physician is to be not only the adviser of the family, but also the counselor of the community, whose word should be heeded as always important and often decisive.[42]

Beecher advocated an enlarged role not only for the physician but also for the institutions of religion and medicine. Prevailing interpretations of nineteenth-century Protestant approaches to social problems have not emphasized the implications of encouraging the physician to participate actively in achieving larger social goals, but this was one theme of the day.[43] What Beecher and others of like mind could not foresee was that the prevention of crime and the effective training of children would soon be subject to a new kind of expert scrutiny based less on the distinctive skills of the physician and more on a collaboration between many other professions—social work, teaching and public school administration, policing, and community organizing among them.[44]

Beecher's hope was more strongly stated by the Reverend Thomas De Witt Talmage, who told the graduating students of LICH in 1888 that "millennium for the souls of men will be millennium for the bodies of men. Sin done[,] disease will be done; the clergyman and the physician getting done with their work at the same time."[45] This lingering mixture of religious and utopian ambitions only increased the expectation that physicians were at the forefront of a great mission to eradicate spiritual and physical suffering and bring about a better society.

By the end of the century, the term "character" was rapidly ceding its place to "personality" as the vernacular through which the moral aspects of the learned professions were to be discussed. In his 1899 commencement address to the graduates of LICH, the Reverend John Douglas Adam contrasted the high nature of "personality" against the low nature of "professionalism":

> Personality is the greatest thing in the world. I mean the inner man, the fusion of the emotional, the rational and the volitional into a unity. . . . Without work personality is buried; it lies like a city of gold beneath the desert sand. And personality will be refined by sacrifice. . . . But the professional life has a great enemy. Its enemy is professionalism. Professionalism is the scourge of manhood; professionalism is the exchange of music for a barrel organ; it is the exchange of a picture for a fashion plate; it is the exchange of life for mechanism. When a man surrenders to professionalism the unripe fruit of his personality is plucked and dried and put in cans and labeled.[46]

Adam's pejorative evaluation of the word "professionalism" echoed the long-standing Protestant objection to the embracing of the authority of office even when the officeholder lacks a virtuous character. The elevating of the professional "office" over the person who occupied that office troubled him, and it would bring into the twentieth century an enduring debate about the relative weights assigned to each in judging what was wrong with medicine. How much did good medicine depend on who chose to study and practice it? And how much were new problems faced by physician and patient alike related to the structure of its delivery, that is, to the ongoing reorganization of the profession?

The Influence of Psychology and Vocational Guidance

Nineteenth-century Protestant America democratized the idea of moral character, insisting on its relevance to all walks of life but leaving the specific details of professional accountability to each respective school of professional training. The clergy's influence on the characterological development of professionals became more and more marginal, for two related reasons.

First, professional success honestly attained was for many decades prima facie evidence of high moral character, and therefore the clergyman's advice was at best redundant and at worst trite and accusatory. By the turn of the century, trust in doctors was increasingly based on respect for their professional training and simply taken for granted, at least publicly; in the public mind, character was increasingly rooted in professional competence. Second, the concept of "character" itself was rapidly becoming associated with individual temperament, a part of personality rather than morality, and those who were working in the evolving field of psychology made personality one of their first major focuses of investigation.[47]

The transition from a religiously defined ideal of character to a psychological approach to personality is foreshadowed in the efforts made by ministers to help young people choose a vocation. The commercialization and elaborate testing methods associated with contemporary career guidance had their origin in a Protestant insistence that the practical conduct of life could be improved methodically; in a sense, the concern with which ministers like Abram Littlejohn had struggled in terms of the spiritual life was given a new scientific orientation by the practitioners of vocational psychology.[48]

At the same time, the maintaining of medicine's high reputation among a growing number of professions required its alliance with them and with other social institutions, a process that occurred alongside continuing debates over the physician's responsibilities beyond medical work itself. The popular authority of the medical profession was, at least in the short term, enhanced by numerous debates over the physician's role, while the idea of "role" itself must be seen in the context of earlier and less publicly visible discussions about trusting doctors in light of Christian religious expectations, both Protestant and Catholic. In brief, the notion of role was articulated in two ways, first in terms of a burgeoning literature about who was qualified to study medicine, and second in terms of what the proper balances should be between technical training and personal character, and between the doctor and society.

During the last quarter of the nineteenth century, anyone who wanted to reach young people who were thinking about the choice of a profession had to speak in practical terms. Edward Everett Hale, a prominent Unitarian minister (and author of "The Man without a Country"), addressed Harvard students about their choice of a profession,[49] and among many other works he published were *What Career? Ten Papers on the Choice of a Vocation and the Use of Time* (1879) and *How to Do It* (1871). The latter book was advertised with the following contents: "How to Talk; How to Write; How to Read; How to go into Society; How to Travel; Life at School and in Vacations; Life Alone; Habits with Children; Life with your Elders; Habits of Reading; Getting Ready." Hale's efforts were devoted to the development of qualities of leadership among the middle and upper classes, and his approach was above all a practical one.

The popularizing of an open consideration of an appropriate choice of career—at least for the educated elite—gave impetus to a new understanding of the division of labor in society. Finding a place in that division of labor required an appreciation of the qualities of aptitude and skill. Such qualities were not unimportant in previous centuries, but a profound and enduring change in understanding about what it meant to find and have a calling began to occur. Protestant theological concerns were rapidly succeeded by an individualistic psychology as the emphasis changed from how to act in accordance with God's will to how to act responsibly in securing a place in society.

An interesting, if eclectic, illustration of this change in emphasis appeared in a book entitled *Vocophy [L. Voco, I Name; I Call] The New Profession: A System Enabling a Person to Name the Calling or Vocation One is Best Suited to Follow*, by Lysander Salmon Richards, published in 1881. *Vocophy* was an early and original example, followed by a myriad of more popular works throughout the twentieth century, of vocational guidance and evaluation. Such guidance, formalized, rationalized, and, finally, professionalized, was offered in a wholly egalitarian spirit. Richards pointed out on the first page of the preface that

> In using the pronoun HE throughout the work, we do not use it with any thought of male superiority or adaptation. No distinction of sex is generally intended in these pages, but convenience prompted the use of HE, instead of HE AND SHE. If any female possesses or can gain the necessary requirements demanded in any honorable trade, profession or occupation, though at present solely followed by man, there can be no objection, whether morally or religiously considered, to her following it.[50]

Richards's subsequent evaluation of "ill-adaptation to pursuits" starts with the clergy and doctors:

> Many might follow almost any other calling with better success. They seem to have chosen it simply to gratify a desire without regard to fitness or ability; and because of this non-fitness for their profession, the country swarms with poverty-stricken ministers. This same is true of physicians, except it does not apparently exist to so great an extent.[51]

Without mentioning the relative crowding in both professions, Richards made observations about suitability in terms of the individual person. Each profession—minister, doctor, lawyer, teacher—was treated to the same assessment from the perspective of individual suitability.

Richards' new system, as he called it, was intended to create a new occupation of vocopher, for whom vocophy would provide the requisite knowledge to advise others in their choice of vocation. Without entirely dismissing the allegedly useful knowledge acquired through phrenology, physiology, and physiognomy, Richards called for a more sustained investigation into the "cause and manifestations of genius and its application to the latent, undeveloped force in individuals."[52]

As to the physician in particular, Richards remarked,

> All can call to mind numerous instances of physicians, in whose care none would trust their lives, and who would better fill some other position. Because they have passed through a medical college, are members of a medical association, and have an "M.D." affixed to their names, it is not a guarantee of their especial fitness for the profession. Ability is not the only requirement for a good doctor; a peculiar organization is demanded, and this is possessed only by a few practitioners.[53]

With obeisance to the theory of evolution, Richards attributed the lack of fitness of many in society to poverty, but he invented his system of vocational assessment with none of the pessimism associated at the time with the "survival of the fittest," an idea to which he nevertheless paid the highest respect.[54] His emphasis on individual fitness was a form of tactical optimism over and against the prevailing sentiments about the various so-called inevitabilities of life.

Having the strong desire to pursue a certain vocation was not in itself sufficient justification for doing so. A millennium of advice of fathers and mothers to their children, from Cicero's *De Officiis* to informal, often humorous guides up to the present moment, confirms this. Richards's unique contribution was to propose a more systematic way to determine an individual's suitability for a given occupation, thus directing the anxiety about the choice of a vocation toward an assessment and evaluation of ability, talent, and suitability. In a manual of possible vocations, including sixty-one occupations in all, Richards offered brief summaries of those characteristics most pertinent to each. Under "The Physician," he wrote,

> Should be a calm, pleasant, neat, polite and quiet gentleman, not absent minded, with no insanity manifested in immediate ancestors, and free from any desire for intoxicating drinks. Must have a thorough knowledge of his profession, and a love for it; be devoted to his patients, and ever ready to sacrifice any moment, day or night, to the performance of his duties.[55]

What distinguished Richards's proposed new system from earlier ideas about a calling or vocation was the absence of any mention of religious influences upon its pursuit. Instead, as in his characterization of the physician, the image of a person "ready to sacrifice any moment, day or night" became, in this era, a part of the practical requirements for the pursuit of a medical career. To be, in effect, always "on call" was the equivalent to being called and having a calling.

Lysander Richards's approach to vocational guidance and choice of occupation presaged the application of widely gathered information about occupations to individual abilities and needs. And even prior to the full-blown development of a social science of vocation, ideas about the concept of a "calling" had been changing. At the turn of the twentieth century, for example, in *The Protestant Ethic and the Spirit of Capitalism*, Max Weber described a religious calling, with its removal from the affairs of everyday life, as otherworldly asceticism, exemplified in the life of the monk. This-worldly asceticism arose, in Weber's view, as a result of the intense focus on the fate of the individual that followed the Protestant Reformation and that contributed to the emergence of thrifty middle classes. Throughout the nineteenth century, the meaning of work was less and less associated with religious teachings, leading Weber to conclude that the "idea of duty in one's calling prowls about in our lives like the ghost of dead religious beliefs."[56] This-worldly asceticism has proven to be a transitional stage between traditional and postmodern meanings of vocational choice and its pursuit. That pursuit, once linked to divine inspiration, was gradually conceived of as a dilemma of the "self" adrift without an anchor in a sea of possibilities.

One stabilizing force that educational reformers in the Progressive Era proposed to enable young people to find meaning as well as earn a living in their future pursuits was a more conventional form of vocational guidance than Richards's, which brought a new vision of professionalism to career choice while at the same time extending its reach beyond the educated elite. "Vocation's" adjectival form, "vocational," symbolized a lowering of expectations about the broader range of commitments that had been part and parcel of its Christian, and specifically Protestant, meaning for professionals. Eventually, as educators used the new guidance tools in the context of public education, the phrase "vocational training" came to connote programs for those who were not destined to pursue higher education. In any event, vocational guidance and training were two different aspects of a new way of looking at the sustained association between the individual and work. And the withdrawal of any mediating spiritual guidance, from whatever religious sources, was one further step in the disengagement of public education from what had also originally been broadly Christian purposes.

Among the earliest advocates of professional vocational guidance was Frank Parsons (1854–1908), first director of the Vocation Bureau and Breadwinners' Institute, Civic Service House, in Boston. Civic Service House was an outgrowth of the settlement house movement, and Parsons's association with it was determined by his lifelong commitment to aid immigrants and the working class in their pursuit of work. His was a strategy designed not to enable people to find happiness in work but rather to ameliorate the more destructive results of industrialization, which contributed to high rates of dropouts, starting in grammar school. Parsons was a reformer who, along with others, introduced the hope of vocational guidance, not only for humanitarian reasons, but also as a means to produce better workers overall.[57] His best-known work, published posthumously in 1909, was entitled *Choosing a Vocation*.

Each candidate for vocational guidance, with the assistance and direction of a counselor, was to pursue a process of "self analysis" in relation to available requirements of a particular occupation, and the counselor was to attempt to fit the person to the most suitable job based on this analysis and those requirements. Parsons referred to the honest comparing of individual aptitude with occupational requirements as a process of "true reasoning." The choice of vocation was to be understood as the attempt to reduce inefficiency, to substitute "chance, proximity, or uninformed selection" for a careful comparison of "aptitudes, abilities, ambitions, etc., with the conditions of success in different industries."[58] Efficiency, an idea rooted in the Protestant sensibility about the virtues of hard work, was the epitome of social morality, that is, a way to create a better society not by the dictates of moral instruction but by the achievement of social cohesion. Through efficiency, each would find the work best suited to his abilities.

In making "this greatest decision of his life,"[59] the candidate, guided by the vocational counselor, would understand his purpose in society, a goal at once meaningful to the social reformer and not overly moralistic from the point of view of the candidate. Parsons opened up a terrain of potentially endless possibilities of individual assessment without recourse to the fatalism of either religious predestination or the "survival of the fittest." Everyone had a potential place in the world, just as Lysander Richards had imagined. In this optimistic era of career counseling—an ingredient of American progressivism—the young were given new ways to think about their "greatest decision," even as that decision became by virtue of more information and more choices, less momentous and less decisive. The idea that one's entire life would be determined by choices made or not made early in life was no longer crucial to finding the most probable path toward success in work.

In 1910, as Parsons and others endeavored to bring vocational guidance to a larger public, the Harvard psychologist Hugo Münsterberg (1863–1916) popularized their efforts in an article entitled "Finding a Life Work" in *McClure's Magazine*.[60] Münsterberg helped Parsons develop tests for his candidates, and he soon developed a correspondence course on vocational guidance.[61] Earlier, the American Women's League had contracted

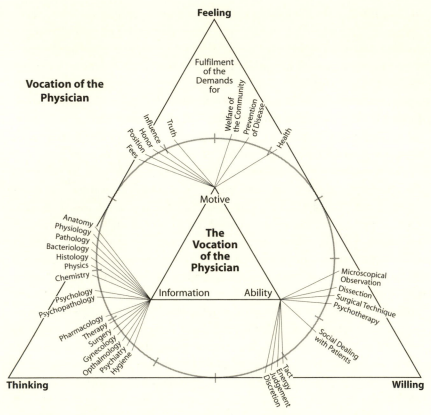

Feeling

Vocation of the Physician

Fulfilment
of the
Demands
for

Welfare of
the Community

Prevention
of Disease

Influence
Position
Honor
Fees

Truth

Health

Motive

The Vocation of the Physician

Anatomy
Physiology
Pathology
Bacteriology
Histology
Physics
Chemistry

Psychology
Psychopathology

Information

Ability

Microscopical
Observation
Dissection
Surgical Technique
Psychotherapy

Pharmacology
Therapy
Surgery
Gynecology
Opthalmology
Psychiatry
Hygiene

Social Dealing
with Patients

Tact
Energy
Judgement
Discretion

Thinking

Willing

From Hugo Münsterberg, *Vocation and Learning* (St. Louis, MO: Lewis Publishing, 1910), p. 233.

with Münsterberg to write a four-volume reading course titled *Vocation and Learning*, which was also published in 1910. A separate chapter was devoted to the vocation of the physician.

Münsterberg noted that medical schools such as Harvard and Johns Hopkins required a bachelor's degree from a "reputable college" for entrance to medical study. The general education of the physician was taking shape in a form that has not changed, except in terms of the advancement of knowledge in different fields, for nearly a century. Münsterberg illustrated his idea of the physician's vocation, dividing it along three lines, motive (related to feeling), information (related to thinking), and ability (related to will). In this psychological rendering of the physician's vocational ideal, the elements related to motive and feeling were focused on the general welfare, while those related to ability and will were concentrated on the patient in particular: "A true physician must be both a friend of mankind and a scholar."[62]

A New Focus on the Doctor-Patient Relationship

The social reformers and professional psychologists who joined simultaneously to give practical and intellectual substance to new ideas about medicine as a vocation were aware of how much it was beginning to matter that the best people be fitted to the best occupations. These were leaders in the formation of a meritocracy against which individual choice and ambition could be measured and evaluated. But even as medicine developed new standards to evaluate the competence of aspiring (and practicing) physicians, concerns about what one might call either the spiritual or the psychological aspects of the relationship between doctors and patients continued to be discussed and debated.

One approach, developed by the British physician Alfred Taylor Schofield (1846–1929), called for the use of an "unconscious therapeutics" in the treatment of patients. Schofield wrote and practiced before the broad influence of Freud and psychoanalysis stipulated an idea of the unconscious as fundamentally tied to repression and sexuality, with potentially negative consequences. Schofield viewed the unconscious in positive terms, as something to acknowledge in its potentially constructive uses in medical treatment.[63] His book *Unconscious Therapeutics: The Personality of the Physician* was indebted to Maurice de Fleury's *Medicine and the Mind*, from which he quoted: "The Church, with its rules of life, its abstinence, its food regimen, and other health laws, has ever been a great hygienist."[64] Schofield's approval was not of the religious influence of the Catholic Church per se but rather of the possibilities for medicine implicit in what various Christian and other faith traditions had known for millennia about the uses of mind over matter. Unlike religious critiques of materialism that had focused on the impure motivations of the practitioner, Schofield's approach rested upon the limitations of the materialist approach altogether.

In his scheme, unconscious therapeutics applied to disease was expressed in four ways between the doctor and the patient. First was the *vis medicatrix naturæ*, "the direct instinctive power of the unconscious mind," "unconscious to both patient and doctor."[65] Second was the "unconscious mind, influenced directly by surrounding forces or other unconscious agencies acting as suggestions . . . generally unconscious to both the doctor and patient, though not always so to the former." Third was purposeful suggestions to the unconscious mind, consciously used by the doctor, "[although] the patient is unconscious of their action." And fourth was the unconscious mind "stimulated directly on the part of the patient by a determination to get well, to shake off illness, ignore pain, etc. These are therapeutic means of which the patient is necessarily always conscious, but the doctor often unconscious."[66]

The power of suggestion, which underlay Schofield's appreciation of how the unconscious was influenced, had many agents. One was the use of such techniques as hypnotism, and another, more important to his overall approach, was the physician's awareness of "all that can be known of the power that he is wielding every day, in being what he is, and looking and speaking as he does."[67] The physician's comportment, for example, the expression on his face alone, could have an unconscious therapeutic effect: "It would be well worth while to write a book on the medical face, first, as seen in the patient as a diagnostic sign of physical and mental disease; and secondly as seen in the doctor as a power for good and evil."[68]

Lamenting the decline of apprenticeship as an aid in directing the formation of the persona of the doctor, Schofield referred to the many works written by physicians about the importance of good manners, appropriate dress, and upright character.[69] Such works appeared in greater abundance at approximately the same time that medical training was becoming more securely a part of higher education. Like Schofield's own work, they only approximated the apprenticeship-like relationship that he noted had been transformed by the formalizing of medical education. In his view, instruction in how the physician could achieve the most unconsciously effective personality was best conveyed by example. In numerous cases, how doctors communicated to women provided some of the most poignant illustrations of the failure of unconscious communication, or in other words, the breakdown of trust. In a long footnote to these observations, Schofield saw further than his contemporaries the implications of the failure of communication:

> As I correct these proofs I come across a terrible case of a lighted life of needless suffering, simply from utter want of understanding on the part of an otherwise clever and successful doctor. He kept pooh-poohing her symptoms and urging her to do what she had no strength to perform, though she had every desire; and thoroughly made her feel she had only herself to blame for her illness. So accustomed are doctors, trained only in the schools, to ignore functional nerve symptoms that, from mere habit, they often pooh-pooh signs of organic disease in mistake, if these be mixed up with them. It was so in this distressing case; indeed the patient despaired of all cure, owing to the feeling of beating against a closed door when telling her troubles to a doctor. . . . I would earnestly press on every doctor who reads these pages to make his patients feel he understands their sufferings; and also to be most careful not to neglect any organic trouble, because overlaid with functional symptoms.[70]

And, then, quoting Dr. Oliver Wendell Holmes—"A smile may be worth 5,000 dollars a year to a man"—Schofield concluded that "we should much prefer to appraise [the value of this kind of professional sensibility] by its therapeutic power to our patients than by the possible dollars or shekels that may accrue to us from it."[71]

Any possible connection between unconscious therapeutics and monetary success was something that Schofield avoided, preferring "the loftier and more altruistic one of our own therapeutic value to our patients."[72] But whether unconscious or not, this tension between behavior and reward, to oneself or to others, was on its way to being made more explicit as a dynamic and essential process of modern society.[73] Schofield recited an inventory of physicians' vices and virtues, all of which were functionally intended to improve or subvert success. Among the vices were "fear, hesitancy, depression, ill-temper, pomposity, verbosity, levity, too much solemnity, artificiality, hurry, impatience, carelessness, forgetfulness, and vanity." Among the virtues were

> dignity, simplicity, brevity, decision, interest, sympathy, candor, naturalness, certainty, cheerfulness, hopefulness, good temper, courage, carefulness, patience, and firmness. Patience in hearing and listening, distinctness in speech and orders, quickness and observation in seeing, and firmness and gentleness in touch, are also helpful adjuncts.[74]

Schofield's register of inappropriate and salutary behaviors for the physician was grounded in a probabilistic understanding of common sense rather than in specific traditions of religious faith, and his unconscious therapeutics represented the effacement of such traditions, but at the same time it represented a claim for the medical efficacy of something beyond mere professional expertise—something intimately related to the issue of trust.

In the end, it was a great benefit of scientific method that a physician's authority could no longer be separated from certain standards of professional competence. But at the same time, as Schofield and others argued, that competence was still based upon the actions of a person whose effects upon others, whether defined as conscious or unconscious, have never been completely amenable to scientific understanding.

Many of Schofield's insights about medical practice were restated several decades later by Lawrence J. Henderson (1878–1942), a biochemist who spent his career at Harvard University.[75] Henderson embraced a broad sensibility about the growing influence of science upon the world. He was instrumental in bringing Alfred North Whitehead to Harvard in Whitehead's later years, and he is remembered, along with others, for introducing the thought of the Italian sociologist Vilfredo Pareto to an American audience. The search for order in all types of systems, from the biological to the social, intensified his determination to put the social role of medicine on the same plane as its scientific role. This search was consistent with deeper elements of his Protestant character, which he summarized well in an unpublished memoir:

> I acquired in childhood and have preserved many of the standards of a respectable, old fashioned Yankee, and perhaps still more a deep feeling that the pattern of behavior with which these sentiments correspond is the decent and respectable way to live. Long ago, I came to realize that patterns of behavior are relative, that they correspond more or less perfectly to the historical, economic and social circumstances of a particular race, class or group in a particular place at a particular time. Nevertheless, my feeling persists that there is something peculiarly valuable about the pattern of behavior of the respectable, hard-working, thrifty Yankees of the kind who were anxious to be fairly enlightened and at the same time fairly "correct," that this pattern of behavior is somehow an absolute; and the fact that I clearly realize the error of this proposition as a scientific theorem seems to leave my *feeling* completely unmodified.[76]

With regard to both his intellect and his feelings, then, Henderson's encounter with both the scientific and social worlds was defined by his character, a predicate to rather than a result of his vocation. His notion of a "pattern of behavior" that was "somehow an absolute" defined brilliantly a new vision of the connection between character and vocation, a connection he would be unable to ignore as he examined the condition of the medical profession during his day.

Henderson's contribution to historical and sociological thinking about medicine came in the publication of three papers, "Physician and Patient as a Social System" (1935), "The Relation of Medicine to the Fundamental Sciences" (1935), and "The Practice of Medicine as Applied Sociology" (1936). Applauding the increased application of science to medicine, Henderson was less impressed with its application to "the personal relations between the physician and the patient." Although it would take another thirty years for public complaints about professional indifference to crystallize fully, Henderson was well ahead of his time when he observed in "Physician and Patient as a Social System" that

> a multitude of important new facts and theories, of new methods and routines, so far absorb the physician's attention and arouse his interest that the personal relations seem to have become less important, if not absolutely, at least relatively to the new and powerful technology of medical practice.[77]

No one was to blame for this development, but it was Henderson's hope that a "science of human relations" would parallel in its potential applications the contributions of the natural sciences. At the same time, he was somewhat dismissive of both sociology and psychology insofar as their advocates "are in general little aware of the problem of practicing what they know in the affairs of everyday life." And, in what amounts to an enduring aphorism, he concluded, "Indeed, skill in managing one's relations with others is probably less common among professional psychologists and sociologists than among the ablest men of affairs or the wisest physicians."[78]

Henderson was saying more about the function of academic "culture" and professional training generally than about the impact of psychological and sociological knowledge on society. After all, within his own university a generation earlier, Hugo Münsterberg had helped to promote the role that psychology could play in the affairs of everyday life. And it was possible to hear the clear echoes of Alfred T. Schofield when Henderson spoke of the special interpersonal skills of certain doctors:

> Sometimes in these favored persons whose perceptions and sensi-
> tivities are well suited to the task, it results in patterns of behavior
> that are among the most interesting and, if I may use the word,
> beautiful that I know. . . . Doctors like [this] have always existed
> and will always exist, but their skill dies with them except when
> their apprentices have learned some measure to imitate them.[79]

Although couching many of his comments in the language of science, Henderson was raising once again what had been for millennia the question of character: in awe of the characterological authority of certain physicians, Frederick Shattuck for example, he was also intent on extracting something from their "patterns of behavior" that could be used for the better training of all physicians.

Following Schofield's formulation of unconscious therapeutics, Henderson appealed to the work of the Italian sociologist Vilfredo Pareto, whose theory of "sentiments" in the doctor-patient relationship played a central part in helping to incorporate the role of unreason into sociological thinking:

> A patient sitting in your office, facing you, is rarely in a favorable
> state of mind to appreciate the precise significance of a logical state-
> ment, and it is in general not merely difficult but quite impossible
> for him to perceive the precise meaning of a train of thought. It is
> also out of the question that the physician should convey what he
> desires to convey to the patient, if he follows the practice of blurt-
> ing out just what comes to his mind. The patient is moved by fears
> and by many other sentiments, and these, together with reason,
> are being modified by the doctor's words and phrases, by his man-
> ner and expression. This generalization appears to me to be as well
> founded as the generalization of physical science.[80]

This use of the term "sentiment" had a strong affinity with Schofield's approach in *Unconscious Therapeutics*, and it is important to see how Henderson reiterated and deepened the practical implications of an approach that acknowledges one person's effect on another, whether conscious or unconscious. In a footnote, he pointed out that in this new view of the physician's task "it is possible to discern more than traces of the methods of psychoanalysis, divested however of the usual theoretical and dogmatic accompaniments, and therefore considerably modified."[81] In other words, just as Schofield and others before him had begun to chart a largely unmapped terrain of human interactions before psychoanalysis, Henderson attempted three decades later to distill from the insights of the psychoanalytic movement certain practical methods that might be discernable beneath the cover of the grand theories of id and ego, Eros and Thanatos.

Although Henderson apparently took no notice of the advice literature about the interpersonal methods of doctoring that preceded his "scientific" approach, his assertions were remarkably consistent with what common sense required but what specific circumstances might subvert. Consider his various forms of advice:

> In talking with the patient, the doctor must not only appear to be, but must be, really interested in what the patient says.
>
> There should be no argument about the prejudices of the patient, for, at any stage, when you are endeavoring to evoke the subjective aspect of the patient's experience or to modify his sentiments, logic will not avail.
>
> Beware of the expression of moral judgments. Beware of bare statements of bare truth or bare logic.
>
> Remember especially that the principal effect of a sentence of confinement or of death is an emotional effect, and that the patient will eagerly scrutinize and rationalize what you say, that he will carry it away with him, that he will turn your phrases over and over in his mind, seeking persistently for shades of meaning that you never thought of. Try to remember how as a very young man you have similarly scrutinized for non-existent meaning the casual phrases of those whom you have admired, or respected, or loved.[82]

The "emotional effect," that is, anxiety, provoked by the patient's illness and a diagnosis was, then, to be countered by the authority—personal as well as professional—of the physician. Henderson's interpretation of the professional responsibility in this regard meant that it was part of the physician's role to be thoughtful and compassionate about the patient's state of mind. Focusing on what effect a doctor's words and demeanor might have, rather than on the exercise of his authority, Henderson did not address the issue of what the consequences might be of a patient's doubt in such authority. But in asserting that "the doctor must not only appear to be, but must be, really interested in what the patient says" he was advocating for a new convergence between person and office.

Henderson also recognized that both the doctor and patient were faced with the inevitable asymmetry of their encounter, which could be made more balanced by the sentiment of trust. In Henderson's view building that trust was mostly the responsibility of the physician, who needed to understand and respond to the inevitable consequences of his actions. But this trust was also predicated on an even deeper assumption about the role of the physician in society: Henderson was careful to point out more than once that the physician should not convey any moral judgment about a patient's condition. The justification for this neutrality is not examined, but the implication for the issue of trust is obvious. If the doctor's motivation was to improve, whenever possible, the health of the patient, then the relationship between the two could not be a purgatory in which moral judgment was interlaced with clinical observation. Although the purity of such separation could be never assured, it represented a practical principle of the sort that required the physician not only *not* to moralize but also to make this a tenet of professional and moral responsibility. And whereas ancient stipulations about confidentiality were intended to define the physician's relation to others besides the patient, Henderson's focus was on the confidential interaction itself. Although not in itself religious, this new emphasis was clearly indebted to a Protestant dispensation that had placed profound emphasis upon the doctor's conscience, seeing it as distinct from, and possibly in opposition to, the moral dictates of the larger society. The deepest trust in particular doctors, before the age of widely available medical information, was anchored in the belief that doctors were agents of no orthodoxy other than their medical vocation, the truth of which was for them to determine as they saw fit.

Henderson's mission to bring the spirit of science to the human relations between doctors and patients was mediated by the continuing debates about what practices were in the best interests of public health, and as the profession of medicine evolved, it could not escape the attacks of critics on both the individual authority of the physician and the corporate authority of medical institutions. The insularity that defined for Henderson the microcosm of the physician-patient relation could not keep out the larger claims of all kinds of moralizers whose missionary efforts on behalf of public health would transform every action and every relation at all levels of human life.

The Influence of a Sociological Perspective

Henderson's contribution helped to define an important direction in what became, in academic sociology after World War II, the subfield of medical sociology, but the term itself appeared much earlier in the title of an article published by Charles McIntire in the *Bulletin of the American Academy of Medicine* in 1894. No "science of sociology," he wrote, could ignore the omnipresence of Herbert Spencer and his evolutionary ideas, or their contribution to the array of related social sciences whose mission was to contribute to the "progress of civilization, and all that relates to society."[83]

The use of the term "medical sociology" only in relation to a subfield of sociology or as an invitation to interdisciplinary synthesis does not do justice to the many ways that at the beginning of the twentieth century physicians were regarded as arbiters of both individual disease and the diseases of society. In this spirit, a physician, James Peter Warbasse (1866–1957), in a work published in 1909, applied the term to a medical view of social problems. Warbasse, who wrote a three-volume treatise on surgery, was also a defender of animal experimentation and a pioneer in consumer activism.[84] He was already in his forties when he adapted the term "sociology" to more distinctively Catholic purposes, parallel to the already extensive, but less publicly noticed, traditions in pastoral medicine. Indeed, it is one sign of Warbasse's incorporation into the larger project of a social science of medicine that he was characterized for his "somewhat flat" treatment, dealing "with the broad social aspects of medicine."[85]

Whether flat or not, Warbasse's *Medical Sociology: A Series of Observations Touching upon the Sociology of Health and the Relations of Medicine to Society* serves as a useful contrast to the ambitions of the founders of vocational guidance. Alfred T. Schofield's work on unconscious therapeutics was an early example of a post-Protestant approach to health and well-being insofar as it recognized the efficacy of trust in the medical encounter but did not attribute such efficacy to any particular grounds of religious faith and doctrine. The same challenge facing Protestant ministers in their efforts to bridge religious insight with medical practice was now well on its way to being transformed into a personal psychology of human encounters out of which more and less effective results could be observed, examined, and eventually even measured.

At the same time, the idea that medicine and the pursuit of good health were necessary for the advancement of civilization inspired broader strategies that could not be accomplished only in the context of the doctor-patient relationship. In the end, Warbasse concluded,

> The influence of medical science upon human progress is destined
> to bring into the circle of happiness all those things which make

for health, for health is one of the most important prerequisites of happiness.[86]

The merging of the pursuit of happiness with the pursuit of health has been a leading preoccupation of advanced societies for nearly a century. Warbasse advocated an idea of morality consistent with progressive goals of education, and he argued that the achievement of "healthful happiness" was a process of enlightenment "in which, if the walk to the office is the more healthful it will be preferred to the ride, in which the harmful tipple [drink] will be declined with pleasure, and in which my friend will value his health more than his pipe."[87] The balancing of choices in life, part of what is now called lifestyle, had a basis not only in moral prescriptions but also in medical predictions about the outcome of various behaviors. Such balancing would not be managed at the level of the individual encounter between physician and patient but rather as the result of the aggregate influence of medical understanding of the public health. This aggregation eventually found its formalization in public health movements, the leading example of which in America in the twentieth century was that against tobacco. No rational crusade against certain types of individual behavior could succeed on moral prescription alone.

Warbasse realized this and attempted to excite moral and medical interest in social problems, that is, those kinds of problems that for centuries had been central to the tasks of pastoral medicine and counseling. It is no coincidence that among the chapters in his book were "The Venereal Peril," "The Instruction of the Young in Sexual Hygiene," "Sexual Morality and the State," and "Sexual Continence." Although he dismissed with some vehemence what he termed the superstitions of the church about human sexuality, he nevertheless echoed the prevalent views about sexual morality, however hypocritically observed, in early twentieth-century America:

> The man who yields to what he knows is wrong and harmful—there is just one thing for him to do, and that is to stop. If he desires to correct his habits, but does not, and is much in a state of sexual excitement, then I should say that one or more of three things is the trouble: he is either suffering from idleness, the prime promoter of vice; his education and knowledge of the simple things are defective; or he has a mental defect which should receive consideration from the neurologists.[88]

Despite these recommendations, Warbasse was far more interested in the control of the consequences of sexual activity—for example, sexually transmitted diseases—than in the control of sexual activity itself. Sex within marriage was part of a larger plan for health, but marriage and health could be undermined by the refusal to keep track of the advance of venereal disease in the larger population. Public health authorities, as distinct from physicians, would be increasingly called upon in an ever more anonymous social order in which the outcomes of one's actions could be made subject to medical diagnosis and eventually testing, (as in the case of contemporary drug use) as opposed to being seen primarily as moral failings.

Warbasse's constructive impulse, which reached well beyond the traditional definitions of the physician's responsibilities, was consistent with the aim of many of the Progressives to improve individual lives by creating and directing institutions that would in various ways guide and direct them. Writing in 1924, Gerald Birney Smith, professor of Christian theology in the Divinity School of the University of Chicago, defined the new Christian physician of public health:

> The Christian physician may most effectually preach the gospel of clean living without using cant phrases or seeming to be unduly pious. The provision for hospitals, the administration of public health, the education of parents to the right of children to be well-born, the understanding of the relationship between physical health and normal appetites and desires, the discovery of the cause of occupational diseases, are some of the enterprises in which physicians must exercise leadership. So prominent is the ideal of ministry in the code of the physician that it may almost be said that his vocational standing may be measured largely in terms of the Christian ideal.[89]

The physician's "vocational standing," that is, moral authority, derived from an ideal internal to professional regulation (what became known as professional "autonomy") and another ideal (i.e., the Christian ideal) external to the profession, but underwriting as well as overseeing it. It is important to notice the equivocations contained in such phrases as "may almost be said" and "largely in terms of" that distinguish the pronouncements of the nineteenth-century Protestant minister from broader theorizing intended to invoke compatibility rather than confrontation.

The theological necessity to define rather than to instruct the "Christian physician" meant a real withdrawal of clerical presence, both Protestant and Catholic, from active engagement in the life of the professions. The new physician would have to find meaning in a vocation through the diverse social sciences and their allied movements in public health.

Two distinct social roles for medicine thus evolved historically: one grew out of the particular responsibilities of physicians and patients to each other; the other was predicated upon a definition of the corporate responsibility of medicine to the larger society. Warbasse appropriated the term "medical sociology" before academic sociology and social epidemiology had secured a professional mandate in their relations to universities, hospitals, and government. He did so with the dual inheritance of pastoral medicine and Protestant ideas about conscience and vocation. Such forgotten figures as Lysander Richards, Frank Parsons, Alfred T. Schofield, Lawrence J. Henderson, and Peter Warbasse presaged the rapid and decisive professionalization of social science. Before an era of social-scientific claims about "professional dominance," the strategies of those seeking to influence the training and practice of doctors were largely constructive, if not effective. After the era of professional dominance—culminating in so-called managed care—that constructive impulse may again have greater importance than has been apparent until quite recently.

The Lingering Question of Character

For nearly seven decades, roughly from 1900 to 1970, the American public would be most impressed with what appeared to them to be an unassailable connection between the character of the practitioner and the high status of the medical profession. The fracturing of this connection, which began in the 1960s, had much to do with the general suspicion directed toward all those in authority, but in the case of medicine, it had as much, if not more to do with the doubts about individual character anticipated in the admonitions of Protestant ministers a hundred years earlier and reinforced in the first half of the twentieth century by a growing body of social-scientific research.

While physicians sought and gained broader popular acceptance throughout the second half of the nineteenth century, in the United States at least, they were not confronted with the same kind of dramatic rivalry with state-established religion as had been the case in England. The debates in America were as much about the science and commerce of medicine, its practical delivery and organization of payment, as about its status among the professions. A decade or more before the famous Flexner Report of 1910, the intraprofessional rivalries that produced different approaches to medical treatment were already abating among college-educated professionals, so much so that trust in medicine also meant a trust in the emerging system of professional, scientific education. The doctor was now part of an institutional arrangement that required undergraduate preparation, professional training, and clinical experience, all of which could be achieved in the broader settings of universities and hospitals.

With both institutional security and little public controversy about its role in society, the medical profession moved to the height of its cultural authority by the middle of the twentieth century. The absence of publicity about physicians, except in their own medical press, was a sign of that authority, which held sway for more than half a century. This was, to be sure, a distinctly Protestant achievement insofar as any "publicity" implied "bad" publicity. In addition to reporting on the events of the day, newspapers, in the Protestant configuration of public announcements, recorded births, marriages, and deaths, and except for the rise of "public interest" stories (including, for example, those about Albert Schweitzer), the medical profession largely avoided public notice.

Signs of concern about the physician's vocation, that is, about the depth and resolve of individual commitment and moral duty, were nevertheless evident in an address delivered to the American College of Physicians in 1949 by Henry Allen Moe, who led the Guggenheim Foundation and who served as president of the American Philosophical Society and was the first chairman of the National Endowment for the Humanities. Moe summarized the enduring tension between character and competence this way:

> All of our science and medicine and all of our technology, while not negligible in any fundamental view of us, are not to be compared in influence with the Sermon on the Mount, the Ten Commandments, the Declaration of Independence, the Constitution of the United States. It is such creative efforts of the mind and spirit, some diffused into our minds and spirits, which make us what we are, free men with free ideas. . . . If those efforts of the mind and spirit that yield results comparatively fast, if the activities that are deemed useful for present progress and power and strength, are exalted and entrenched, and if those activities which determine the character of people are denigrated, then—as a long-term proposition—the structure of freedom, the structure of liberty and order under justice, of every life, will fade. There are signs that this is a great twentieth-century problem.[90]

Moe's effort to caution doctors about the dangers of denigrating "those activities which determine the character of people" was not widely shared among members of a profession that did not intentionally disassociate itself from the American civil and religious character of its authority. At the same time, the profession was regarding its own success less than ever in terms of vocation and more in terms of career.

The pharmaceutical firm of E. R. Squibb & Sons lent its name to the publication of *The Physician and His Practice* (1954), edited by Joseph Garland, M.D. (the editor of *The New England Journal of Medicine*). Garland described the book, a collection of articles, as "primarily a source book of information regarding his [the physician's] career":

> A proper emphasis is placed on the character and personality of the physician and the standards that are expected of him—and of his

wife—in relation to the two important circles in which they move: the intimate family circle and the larger community one.[91]

C. Sidney Burwell, formerly dean of the Faculty of Medicine at Harvard Medical School, opened the volume with a summary account of the "Evolution of the Doctor." Heralding the enormous gains of medical science during the first half of the twentieth century, Burwell did not call for higher standards of educational or technical competence among physicians but rather took them for granted. He emphasized instead qualities of physicianhood that were associated more with caring than curing:

> At a time when medicine has so much to offer patients, it is a tragedy of the first order when its effectiveness is interfered with by defects of character or by bad manners. The role that manners play in the practice of medicine is a large one. Effective contact with patients and their families is largely a matter of good manners, which demonstrate the physician's concern for his patient and his effort to understand him. Counter demonstrations of rudeness, lack of consideration, or an obvious desire not to understand are guaranteed deterrents to effective practice. Good manners are a firm foundation of effective communication between doctor and patient. They can also be a firm foundation for effective understanding among doctors. Integrity of purpose and good manners will together solve most of the problems in medical ethics.[92]

Today's observers of medicine would regard Burwell's assessment, particularly of the "integrity of purpose" and "good manners," to be quaint, if not antiquated. Yet Burwell, however unwittingly, was reciting an inheritance that had long since become the basis for how physicians, especially those at the top of their profession, defined and maintained their relation to the public. "Integrity of purpose" recycled and conveyed convictions about duty, and it shifted the burden away from the outcome of treatments to the beneficent intentions of the person who offered them. "Good manners" were, above all, intended to diminish any sense of indifference on the part of the doctor that a patient might experience. Indeed, Burwell's concern was that something might be lost as new research and a growing number of professional journals expanded the horizons of medical knowledge. What was a unique pain for a patient was in danger of becoming, for the physician, just a symptom in a larger taxonomy of diagnosis and treatment—and all attempts at classification (in any field) deny the seemingly inexhaustible and unique character of individual experience.

If concerns were expressed by physicians about the general education of fledgling doctors, they were not about medicine's association with the great traditions of civil and religious authority embodied in such things as the Sermon on the Mount, the Ten Commandments, the Declaration of Independence, and the Constitution of the United States. Instead, one distinctive aspect of the legacy of such concerns was taken up in calls for physicians to be more deeply educated in the humanities.[93]

These were not calls for the continuing education of physicians, but rather for early, that is, undergraduate preparation for the study of medicine. In his presidential address before the American Surgical Association in 1952, Dr. Daniel C. Elkin conceded the physician's social responsibility but went further: "He should concern himself with the problems of man and society, but he cannot do this if his thinking and awareness do not go beyond the confines of a single field of endeavor." Elkin emphasized this point by quoting from "A Case for the Study of the Humanities in the Making of a Doctor," just published by Stanley Elwood Dorst in *Annals of Surgery:*

> How well has modern education in America nourished and cared for our spiritual heritage? How has it taught our youth to distinguish the liberal, humane, life-giving forces from the evil, life-destroying forces? How well has our education disciplined us to live while training us to do?
>
> The lesson should be clear; the modern barbarians do not destroy science and technology, they do not wipe out the machine values, but instead convert them into terrible forces of evil and death so that those who would resist their mad rush must out-do them in ruthlessness. What they do destroy with devastating thoroughness is liberal culture of the people. They destroy their roots into the past, their libraries, their free press, their religion, their belief in the essential dignity of man. In short—destroy the education which makes men free.[94]

That "liberal culture of people" was an essential ingredient of the post-Protestant idea of medical vocation. Elkin's criticisms were not of the physician's moral character but rather his "educated" manner: "I am greatly concerned, as I know many of you to be, over the quality of scholarship manifested by our physicians. Many of you have served on editorial boards and no doubt have been struck by the ignorance, indeed actual illiteracy, of many doctors in the basic knowledge of our own tongue."[95] And with an almost breathless (and slightly overblown) call to arms, Elkin concluded, "We have an obligation to demonstrate that there are things other than [technique] in surgery, science in medicine, and knowledge in life."[96]

The kind of crisis in confidence that was being announced had everything to do with World War II, although the lapses into barbarism that marked the European descent into totalitarianism were difficult to find, even by way of analogy, in America in 1950. If the rising generation of doctors was more ignorant, less grammatical, less cultured, and even ungrateful, the proposal for a more humanistic education was about all that leading physicians could offer in light of a new and careful separation between religion and the medical profession that was evolving to accommodate America's growing religious pluralism. The "liberal culture," whose historically religious predicates served as touchstones for debates about core values, struggled with the task of shaping the physician's professional identity specifically in terms of moral character.

The identity of the physician was thus contested in several ways. Certainly the pursuit of career was an occasion for reflection about success and failure, two further elements in the definition of liberal culture. Professional success and failure were visible signs that achievement mattered even in a society that had also long been the subject of clerical criticism about its abiding materialism. The type of materialism that ministers preached against in the nineteenth century was rooted in spiritual impoverishment. It was the kind of materialism that led physicians, in particular, to separate their divinely inspired obligations from their purely technical abilities.

During the 1960s, the American Medical Association established a Department on Medicine and Religion and instituted a special program on their relationship in conjunction with its annual conventions. The second of such programs was offered as part of the 113th Annual Convention in San Francisco in 1964. In its advertising for the program, the *Journal of the American Medical Association* noted, "Physicians who plan to attend are encouraged to bring their wives, and doctors in the San Francisco area are also encouraged to invite their clergymen."[97] Rabbi Abraham Joshua Heschel was invited, along with Dr. William C. Menninger, M.D., to speak on "The Patient as a Person." Heschel's address, published later in *Ramparts*, was a strong challenge to the professional sensibilities of attending members. He delivered what amounted to a jeremiad, anticipating many of the complaints against doctors that would be made more loudly and more publicly in the coming decades. This critique was set forth in a series of aphorisms that centered on the dangers of careerism:

> The mortal danger faced by all of us is to succumb to the common virus of commercialism—the temptation to make a lot of money.
>
> The motivation to dedicate one's life to the great calling of medicine has its source in the depth of the person. Yet a great calling, whether teaching, healing, or writing, is a jealous mistress; she requires complete devotion, supreme appreciation. Medicine, teaching, and the ministry are not sinecures; nor are patients, students, and parishioners shares to be traded at the stock exchange.

May I suggest a therapy for the virus of commercialism: a personal decision to establish a maximum level of income.

Luxuries are expensive, but making money is even more expensive. We pay for it dearly. Making money may cost us values that no money can buy.

The flesh is weak, temptations are strong. But the sign of intelligence is the capacity to delay the satisfaction of desire and above all to exercise preference, to make an option, when the integrity of one's vocation is in danger of being corrupted. . . .

Striving for personal success is a legitimate and wholesome ingredient of the person. The danger begins when personal success becomes a way of thinking, the supreme standard of all values. Success as the object of supreme and exclusive concern is both pernicious and demonic. Such passion knows no limit. According to my own medical theory, more people die of success than of cancer.[98]

Heschel's admonitions about the corruption of vocation were Protestant in tone and substance, but they derived their special force from prophetic Judaism.[99] Unlike the many clergymen who were determined to find ways to accommodate the clear and present realities (rather than dangers) of what success in the medical profession might mean, Rabbi Heschel used the occasion to raise once again the question of the character of the physician, and in particular he lamented the loss of a more sustained personal relationship between doctor and patient. The doctor's "attitudes are either sensitive or cruel, human or inhuman; there is no middle course. Indifference is callousness."[100] And he noted that access to the doctor was changing as well:

It is terribly embarrassing to know that some individual doctors seem to think that it is highly improper for a patient to get sick during weekends. (Night calls are as fashionable as horse and buggy.) The patient is haunted with fear, but some doctors are in a hurry, and above all impatient. They have something in common with God; they cannot be easily reached, not even at the golf course.[101]

The *Journal of the American Medical Association* reported on the session, entitling its piece "Psychiatrist, Rabbi Agree on Importance of Warm Physician-Patient Relationship," and quoting various excerpts from the talks by Menninger and Heschel, but in Heschel's case, the quotations were highly selective. If the assembled audience was not persuaded by Rabbi Heschel's remarks, the only evidence in the pages of *JAMA* came in the response by Dr. Edward R. Annis, M.D., president of the American Medical Association, who presided over the meeting and offered informal comments. *JAMA* reported that "Annis denied that the doctor-patient relationship has declined with the rise of modern medicine." Instead, the laments for the era of the old family physician needed to be put in perspective:

> Time and compassion were about the only remedies doctors once had for many illnesses. "He gave unstintingly of what he had," Annis said. "But the patient died." Today, the doctor may not be around long enough for the patient to remember his face, Annis said. "He prescribes a remedy and is gone—but the patient lives."[102]

Although the special program had been entitled "The Patient as a Person," Rabbi Heschel shifted the focus—at least as evidenced by Dr. Annis's remarks—to the doctor's vocation. He pointed to such qualities of bad character as indifference, something that Annis was quick to counter with his appeal to what has generally come to be known as "outcomes," that is, the results of a medical action as distinct from a judgment of the person or persons overseeing and producing those results. Annis recast indifference as a rational impersonality and defended it over and against indifference (which, he conceded, was, in a technically well trained doctor, a sign of incompetence). But Heschel bemoaned something other than the lack of humanistic training of doctors, touching upon a growing professional arrogance or hubris that was bound to be exposed when mistakes were made. Although he did not state it this way, his fusion of indifference with impersonality can also be seen as an attempt to maintain the grounds for forgiveness when mistakes were made. Subsequent developments in malpractice litigation were not least of all the result of the changed circumstances that Edward Annis defended. Remembering the doctor's face meant acknowledging his humanity as well.

In retrospect, Heschel's appearance before the leaders of the American Medical Association seems to have been an odd choice, given the legions of less prophetic-minded clergy that could have been invited, but this was an era when medicine had begun to open its door to people of many different backgrounds, and to women as well. The following year's annual convention was a tribute to the insight that if medicine and religion were to cooperate, they first had to *appear* to cooperate. Heschel had overwhelmed his audience, leaving the prospect of cooperation uncertain. In 1965, the "Medical News" headline in JAMA, announcing the third annual Medicine and Religion Program, put things back on track: "MDs, Clergymen: Both Vital to 'Healing' Ministry." The Reverend John E. Hines, leader of the Episcopal Church, delivered remarks along with Howard A. Rusk, M.D., director of the Institute of Physical Medicine and Rehabilitation at New York University–Bellevue Medical Center.

Rusk observed,

> In these days when the science of medicine is advancing at such a
> pace that it is almost impossible for the practitioner to hope to keep
> up with even a portion of the scientific advances, it is fundamental
> that we remember that we are doctors first and scientists second.

This image "that we are doctors first and scientists second" was a re-
cycling and reiteration of the nineteenth-century claim that a physician, in
order to be a good physician, had to be a good Christian first. Rusk succeeded in modifying this ideal to its present form, in which being a "good
person" is the predicate to the authority to minister to the sick—or in more
contemporary vernacular, to care—even though a specifically Christian ref-
erent was no longer cited, at least openly.

Instead, citing the physician's experience in overcoming the illness and
suffering of his patient, Rusk concluded,

> I believe that this basic and inherent desire of man to do something
> for his less fortunate fellow transcends religious dogmas, political
> beliefs, and geographic barriers. If we could only use this universal
> language, we would have a tool to unravel the babel of tongues and
> an instrument which would penetrate any iron curtain or closed
> boundary.

Here history intruded itself again in the form of an acknowledgment of
the Cold War. More importantly, in this context Rusk's idealistic misread-
ing of the story of Babel revealed an agenda for medicine that would carry
its mandate far beyond the confines of the physician-patient relation: "If we
could start to work here together in a program where all of us have the same
goals, it is more than possible that, with God's help, we would find the solution for living together in peace."[103]

> Bishop Hines, for his part, remarked on the nature of the fragmented
> patient: Sooner or later—and it will more likely be sooner—the
> physician will have to enter into a "depth relationship" with some-
> one for whose very existence he is responsible. He may try to evade
> this relationship, and there are avenues which appear open to him
> to do so, namely "treating the fragments," overspecialization, and
> so forth, thereby giving partial service to the whole patient.[104]

The recognition of what already several years earlier had been heralded
as "an impending crisis," that is, the demise of family practice along with the
increase of specialization, was commonplace by the mid-1960s.[105]

Here was an instance, unlike the present era of managed care, where
accountability was stated less in terms of structural variables and more in

terms of the physician's character. Bishop Hines lamented the loss of such accountability, criticizing the image of "the technically proficient robot."[106] Both Heschel and Hines sought to influence a realm that in one sense no longer existed. Doctors, historically, came to medicine already possessed of certain character. It was not something that was conceived of being made or, for that matter, remade by education or by structural changes in the delivery of services. If religion had a role to play in the national story of medicine as a profession and career, it would not be in the form of admonishing or exhorting physicians to do better. By the end of the 1960s, the shaping of the conversation that permitted religion a place at the table was made by the intellectual social movement now called bioethics.

Within a few years during the turbulent 1960s, the AMA's effort to forge a cooperative effort between religion and medicine lost its force as the public became accustomed to hearing straightforward questions raised about life and death and about the doctor's responsibility in both. At the AMA convention in 1968, the Medicine and Religion Program was headlined in *JAMA* "When Do You Pull the Plug?"[107] This was not a rhetorical question, and its rising public visibility would in subsequent years make it a matter for public, democratic, and legal deliberation rather than one for only doctors and clergymen to ponder from above the fray. Such a question marked the symbolic end of the unassailable character of the physician's popular authority. The Medicine and Religion Program held out the promise for a publicly visible and substantive cooperation between physicians and the clergy at a moment when the authority of all professions was under attack. It was inevitable that the kinds of questions being pressed would not be substantively settled within or among those two same professions once so intimately connected. With the government's increasing role in the management of medicine, first with Medicare and Medicaid, and then with various governmental commissions in pursuit of answers to bioethical questions, the separation of church and state would make cooperation between the professions appear ever more peculiar and inappropriate.

PART TWO

Beyond the Golden Age of Trust in Medicine

By his means the medical man preserves the life of the mortally ill man, even if the patient implores us to relieve him of life, even if his relatives, to whom his life is worthless and to whom the costs of maintaining his worthless life grow unbearable, grant his redemption from suffering. Perhaps a poor lunatic is involved, whose relatives, whether they admit it or not, wish and must wish for his death. Yet the presuppositions of medicine, and the penal code, prevent the physician from relinquishing his therapeutic efforts. Whether life is worth while living and when—this question is not asked by medicine.

—Max Weber, "Science as a Vocation," 1919

CHAPTER 5

The Growth of Popular Distrust in Medicine

Introducing a 1963 issue of *Daedalus* on "The Professions," Kenneth S. Lynn cheered, "Everywhere in American life, the professions are triumphant."[1] In the following few years, this glacial confidence about professional triumphalism receded rapidly, and the decade of the 1960s is now remembered for a steep decline in public trust in all professionals.[2] The decline in confidence in medicine in particular had as much to do with negative publicity about medical outcomes as it did with specific complaints about individual physicians. It appears to have had very little connection with any real concerns about the remarkable progress of medical science except in the public perception of the changing balance between humane care and technological control.[3] The general disavowal of institutional authority during the 1960s did not initially serve the interests of one professional group over and against another. Rather, the types of concern identified by a century's worth of Christian thinking about the individual character of the practitioner were initially reiterated as challenges to all forms of individual and institutional authority.[4]

Nineteenth-century meditations on medical vocation and responsibility—on physicianhood—by Protestant ministers and Catholic moralists were brought up once again in twentieth-century analyses of professionalism and professional power, in particular by social scientists but also by journalists. During this time, the status and voice of the patient was not as ignored as revisionists would have us believe, but it was also not balanced against the rising influence of medicine upon nearly every sphere of human life. What has come to be called the empowerment of the ill patient dramatically recast this balance, creating the active vocation of patienthood. The patient with the disease, rather than the physician with the diagnosis or treatment, would henceforth become identified with numerous self-help movements, leading to a further decline in medical authority, if not power, in America.

The larger social and cultural contexts in which this decline in authority occurred have been amply documented in work on new social movements, in particular the women's health movement, about which more will be said below. In one important sense, the so-called revolts of the 1960s can be seen as the culmination of, rather than the exception to, a long history of the balance of power between doctors and patients, tipping too far at times in one direction or the other. Following thirty years of calls for a greater voice for patients in determining their choices about treatment, an inevitable asymmetry was bound to be revealed nevertheless. Writing in 1994 in the *Wall Street Journal* under the headline "Breast Cancer Patients Get More Assertive by Doing Research and Asking Questions," Laurie McGinley noted that "with the help of a growing body of medical information and data available to the public, cancer patients are helping to make decisions that traditionally have been made almost exclusively by doctors." Further, "Advocates say women who are managing their disease aren't trying to take their doctors' place, but they also say there is no substitute for personal vigilance."[5]

The changing valences of trust can be identified here, first, in terms of the patient's challenge (e.g., "more assertive") to the tradition of medical decision-making, and, second, in the exhortation of (e.g., "no substitute for") personal vigilance. Both the degree of assertiveness and the extensiveness of personal vigilance in popular terms have been wildly overestimated in their organizational impact on the physician-patient relation, yet profoundly underestimated in their psychological influence on the nature of communication in medicine generally.

If any specific influence can account for the changed character of trust between physicians and patients during the second half of the twentieth century, then the role played by advocates of women's health must rank very high. Medical innovation and error in the treatment of women's health has resulted in several widely publicized and litigated instances of iatrogenically induced harm, that harm caused inadvertently by medicine (e.g., the negative effects of "the pill," DES, Thalidomide, the Dalkon Shield, mastectomy/lumpectomy, and silicone implants, among others).[6] The discovery of these iatrogenic harms was confirmed by epidemiology, which, in alliance with a growing interest in women's health that came with calls for "women's liberation" throughout the 1950s and 1960s, did much to alter public accounts of the interactions of physicians and patients.

All insights about physician-patient communication correspond to the problem of how any expertly trained elite communicates its knowledge to anxious laity. In this sense, the problem of moral and cultural authority returns with new urgency. Contemporary women's health advocacy has transformed expectations about women's participation in the maintenance of their health. This now appears to be empirically indisputable. The changing status of women in American society, along with their increased number in the medical profession, has created a new kind of patient with more informed expectations about risk and responsibility. The appearance of this new patient has greatly affected both men's and women's attitudes toward their health.[7]

Communication and Trust

Before describing the especially important role that second-wave feminism has played in redefining the communication between physicians and patients, it is important to acknowledge the less politically visible efforts of researchers who have also responded to similar currents of distrust created by the structure of the "delivery" of medical "services" and failure of such communication. Because physicians and others explicitly recognized early in the twentieth century that communication between doctors and patients was a problem beyond the formal pronouncements of a code of ethics, it is also important to note the continuities that endure between earlier and later efforts to enhance that communication.

In 1985, Eric J. Cassell, a physician, published a two-volume work on the sociolinguistic nature of communication between doctors and patients. In his introduction to Cassell's work, the medical historian Stanley Joel Reiser asserted that "the patient's role as narrator in the drama of illness has declined in the twentieth century," due largely to the fact that the technologies of diagnosis made such narration superfluous if not epiphenomenal. The investigation by medical scientific method was pitted against the suspect subjectivity of patients whose complaints required outside audits of one sort or another. In one respect, there is nothing new in this problem. What appears to have made it more noticeable was its intensification, with the appearance of ever more sophisticated and refined technologies of diagnosis that were utilized in ever larger and more bureaucratic hospital systems. Echoing the framework of Lawrence J. Henderson, Reiser concluded that although the analysis of communication could not achieve the exactness of the examination of a biochemical event, some analogous effort was nevertheless in order. Again, why it was in order was taken for granted, based presumably on forces outside the realm of science that were not identified.[8]

Cassell's work appeared nearly simultaneously with other studies of the linguistic dynamics of physician-patient interaction. In contrast to slightly later works that viewed all such micro-encounters as reflections or consequences of the larger political economy of American health-care, embodied in such micro-encounters, Cassell offered a disinterested account of the complicated role that language and gesture invariably play in how patients and doctors understand one another. Following in the tradition of Lawrence Henderson, Cassell's disinterest acknowledged also that times change, that the nature of interactions change, and that the expectations of patients and doctors alike change.[9] But he did not extrapolate from micro-encounters to formulate generalizations about the larger social order. In opening his study, he told the following anecdote:

> During the 1930s my grandmother saw a specialist about a mela-noma on her face. During the course of the visit when she asked him a question, he slapped her face, saying, "I ask the questions here. I'll do the talking!" Can you imagine such an event occurring today? Melanomas may not have changed much in the last fifty years, but the profession of medicine has.[10]

The more interesting part of Cassell's account is not his or anyone else's understandable reaction to his grandmother's humiliation but rather to his question, "Can you imagine such an event occurring today?" That a doctor "today" could no longer slap a patient's face with impunity was supposed to be evidence of a changed expectation between doctors and patients about their interactions. But Cassell's incredulity itself has a sociohistorical context, since it is not obvious from his anecdote whether his grandmother's doctor's behavior was typical of such arrogance on the part of doctors or exceptional for its time and place. It is more obvious that Cassell's incredulity was typical of many patients who have come to expect nothing less than the right to be heard, understood, and attended by the physician, whether or not they feel that they can always achieve this. The growing confidence of patients along with the declining image of imperial physicians provided renewed justification for analyzing communication between them. In an earlier era, the assumption was that communication was first and foremost therapeutically important. In the next era, the dignity and rights of the patient were put front and center. In both eras, the matter and manner of communication were personally fused but also analytically distinct, permitting the kinds of interpretive efforts that Cassell and others pursued.

This sociohistorical context that gives different anecdotes a stronger or weaker moral resonance does not make what is morally commendable or condemnable unrecognizable. Both Sophocles' *Antigone* and public anxieties about the uses of corpses in medical teaching and scientific research, for example, morally enrich any context in which questions are raised about respect and disrespect for the dead and the obligations to them.[11] The doctor-patient relation has endured for millennia as a relation of authority because each changing context of understanding between two people leaves more than traces, if not a blueprint, of what each ideally expects from the other, whether or not such expectations are satisfied. This dynamic led Cassell to observe that the demand for truth-telling always has clinical as well as contextual dimensions.

The clinical dimension was obvious to him:

It is important to realize that in years past, when physicians were not truthful with their patients, neither they nor others considered the doctors to be "liars." It was widely believed that telling patients the terrible facts of their diseases was bad for them; the truth would harm them. I remember this dialogue from almost twenty years ago: the surgeon had found an inoperable carcinoma of the stomach, and when asked by the patient what the operation showed, the surgeon said, "Well, George, we did a lot [of] cuttin' and shnitten and pulled out some bad stuff, and you're gonna be okay." I cared for George until his death, some months later. The day before he died, and *only* the day before he died, he said, "Ya know, Doc, I sometimes wonder whether I'm getting better!" That was not an uncommon occurrence in those days. We do not know, however, whether patients were being any more truthful with their physicians than vice versa. I remember too well instances where patients demanded the truth and then, after being informed, became depressed to the point where caring for them was extremely difficult.[12]

For Cassell, the point was not the act of telling the truth, but what therapeutic function the truth could serve, thus hearkening back to ideas put forward by Alfred Schofield and Lawrence Henderson, among others. Putting the medical interest first was consistent with Cassell's commitment to the idea that the principal aim of medicine was to heal patients. It seems obvious that such a commitment orders interests and thus creates and nourishes trust in authority. More important, Cassell's commitment to this priority led him to conclude that the physician-patient relation should never be seen as tentative or uncertain even though the nature of the information conveyed in it may be wrong:

Strange as it may seem, for information to serve the functions that I am describing . . . it is not necessary that it be correct. . . . The basic point is that the information must be credible to the patient. Believability requires not only that words be plausible but that a speaker be worthy of trust. Both criteria are met best by someone (the physician) considered an authority by the patient, who is speaking what he or she believes to be the truth in a language that can be understood by the patient.[13]

Of course, the specter of malpractice may hover over such remarks. But to "be worthy of trust" is not and cannot be, finally, a matter dictated or resolved by law or science. Cassell's work, which was intended to help the medical student and young practitioner pay closer attention to communication, belongs in the long tradition of medical vocation in which the priorities of commitment were well established.

On the other hand, Cassell and many after him were aware of the social contexts in which information was communicated. He did not deny these contexts so much as subordinate them to those clinical perceptions about the efficacy of certain therapeutic functions, including communication. Yet others, especially social scientists, started from the assumption that the clinical realities were always subordinate to their social contexts. Eliot Mishler, a pioneer and leading authority on doctor-patient communication, described very well the appearance of new critics of medicine:

> [The] assumption of the relative autonomy of medicine and its neutrality with regard to conflicting interests and values within society is challenged directly by the new critics. Their argument begins with the counterclaim that medicine is not insulated from the larger society but is embedded within and responsive to socio-cultural, economic, and political forces.... Not only is medicine influenced by society, but medicine has consequences for society. Even more specifically, because these critics view society as an arena of conflict over power and resources, they assert further that the health-care system not only pursues its own special interests but, at the same time, aligns itself with dominant groups and classes in the society, thus serving their special interests as well.[14]

Mishler's reference to the new critics, in 1981, took special notice of the work of Ivan Illich, who published *Medical Nemesis: The Expropriation of Health* in 1975. The debate initiated by Illich and others is worth revisiting because it has been caricatured and effaced in substantial ways in light of the dramatic transformations in physician authority over the past quarter century.

The New Critics

Ivan Illich was never easily absorbed into the frameworks of social protest that achieved notoriety as the baby boom generation came of age in the late 1960s and early 1970s. At one time a parish priest in New York and then a recluse of sorts in Cuernavaca, Mexico, or at least self-exiled sufficiently that his later writings were greeted with less enthusiasm, he indicted modern industrial societies for their oppressive institutions, including education, urbanization, and medicine.[15] He was unsparing in his critique of modernity, but it was not first a political-economic critique, although for many that may have been its most important aspect. Such critiques of inequality find fault principally with the economic organization of medical practice, or as Mishler described it, with a medical profession that "aligns itself with dominant groups and classes in the society." Instead, Illich should be regarded as one of the last important religious critics of medicine in the great admonitory traditions that evolved in their special ways within both Protestantism and Catholicism. He is also among the first and most important postreligious critics who have made their special mark on the public understanding of the doctor's diminishing authority.

In the memorable opening lines to *Medical Nemesis*, Illich proclaimed, "The medical establishment has become a major threat to health. The disabling impact of professional control over medicine has reached the proportions of an epidemic."[16] Like a latter-day Luther, Illich proposed a "laicization of the Aesculapian temple" that "could lead to a delegitimating of the basic religious tenets of modern medicine," and enabling the "layman in medicine . . . to acquire the competence to evaluate the impact of medicine on health care."[17] The key to unlocking the power of the people to regain control of their lives was in their recognizing the deleterious impact of what Illich called iatrogenesis, adapting the medical term of harm caused by medical treatment to the ills created by a debilitating dependence on modern expertise:

> Built-in iatrogenesis now affects all social relations. It is the result of internalized colonization of liberty by affluence. In rich countries medical colonization has reached sickening proportions; poor countries are quickly following suit. (The siren of one ambulance can destroy Samaritan attitudes in a whole Chilean town.) This process, which I shall call the "medicalization of life," deserves articulate political recognition. Medicine could become a prime target for political action that aims at an inversion of industrial society.[18]

Illich's polemic, brilliantly captured in the image of "the siren of one ambulance," struck deeply at the culture of affluence with its rising expectations and living standards throughout the world. Unlike conventional Marxist accounts of the political economy of suffering, Illich's was a transcendental critique of the human condition defined by the web of industrial prosperity and waste. In this sense, he appealed to those attracted to the "early" Marx, whose yearnings for a new world were not yet stated in terms of the harshness or deleterious results of class warfare. Illich, too, avoided the conventional account of prevalent class divisions and instead heralded postmodern critiques of society that raise omniscience to a new level, one above the material struggle for power.

Three types of iatrogenesis were produced in advanced industrial societies: clinical, social, and cultural. By the mid-1970s, the "role" of medicine in the maintenance and promotion of health was broadly discussed, inspiring much of the criticism of doctors as distant, arrogant, and uncaring. A thesis about medicine's role developed around the assertion that much of the improvement in the public's health, as measured by morbidity and mortality rates, was due to the general decline in infectious diseases that preceded their prevention and treatment by medical doctors. In other words, environmental determinants, as distinct from clinical protocols, were largely responsible for improved health. Purer water, safer food, cleaner dwellings, more widely available education, all contributed throughout the nineteenth century to a continuing reduction in disease and death caused by infectious diseases. This was half the thesis of the work of Thomas McKeown, who posited also the increasing importance of behavioral determinants of disease, that is, actions by individuals that were likely to affect their long-term health, especially the use of tobacco and alcohol and the approach to diet.[19]

Clinical iatrogenesis was attributed to specific kinds of medical actions, which Illich readily admitted were as old as the profession itself ("Doctor-inflicted pain and infirmity have always been part of medical practice").[20] Doctors' mistakes once again drew attention, but under different assumptions about their meaning to the public. Illich, however unwittingly, drew upon fresh anxieties about the guarantees of the effectiveness of all medical treatments. The increase in malpractice suits during the 1970s and 1980s reflected the distrust of the profession as well as the demands for even higher levels of quality in medical care. These demands were the consequence of the increase in medical specialties and subspecialties, creating more insistence on effective treatments and less tolerance for error. Illich capitalized on a type of anxiety that came of prosperity and improved medical science. By rolling out sensationalized statistics about medical harm, he used and was used by such anxiety. He was naive about the dialectic of sensationalism and refutation in which the anxiety persists long after evidence is presented to refute the reasons for its onset. Some of his illustrations of such harm would in subsequent years be refuted.[21] The enduring significance of his use of medical information in his book was its decidedly confusing nature, no doubt to practitioners and patients alike.[22] But it was also true that the increased presence of government agencies (e.g., the Food and Drug Administration and the Federal Trade Commission), trial lawyers, and expert witnesses gave a public visibility to distrust about doctors' motives and actions that greatly altered how secure either doctors or patients could feel within the bureaucratic systems created by modern medical science.

The purpose of introducing clinical iatrogenesis first was to lay the grounds for two other, far more systemic, dimensions of harm. A "second level" impact of medicine, termed social iatrogenesis, was medicine's reinforcing of "a morbid society that encourages people to become consumers of curative, preventive, industrial, and environmental medicine."[23] What doctors did was, in effect, reinforced by this consumption, but they were then less culpable for the situation in which they and everyone else found themselves. Social iatrogenesis was a kind of false consciousness created by overmedicalization, which resulted in medically defined exemptions from work for those who might otherwise assert their political will as workers.

A "third level" impact of medicine, termed cultural iatrogenesis, destroyed "the potential of people to deal with their human weakness, vulnerability, and uniqueness in a personal and autonomous way."[24] Calling this the "ultimate evil of medical 'progress,'" Illich objected to the pursuit of "better health" "as if it were a commodity."[25] All three levels, then, would appear to be systems within systems, each interlocked and each reinforcing the inevitable harm caused by the other. Illich's proposed way out of this "self-reinforcing iatrogenic loop" or "nemesis" was surprisingly counterintuitive. Instead of calling for overhauls of any particular system of medical care delivery, he insisted that the "*reversal of nemesis* can come only from within man and not from yet another managed (heteronomous) source depending once again on presumptuous expertise and subsequent mystification."[26] Illich left behind the policy debates of the welfare state in which the allocation of resources was paramount, and he reiterated what should best be called an appeal to spiritual transformation. Quite apart from his Marxist rhetorical trappings was a mission to heal expectations as much as to transform social realities.

In this spirit, Illich aligned himself with the conservative Presbyterian theologian Paul Ramsey, whose work helped to shape debates in contemporary bioethics:

> Paul Ramsey [in] *Fabricated Man: The Ethics of Genetic Control* . . . argues that there are things we can do which ought not to be done. To exclude these things is a necessary condition for safeguarding man from total abasement by technical control. Ramsey reaches this conclusion about specific kinds of medical techniques. I make the same argument, but about the global intensity of the medical endeavor.[27]

Illich ignored the evolutionary distinctions of sin, crime, and sickness by asserting that "Medicine is a moral enterprise and therefore inevitably gives content to good and evil."[28] And, "Morality is as implicit in sickness as it is in crime or in sin."[29] Against the secular view of the diminishing influence of religious and moral ideas on human affairs, Illich resurrected the ghost of strong moralism. Medicine was and would always be a moral enterprise.

The irony of Illich's thesis was that in its manifest, radical indictment of modern medicine, it proposed what would be construed by many as anti-progressive themes. Ramsey, for example, saw the liberalization of abortion laws as the beginning of the end of a distinctive medical morality.[30] Illich addressed specifically treatment decisions at the end of life and the incredible lengths to which medicine would go to sustain life. In the quarter of a century following Illich's *Medical Nemesis*, first Karen Ann Quinlan, then Nancy Cruzan, Jack Kevorkian, and finally (until the next unexpected, celebrated case) Terri Schiavo became exemplars of the disestablishment of medical supervision at the end of life.[31] Illich was, in this sense, ahead of his time, proposing a counterrevolution but on principles that were anything but libertarian.

In fact, Illich's central principle of empowering individuals was what drew the loudest criticism. As H. Jack Geiger, who from 1965 to 1972 directed urban and rural health centers at Columbia Point, Boston, and Mound Bayou, Mississippi, and who was to become a leading figure in both Physicians for Human Rights and Physicians for Social Responsibility, wrote in the *New York Times Book Review* in 1976,

> Real change in the distribution of resources and power would be approached, if at all, through an individualist ideal of personal action, and enlightenment—a kind of spiritual recognition of the limits of growth and material progress—substituted for economic reform. The polemic that began with such a sociocultural bang ends in a political whimper.[32]

This "spiritual recognition" was all well and good for those who, like Geiger, sought to influence the shape and future of major social institutions, but useless for the task at hand. Describing Illich as a Luddite sealed the judgment against him as one who was hopelessly behind the times.[33] But what Illich's critics did not recognize is that the changes in attitude and practice, specifically on the matter of end-of-life decisions, would become more important to challenging the power and authority of medicine than any proposal for the redistribution of health resources has been in the meantime.

It has been pointed out that Illich's various theses in *Medical Nemesis* were already stated before him. H. Jack Geiger quoted from a physician's review of the book: "There are already more radical thinkers within the ranks of medicine than Illich, and they understand more about biology."[34] But this standard put-down did not take up the implications of Illich's call for a spiritual resistance to medicalization. Somewhere between having nothing to do with the health system and complying completely with its dictates, an image was taking shape of a new type of patient. Illich's critique is mostly remembered for his apparent endorsement of suffering, pain, and tangentially, individual responsibility so that this image may not be as apparent.[35]

Yet in the formulation of cultural iatrogenesis, Illich offered the following observations about suffering: "It is a symptom of such iatrogenesis that the term 'suffering' has become almost useless for designating a realistic human response because it evokes superstition, sadomasochism, or the rich man's condescension to the lot of the poor."[36] In calling for "the need for an art of suffering and dying,"[37] Illich identified a process already under way in which public notice of and debate about medically mandated confinements to life-support systems in hospitals would be replaced by an explosion of narrative accounts of human suffering and dying. Writing before the appearance of AIDS, Illich's work is all the more prescient. While imagining Ivan Illich on a health care task force is nearly impossible, those of his detractors who analyzed everything but "soul sickness" would eventually earn their reputations as policy wonks scheming behind closed doors to fix the brokenness of existence with dollars and brains, but failing nonetheless.[38]

"Patienthood" and Self-Help

Social-scientific literature on the physician-patient relationship that appeared from roughly midcentury to the 1990s paralleled the Illich-like jeremiads, journalistic inquiries, and self-help guides.[39] The sociologist Talcott Parsons's pioneering discussion of themes in the sociology of medicine in *The Social System* (1951) was deeply stamped with Protestant ideas about individual responsibility, on the part of physicians and patients alike. His formulation of the "sick role" captured all of the human tensions that were naturally a part of being ill and of treating illness. These tensions were diffused in a series of institutional expectations that enabled the patient and the practitioner to negotiate their respective ways through the uncertainties that each had about the outcome of those negotiations. Parsons articulated a normative faith for medical practice in a Protestant vernacular that contained little explicitly in the way of religious ideas or language, but whose tenets included specificity of function (i.e., expert in a specific domain of knowledge), affective neutrality (e.g., scientifically objective and nonjudgmental), and suppression of the profit motive in the provision of treatment. Each of these tenets was a theoretical guide to how the doctor-patient relation was possible and why that relation was sociologically determined by the growth of scientific knowledge and technical expertise and by the dedication to a vocation.

Both expertise and dedication reassured patients that the doctor acted first and foremost in the patient's best interest, based upon long training and a commitment that transcended monetary reward. The "sick role" was also a description of the expectations incumbent upon the patient, who, by entering into this inevitably asymmetrical relation, understood that caring and curing were not always synonymous. But "care" symbolized a fiduciary responsibility and communicative trust on the part of the physician against which any failure to "cure" had to be measured.[40]

Parsons's normative description of medical practice in 1950 was remote from the popular perception of physicians that would follow general challenges to institutional authority several decades later. Young practitioners (in the genre of physician autobiography) and social scientists (by way of ethnographic study) examined and confirmed this popular perception throughout the 1970s and 1980s. They passionately contended that the rites of passage to physician-hood, especially during the resident years, brought out the worst in doctors, forcing them into a structured indifference toward patients and a nearly hostile contempt for attending physicians who oversaw residency programs. Patients, and especially those with the least financial means, were said to suffer most.[41]

Critics of Parsons's "sick role" argued that the ideal typical physician-patient relation could not be judged apart from the diverse social contexts in which it was played out. Patients with acute symptoms amenable to specific therapies were significantly different from those whose symptoms were either nonspecific or chronic and less responsive to standard therapies. Doctors practicing alone with long-term, stable patient populations were not the same as doctors moving in and out of medical groups whose patient populations were constantly changing. In other words, Parsons's depiction was accurate insofar as an illness was assumed to be either temporary or controllable (for example, diabetes), and the doctor-patient relation was believed to be a personal, mutually informed encounter between people known to one another.

Parsons was also chided for uncritically reflecting a "middle class" portrait of medical work. His portrayal was more hopeful than class-determined. He took for granted that more or less obvious distinctions could be made between diagnosis of real illnesses and malingering as well as between competence and incompetence. Challenges to his perspective were largely criticisms of his worldview, thoroughly Protestant in tone and character, and infused with both an individual ideal of moral responsibility as well as a narrow corporate ideal of professional obligation. These were ideals that would be overshadowed by calls for some form of nationwide health care system, in the form of Medicaid and Medicare, and eventually a universally accessible system. At the same time, Parsons's reiteration of the ethical and humane characteristics of physicians was, in little more than a decade, no longer rhetorically useful. In social science and popular culture generally, the admonitory voice that criticized doctors was heard well above the exhortative one that encouraged them. The exhortation of physicians would be transformed into the "empowerment" of patients.

The new image of the patient assuming greater responsibility for his or her individual health while demanding greater accountability from the system in which such responsibility was required was articulated early on and indirectly by Carol Hanisch's formulation, "The personal is political."[42]

It is precisely the convergence or conflation of these two ideas, depending upon one's point of view, that did so much to heighten public awareness of certain dissatisfactions about the evolving American health care system. This idea was translated into social science research agendas whose implications have yet to be fully assessed, seeing how much these agendas continue to inform present debates. In matters where personal discomfort, anxiety, and illness were paramount, the assertion of an encircling horizon of constraints that limited personal control became a political rallying call to transform the physician-patient relationship.

Popular and professional literatures that address the nature and problems of women's health are a systemic feature of contemporary America. That is to say, the cultural preoccupation with health and well-being is impossible to understand outside the popularization and professionalization of the concerns of women in particular. The transformation in attitudes of younger physicians that has been noted in recent years is directly tied to the challenges to professional (and male) dominance during the past quarter century.[43] Now, of course, that conceptualization of "dominance" has shifted almost entirely to the role that business has come to play in medicine. This was not always the case.

The 1973 publication by Simon and Schuster of *Our Bodies, Ourselves*, by the Boston Women's Health Book Collective, signaled a constructive but not unprecedented attempt to establish guidelines for women about their health. In previous decades, such work had been authored by physicians and nurses, and also by advocates of birth control. What distinguished this publication from previous efforts was its close proximity to the rhetoric of consciousness-raising, which borrowed heavily from the traditions of psychoanalysis, Gestalt psychology, and Marxism. If the personal was to become political, then consciousness-raising required the capture of individual hearts and minds—gain control of your body and you will be in a better position to gain control of the world around you. In keeping with the insights of Ivan Illich, this was not so much a call to join or identify with a particular movement as a call for individual self-examination and personal transformation by way of a book. In 1971, pursuit of this self-understanding required reading 136 pages; by 1998, the book approached 800 pages.[44]

The origins of the Boston Women's Health Book Collective are described in the preface to *Our Bodies, Ourselves*:

> In the beginning [1969] we called the group "the doctor's group." We had all experienced similar feelings of frustration and anger toward specific doctors and the medical maze in general, and initially we wanted to do something about those doctors who were condescending, paternalistic, judgmental and non-informative.[45]

This was a remarkably prescient sentence; especially regarding the charges that doctors were judgmental and noninformative. Of all the changes in the doctor's persona that have occurred subsequently, the retreat from being judgmental and the new candor, indeed necessity, about being medically informative have become central to a new kind of physician-patient relationship.

The impetus for creating this new relationship was never too far removed from commonsensical ideas about the interactions between doctors and patients. Sociologists made the implicit or taken-for-granted aspects of interaction more explicit in detailed analyses of conversations between doctors and patients. In her careful account of such conversations, the sociologist Candace West described, among other kinds of interactions, "turn-taking between physicians and patients; the organization of questions and answers, repairs of misunderstandings, and sociable commentary in medical discourse."[46] In one respect, these typical interactions reflected problems in all sorts of human encounters, other than medical ones. Talcott Parsons had described general expectations about the responsibilities of licensed practitioners and patients in their care. But the generality itself was an easy target for criticism by social scientists and others who found the basis for these responsibilities to be built upon the asymmetrical relations and unequal power of those involved. The assumption that power corrupts was easily assimilated to all social conditions of inequality, especially ones in which the structured interactions were between men and women.[47]

The sociologist Sue Fisher's *In the Patient's Best Interest: Women and the Politics of Medical Decisions*, published in 1986, was representative of the social-scientific research paradigm in which personal experiences served as the catalyst for analytic investigation of physician-patient interaction. As Fisher related:

> *In the Patient's Best Interest* grew from my own experience, from conversations with friends about their experiences, and from hundreds of hours spent in the examining rooms of two teaching hospitals. The analysis it contains was sharpened as I read analyses by feminists scholars of the sexual politics evident in every aspect of our lives. The truth of it was honed by my deep concern with the fabric of women's lives and therefore of necessity with the quality of medical care available to them.[48]

Fisher's work was not "activist" in a straightforward political sense—she did not intervene directly in the negotiations between doctors and patients of which she disapproved:

> At first I was angry and silently expressed my anger alternately at both doctors and patients. Individual doctors were seen as inept and specific patients were seen as passively going along with whatever

the doctors recommended. When I caught myself blaming individuals for problems my reading and experience had shown me were structural, my dilemma increased.[49]

Fisher's dilemma, simply put, was that from her point of view, informed as she was about various decision-making processes about women's health, patients and doctors were not free to make informed decisions or give informed recommendations, at least not at that time:

> Each time I compromised my feelings in the examining room, I renewed my commitment to sharing the backstage knowledge I had gained by demystifying the delivery of health care and displaying how medical decisions are accomplished in interactions, as well as how they are shaped by social and political forces.[50]

The freedom to make informed decisions (on the part of patients) and recommendations (on the part of physicians) was never fully realized, but the sociologist was invested with a kind of heuristic authority that would reveal, however indirectly, the "backstage knowledge" and mystifying nature of the *real* authority that was being criticized. The dilemma for Fisher and many others was not the by now pious doubts about value-neutral social science or the complexities of assessing the results of conversational analysis, but the long-term implications of feminist analysis in redefining the physician-patient relationship.[51] Long after the arcane arguments about theory and methodology accrue as citations in a voluminous social-scientific literature, patients still seek assistance and assurance in their visits with doctors.[52]

Fisher's effort to shadow medicine for its own good and for the good of patients is not new. It recalls the many efforts on the part of Protestant clergy in the last century to guide patients and physicians in their inevitable difficulties. One decisive difference that distinguishes Protestant clerical assumptions from post-Protestant feminist insights is the change in valence about trust. Feminist distrust was not unwarranted, but neither was clerical trust in its own time. The social-scientific observation that medicine had its own "interests" could be generalized to all relations in authority, and so it was, perhaps, more in the case of medicine than any other occupation. The freshness of the feminist critique was in part due to a new willingness among patients to raise questions about their health and about their responsibilities in taking care of it. Doctors, including women doctors, were, as Fisher rightly appreciated, caught in the same "structural" transformations as patients. The mediating authority was no longer confined to the physician's specific clinical experience but rather to a much more sophisticated appreciation of risks generally, which in turn was heightened by the thousands of continuing studies of women's health in particular.[53]

A focus on the dynamics of interaction was only a point of departure in the more ambitious agenda to transform the structure of health care delivery in the United States. That agenda was finally intended to alter the structure of professional dominance itself, by leveling the status hierarchy in health care while simultaneously empowering patients to recognize their new "agency" as consumers of health care. In the heyday of this more radical ambition, terms such as "patient" were belittled as linguistic markers of subordination. Although the radical qualities of this ambition faded, their residues gave new strength to the attention paid to the plight of the patient.[54]

Narratives of Patient Experiences

One of the interesting aspects of professional sociological work on the physician-patient relationship is its relevance to the practical and pressing problems of being a patient. The work of Sue Fisher, for example, as significant as it may have been in inspiring new agendas in the field of medical sociology, was but a small indication of the powerful dynamics at work in the transformation of medical authority during the past quarter century.

In this respect, sociology is not all that different from anthropology in the relatively recent growth of literature that has brought these fields more directly in contact with the everyday practice of medicine. In 1958, Raymond Firth, who headed the anthropology department at the London School of Economics, observed,

> Very recently anthropologists have been brought into relation with medical work, especially in what have been called the underdeveloped areas. But I am reminded here of a remark of Jean Cocteau about poetry, when he was installed not long ago as a member of the French Academy. He said characteristically, "I know that poetry is essential. But I do not know what it is essential for." Now much the same is still true of ideas about anthropology in relation to medicine.[55]

Firth's point was consistent with the broad hesitation embraced by many about interfering too precipitously in the doctor's world. But it also presaged the growing frustration of many others with what was perceived to be a new mandate about health and well-being that required more of physicians than they either recognized or were able to provide. Firth importantly called attention to the Constitution of the World Health Organization adopted in 1946, which declared that "health is a state of complete physical, mental and social well-being, and not merely the absence of disease and infirmity."[56] He regarded such a statement as an organizational optimum, not a norm, but the interesting question is how the acculturation of this optimum idea spread so rapidly, in less than several decades, to define the expectations about health and well-being of large segments of affluent populations in all advanced nations.

The answer must be developed along two lines, the first of which assesses the personal diminution of authority of physicians as they accommodated themselves to a myriad of self-help movements in and around medicine during this time. The growing emphasis on women's health in particular, which helped to redefine expectations, if not always realities, about health and suffering, literally transformed the everyday news about medicine. The second line concerns changes in the nature and meaning of illness itself at a time when advances in diagnosis and treatment were achieving enormous publicity as well. In certain respects a competition for attention has ensued, pitting medical breakthroughs over and against the lived worlds of the ill patient. Self-help movements have been encouraged by religious and missionary ideas, and it is no coincidence that illness and disability are increasingly construed as kinds of vocation because of such encouragement. An extensive literature of witnessing to illness has appeared during this time, not all of which to be sure was inspired by criticisms of the treatment of women by physicians.[57]

In scholarly efforts at depicting the lived worlds of illness, the implications of constructing and communicating narrative accounts of these worlds have moved toward a justification of existence in being ill by way of a reassessment of others' responsibilities and duties toward those who are ill. And unlike the jeremiads of previous decades by such figures as Ivan Illich, the turn toward narrative, sometimes described as postmodern, in many respects reflects a kinder and gentler approach that substitutes the more amorphous critique of social systems with an exquisitely refined critique of social interactions.[58] In this transforming of the rhetorical stakes, a torrent of published personal accounts of illness has been unleashed, what the sociologist Arthur W. Frank called an expression of, and a need for, a multivocal clinical ethic.[59] Such witnessing has drawn deeply from religious and "spiritual" ideas of personal transformation.

Frank's ambition to empower patienthood with a sensibility of mission was intentionally nonconfrontational. Rather than depict doctors or the normative expectations of the community as inevitably shaping and defining how illness should be understood, Frank called for a defiance of conventional expectations altogether. The idea of a narrative—a story or account of illness—was an antidote to the overly technological and role-specific aspects of caring about and for an ill person. Suffering was not simply an experience; it was the basis for a special communication of experience, if only those suffering less would listen. The problem was that the specific narrative of illness, that is, the specific worldview about the perception that the ill had of illness, could limit how well such communication was accomplished. Frank portrayed three such worldviews: restitution, chaos, and quest.

In the restitution narrative, illness is not memorable, because its duration is short and the ill person follows the doctor's orders and gets well. Frank is impressed with the power of this kind of narrative, empirically the most common of all:

> The restitution narrative has its proper sphere: images of health can model behavior that many people can adopt and adapt. The problem arises when the ill person does not find restitution, or when someone who can only tell restitution stories encounters another whose health will not be restored.[60]

Restitution narratives symbolize the achievement of modernity, in Frank's assessment. They are the proof of medical progress, though he laments that the costs of treatment for some illnesses may preclude some from obtaining help. This has always been the case to some extent, and Frank seeks to indict the objectivity of progress for its complicity in the inequalities it inevitably creates.

Perhaps it is better to put such progress in the broader context of democratization itself, where demand for proven treatments cannot go unheard for very long, as is the case in the response to AIDS in Africa or the push toward realizing the promise of stem-cell research. Nevertheless, Frank has an important point to offer that the restitution narrative does not account for all who are ill, a point that shifts attention away from the structure of modern society and its narrative of recovery and survival to the more intimate realities of illness among others. He concludes, "The tragedy is not death, but having the self-story end before the life is over."[61]

A second narrative, the opposite of restitution, defines the abyss of illness as it spreads chaos in the normal ordering of life. The loss of control is paramount, until some semblance of control returns, whether or not illness is defeated, and the possibility of reporting the "chaos narrative" in such a state is limited, if not impossible. Frank's determination to describe how such a narrative of the sheer experience of pain and the disorientation of illness is beyond reporting lead him to explore narratives of the Holocaust as a basis of comparison. He cannot be begrudged his recognition of the powerful resonance between the specificity of historical experience and the universality of human pain and despair beyond speech. But he pushes this recognition to an image of total chaos in which many reasonable human responses such as defiance or the acceptance of help from others are deemed extraneous, even irrelevant. That the implications of the chaos of the Holocaust did not end for those who survived it marks something greater, of course, than the "discovery" of the many clinical realities of posttraumatic syndromes. What Frank proposes, as a kind of postmodern understanding of illness, is how the experience of chaos informs a middle ground, the quest narrative, between itself and routine restitution, one that may become the basis for a new ethic of human encounter.[62] It is a remarkable ambition for narrative accounts, with broad public attraction, allowing as it does for the entry of less often heard voices in the drama of illness. Yet even as the impulse to write autobiography on the basis of public achievement is rivaled by the new call to formulate a narrative on the basis of the experience of illness, a hierarchy of witnessing may emerge where not all suffering may be assumed to be equally compelling.

Because the restitution narrative accounts for the routine triumphs of medicine and because the chaos narrative is beyond communication, Frank introduces the quest narrative, which accepts illness and seeks "to *use* it."[63] He observes that "involvement in patient advocacy is one enactment of a quest story; making significant vocational and personal changes in one's life following illness is another."[64] Citing Joseph Campbell's *The Hero with a Thousand Faces*, Frank carefully remarks, "If the idea of 'journey' has become a New Age spice sprinkled indiscriminately to season almost any experience, pop psychology could have done worse. The journey may be a fad, but it nevertheless represents a form of reflexive monitoring."[65]

"Reflexive monitoring" in an older rendition is what might have been called coming to terms, that is, finding a way to express intellectually and emotionally the meaning of one's situation or condition. The postmodern vocation of patienthood derives much of its contemporary force precisely in the mutual reinforcement that self-expression gives to the authentication of experience. At the same time, self-help is not at all a lonely quest.

The possibility of finding others with similar conditions to whom one can turn for support is something that was, in fact, initially created by the conditions of medical research itself. Over forty years ago, Renée Fox described how physicians and patients "came to terms" with their mutual ignorance about disease and its treatment. Fox assumed that reflexive monitoring arose in the shared reality of physician and patient. Frank does not. Instead he believes that, in many instances, "medical care becomes the health care industry."[66]

The quest narrative is, in fact, least of all about the physician-patient encounter. Illness itself is not only existential in that sense, it is also authentic beyond the terms of therapeutic intervention. In recent years, the appearance of a variety of physically and emotionally debilitating illnesses with unspecified organic sources, among which is chronic fatigue syndrome, is indicative of the powerful quest for cure at a time when the quest itself may have significance far beyond what treatment, whether successful or not, may be available. In nearly the reverse sense, the almost universal treatment of depression and other forms of mental instability with medication has superseded the older quest for cure that was established through conversational and thus more intimate encounters between doctors and patients. In the latter case, quest is transformed in terms described, for example, in Peter D. Kramer's best-selling book *Listening to Prozac*.[67]

The Conundrums of Litigation

Despite the broader public acknowledgment of the inevitability of illness and death, and thus the remarkable and diverse responses to it in narrative accounts and self-help movements, the wish for a world in which no mistakes are made and all actions are accountable is stronger and more durable than ever. This must be because as powerful as images of human finitude may be, expectations about scientific and technological achievement are even more powerful. In her memoir of inexplicable loss, *Wrongful Death: A Medical Tragedy*, the literary critic Sandra M. Gilbert sought understanding of her sixty-year-old husband's death following surgery for prostate cancer. In the course of her investigations, which included a malpractice suit and subsequent out-of-court settlement, she discovered at least one of the unintended consequences of rising expectations about medical performance: it is often impossible to find out what really happened, once parties in a lawsuit agree on a settlement.

When Gilbert initiated legal proceedings, her search for accountability was complicated by the many interested parties' concern for their own legal and financial vulnerability. Referring to the surgeon who had been deposed by her lawyers, she asked, "But did he say anything about what *did* happen? Why did *he* think my husband died? What was *his* opinion?"[68] These are questions that draw on personal trust, the absence of which must be taken for granted in conditions of legal deposition, though Gilbert seems throughout her narrative to remain unaware, or at least unconvinced, of the different worlds in which the actions of doctors are interpreted and evaluated. Her lawyer, Dan Kelly, promised her and her three grown children that he would show them "the dark side of the moon," a reference to medical horror stories, but also to a legal system that permitted plaintiffs the right to sue only on conditions set by the system itself.

Kelly told the following story:

"A guy from down the Peninsula came to me. Wealthy man, good Catholic. A big contributor to a Catholic hospital down there. A patron, a benefactor. And his wife went in there for routine surgery.

Never mind what. Woman in her fifties. Came out of the OR in a coma. Lived for a month or two in a nursing home, then passed away."

"Terrible." I frown sympathetically. So do the kids.

"Happens all the time. These things happen all the time," Kelly responds. "But the doctor could have leveled, could have made it better. This man and the doctor, they belong to the same club in San Francisco. The guy takes the doctor out to lunch at the club once, twice. Each time, he looks at the doctor and says, 'What happened, Doc? What happened to my Mary?' 'I don't know,' says the doctor. 'It was God's will, Frank. These things are mysterious. Who knows what happened. It was God's will.'"

Kelly snorts. "God's will! Well, the man came to me, had to find out what happened to his wife. And we deposed the people who were in the OR, found out what everyone knew all along. The perfusion machine—that's a machine that keeps the patient breathing during surgery—the perfusion machine ran out of oxygen. Someone forgot to fill it. And you only have two minutes in a situation like that, then she's brain dead. Comes out of there comatose."[69]

Gilbert slowly realized that the thing she desired most, a full accounting, might not be possible to obtain: "And why *don't* physicians 'level' more, I wonder. Pride? Self-deception? Or, in fact, the fear of precisely the kind of lawsuit that Kelly says this doctor could have avoided by telling the truth?"[70]

Gilbert discovered in the process of coming to terms with her husband's death that the multiple realities of medicine were not necessarily understood or accepted in the same way by all physicians, thus diminishing the force of generalizations about the "entire" profession. A physician, Dick, who helped her to interpret the transcript of the deposition of her husband's surgeon, a principal villain in her narrative, revealed something about the timelessness of insensitivity:

Q. Were you involved at all with the resuscitative efforts of this patient?

A. I arrived when he was just terminating. I arrived before he terminated, but he had not responded at that time.

Trying to control myself, I turn to Dick with one eyebrow ironically raised, impersonating a tough-cool-cookie Lauren-Bacall detective lady. "Terminating," I say viciously (though why I should be vicious to Dick I can't imagine). "I suppose that's the sort of language you as a physician are used to."

He looks back at me sadly. "Not at all," he says. "Not at all. I find it just as offensive as *you* do. But maybe that's the way these guys think they have to talk for the record. Maybe they talk differently among themselves."[71]

Was the surgeon as heartless as his talk "for the record" suggested? Or was he caught in a structure of legally constructed insensitivity that made his own "feelings" irrelevant? Gilbert's attempts to sort all this out were both naive and understandable. Trust requires compelling candor, acknowledgment of perplexity, and a willingness to admit one's faults. But how is this to be accomplished in an era of growing skepticism about medicine? What does it mean to say that an explanation is sincere or cynical? And what is inevitably given up whether one chooses to trust or distrust?

In a review of Gilbert's memoir, the novelist Lisa Alther expressed sympathy for her plight but echoed the physician's frustration about the book's implications for the humane practice of medicine:

> Speaking as someone who spent much of her youth diapering three siblings who are now doing microsurgery, I had to wonder as I read Gilbert's account where modern America ever got the idea that physicians should somehow be more competent than the rest of us. Shouldn't this assumption have been swept out to sea along with the corpse of God and the authored text? When we writers make mistakes, we erase them with our delete buttons. When doctors make mistakes, they get labeled "oafish." Yet I also remember all the trips canceled because of my father's patients, all the family dinners presided over by his empty chair, all the sleep interrupted by desperate phone calls. I remember my father crying in his armchair over a patient who had died that day on the operating table. I remember, too, my siblings' exhaustion from long hours on duty at urban medical centers, their terror at having lives depend on their split-second decisions, their despair after sleepless nights spent mopping up after other people's brutality, addictions and misfortune.

Alther's characterization of doctoring as still a demanding vocation, something that could be admitted into contemporary discourse in terms of the family "stress" it created, added another element to the difficulty of pinpointing the real nature of Gilbert's plight. Alther was willing to go so far as to conclude,

> I have to ask if our society's current rage at the ghastly errors doctors occasionally commit might not actually be, in part, rage at our own helplessness, facing down death as we must at every moment—and ultimately failing.[72]

In addition to noting the therapeutic function for Gilbert of writing about her ordeal, Alther returned to the theme of family, that haven in a heartless and godless world, as one source of great strength in Gilbert's encounter with death. In this regard, directed rage with the support of a loving family is a form of self-help, perhaps the best example of postreligious faith that can be attained, at least among most academic elites, in a world in which previous forms of faith have been "swept out to sea along with the corpse of God."[73]

CHAPTER 6

The Evolution of Bioethics

What remains of trust in doctors owes its contemporary force to two re-markable inheritances, from Protestant deliberations on character, office, and profession, on the one hand, and from Catholic deliberations on medically and morally complex cases, on the other. The criticism of the office (i.e., the Protestant inheritance by which "character" as distinct from "conduct" defines the authority of each practitioner) can be distinguished from the criticism of conduct (i.e., the Catholic inheritance by which particular actions are scrutinized and judged). Put another way, physicians are still criticized more for what they do in relation to their medical work than for who they are in relation to their profession. They are legally and financially answerable for the consequences of their medical actions rather than their bedside manner, though endless, and perhaps permanent, disappointments are expressed about the latter. Those disappointments about demeanor do inspire malpractice suits, but they must be linked to legal questions about competence. Trust in the person of the physician, the Protestant inheritance, formed the cultural basis that once inhibited lawsuits, which increased as public confidence in the corporate enterprise of medicine declined. Litigious pursuits were aimed more at actions and results rather than deterred by assurances and promises.

Both Protestant and Catholic inheritances have been recycled through a broader process of cultural transformation that has left many physicians uncertain of their vocation. A historically Protestant insistence that manner always reveals motive has only cynical appeal in an era when the big stakes are on the manner of delivery of services and related economic motives.[1] Physicians are more uncertain today about the meaning of their vocation, despite immense scientific and technological progress, because their historic authority is no longer what it once was, either personally, professionally, or culturally.[2] But even as this authority has waned, the profession during the past half century has sought to maintain its visible commitment to those ideals embodied in the idea of vocation.

Over this time, appeals to and assessments of specific traits of character gradually disappeared, leaving only traces of embattled conscience, psychologized as stress. Instead, a strong determination to give the medical career a solid professional and business foundation in what came to be called medical economics paralleled professional efforts to publicize the physician as caring and competent. At the American Medical Association meetings in San Francisco in 1950, Louis de Rochemont's documentary film, *M.D.—the U.S. Doctor* was debuted, first of a new series known as "The Reader's Digest on the Screen." Described in the pages of the *Journal of the American Medical Association*, the thirty-nine-minute film "depicts the state of the nation's health by reviewing medical progress, tracing the education required for a physician, highlighting the work and interests of the American Medical Association, revealing how research surges onward and describing the life of a rural practitioner."[3] Publicity through media channels was rapidly to become the major strategy for maintaining the "public image" of the profession.

Along with efforts to maintain better public relations, administrative leaders in medicine recognized how the problem in communicating medical progress was related to the explosion in information that made such progress possible. When *Current Medical Digest* published its first issue in October 1933, its editor, Samuel M. Wagaman, described an image of doctoring that seventy years later requires little qualification: "Busy practitioners, with insistent demands upon their time, have little opportunity to select or the facility in translation of such literature as is essential to familiarity with the trend of contemporary medical thought."[4] The idea that doctors were overwhelmed by the growth of knowledge influenced the profession's approach to communicating its goals to the public. The power of the AMA was not simply economic but also decisively cultural, aiding the profession in gaining the public trust for a considerable period of time.

Beneath these multiple layers of scientific and professional growth, new calls to the physician's conscience were raised among a generation of physicians, white, male, and Protestant, who took for granted that they were trusted by virtue of their professionalism as much as by their demonstration of skill. The medical profession's moral authority, that is, its capacity to be morally persuasive either individually or collectively, was undermined by various cultural and legal challenges that marked the 1960s and that led to a general decline in expectation about the physician's duty with respect to ever more intimate matters. A revival of the form of Catholic casuistry of the past—pastoral medicine—appeared coincident with a spiritual exhaustion in the meaning of the physician's career.[5] But in the afterlife of the admonitory traditions of Christian morality, the casuistical content was literally reinvented.

The Decline in Protestantism's Moral Authority

By the middle of the twentieth century, the physician's vocation found its post-Protestant vernacular in the professional focus on the "medical career," leaving little of the Protestant and admonitory inheritance about individual character as part of the meaning of that career. The long-standing assumption that the 1950s were a peaceful prelude to the disruptive 1960s cannot be maintained with respect to the types of challenges that were already forming soon after World War II in the larger society over such matters as sexual mores. Oliver Wendell Holmes's *Elsie Venner*, which a century earlier had exposed the tensions between religious and medical authorities in New England, was superseded by a new, and more vivid, contrast between individual and community authority over matters of privacy and rights. Grace Metalious's best-selling novel of 1956, *Peyton Place*, another New England "exposé," titillated while it subverted the authority of community over and against the rights of individuals.[6]

To be effective, Metalious's mocking of moral hypocrisy required a central figure in authority, not coincidentally, the town doctor, Dr. Matthew Swain. Faced first with the decision of whether to perform an abortion for his patient who is accused of killing her stepfather who raped her, Dr. Swain must then breach confidentiality (and risk his own career for being possibly implicated in performing a criminal abortion) in order to avert a harsh verdict against her. In the 1957 film by the same name, the physician is placed at the center of the drama's conclusion. Dr. Swain's righteous indignation over the community's unwillingness to face up to its gossip-ridden, rumor-mongering ways is the only note of condemnation in the entire film that is not suspect. The legacy of Puritan hypocrisy was at last exposed and exhausted, and the physician was, by his actions, appointed the guardian of the community's conscience. The busybodies of Peyton Place were no longer, even ostensibly, the guardians of moral rectitude, but were instead depicted as the suppressers of and whisperers about uglier treacheries, including abuse, rape, and abortion. In the impending era of sexual liberation, the resort to abortion, the exposing of abuse and rape, and the fights against sexual discrimination and harassment would all supplant an earlier reticence, later condemned as a form of denial, about such matters.

The seeming inevitability of those changes can be illustrated in the deeper binds in which the guardians of moral rectitude found themselves when challenged by the dual powers of the marketplace and of a citizenry made restless by the seeming hypocrisies of social and sexual conventions. After its release in paperback, *Peyton Place* was banned in the state of Rhode Island. The United States Supreme Court, in 1963, ruled against the Rhode Island Legislature's empowering of a commission "to educate the public concerning any book ... or other thing containing obscene, indecent or impure language, or manifestly tending to the corruption of the youth as defined [in other sections] and to investigate and recommend the prosecution of all violations of said sections." The Rhode Island Commission had been given no specific authority to prosecute, but the Court's majority, reversing the opinion of the Rhode Island State Supreme Court, left the clear impression that the commission's power to intimidate was unacceptable.[7]

In his opinion, concurring in the judgment brought in by the majority, Associate Justice Tom C. Clark observed that the legal challenge had been the result of "certain inept phrases in the notices sent out by the Commission" about obscene materials. But he criticized the Court for dropping a "demolition bomb on 'the Commission's practice' without clearly indicating what might be salvaged from the wreckage."[8] Clark's observation was poignant in its implications about the commission's authority to denounce a book as distinct from any power to curtail and prosecute the distribution of materials it deemed harmful to the young. Nevertheless, the Rhode Island Commission's feeble and ill-guided attempts to address profound changes in American mores were decisively resisted, setting the stage for further judicial rulings, for example, on prayer, birth control, and abortion that would challenge the credibility and effectiveness of public institutions and professions.

The increasingly cumbersome efforts at stemming the tide of alleged indecency were symptoms of, rather than solutions to, the emerging problems of authority in a host of moral matters that no longer seemed as clear as they once had under the Protestant dispensations of character and culture. The idealizations of personal character and public culture could not withstand the powerful assaults from above and below out of which arose a nonjudgmental, if not purely relative, standard about individual moral conduct. The declining significance of Protestant authority, exemplified in the caricaturing of an older Protestant judgmental authority, created a vacuum of sorts within specific institutions and professions. Medical economics, the mid-twentieth-century inheritance of Protestant insistence about the links between character and conduct, was easily caricatured as blatant self-interest (thus impugning character without necessarily invoking other aspects of it), opening the way for a return of medical ethics as a new apologetics for medical conduct in distrustful times.

The Influence of Catholic Pastoral Medicine on Bioethics

Sociologists and historians study the nature and changing character of normative or cultural consensus. Historians, and in particular social historians, in recent decades have been interested in how consensus is challenged and transformed.[9] So, too, have sociologists regularly studied the dynamics of such changes, sometimes melding their commitments for change with their understandings of it. Over this same time, some sociologists have come to view consensus as intellectually uninteresting, unless it is a kind of pathological consensus of the sort that raises public anxieties, for example, in connection with cults, whether they are religious or political. And many historians and sociologists have developed an animus toward *understanding* nonpathological consensus and long-standing traditions as well as the stability and endurance of social institutions and social forms over long periods of time.

Despite this contemporary animus, the canonical history of sociology is fully indebted to an early and sustained focus on the stabilizing forces of religion. Auguste Comte, who coined the word "sociology," hoped to make "sociocracy" the final, stable form of human civilization. Sociologist-priests would gather positive knowledge about the best forms of social organization, and they would establish themselves, on the basis of such knowledge, as infallible keepers of social order. T. H. Huxley, the great Victorian polemicist for science, was among the first to notice that Comte's Religion of Humanity was "Catholicism *minus* Christianity,"[10] and that formulation remained relevant over decades. In 1960, for instance the Swiss philosopher Hans Barth, in his neglected work *The Idea of Order*, remarked (without attribution to Huxley) that "The philosophical and political system of positivism is a Catholicism without Christian content."[11] Finally, the most arresting observation about Comte's legacy comes in F. A. Hayek's *The Counter-revolution of Science*, first published in 1952, in which the Comtean ambition is regarded as a precursor to twentieth-century totalitarianism.[12] Even as the debates about the political implications of totalitarianism have receded, the meaning of Huxley's phrase has implications for our understanding about how the remarkable cultural achievement of the establishment of the field of bioethics came about in the United States and elsewhere.

From the perspective of the historical development of religious influences on medical matters during the past century, bioethics can indeed be seen as "Catholicism without Christian content."[13] Like sociology, bioethics has sought, quite appropriately in the minds of most bioethicists, to distance itself from the claims of institutional and collective forms of religious authority. When Daniel Callahan wrote *Abortion: Law, Choice, and Morality*, he did not seek the *nihil obstat* or the imprimatur of the Catholic Church.[14] John T. Noonan, a federal judge in California who is remembered in the abortion debate for his work on drafting a human life amendment to pending legislation in the late 1970s, did not publish such work under the church's imprimatur.[15] This is not to imply in any way that either Callahan or Noonan had abandoned Christianity. Rather it is a sociological observation about the care they took to maintain a relative distance between their work and the dogma of the Catholic Church. Church doctrine does exist on many important bioethical subjects, but is, by virtue of its provenance, at odds with one specific secular mission of bioethics, which is to seek recognition outside the realm of religious traditions and serve as mediator and expert in complicated medical-scientific, legal, and public controversies.

The Catholic sources that relate to debates in bioethics have been, sociologically speaking, influential in *how* deliberations are conducted rather than in *what* answers are reached. Both Callahan's and Noonan's efforts are related to but distinct from the tradition of pastoral medicine out of which they arose. The definitive work on this tradition and the earlier traditions of Catholic reasoning on medical morality has already been described in greater detail in chapter 2; in *The Emergence of Roman Catholic Medical Ethics in North America: An Historical-Methodological-Bibliographical Study* published in 1979,[16] the author, David F. Kelly, gives a detailed account of the influence of Catholic teaching as recently as forty years ago and the continuing efforts by Catholic moralists since then, including Callahan and Noonan, to contribute, in ways that go beyond reiterating the church's doctrinal and pastoral teachings, to the resolution of the many questions that the new powers (along with new doubters) of medicine are raising.

The Catholic roots of these contributions begin and end in the effort to create a pedagogy for answering morally complex medical questions for both Catholic and non-Catholic institutions. Father Charles J. McFadden's *Medical Ethics*, published in 1946 by the medical publisher F. A. Davis, was intended initially for the moral instruction of nurses; by its third edition in 1955, the entire text had been expanded and "adapted to suit the needs of pre-medical students, medical students, doctors, and nurses."[17] By then, Father McFadden realized that his work was part of a larger effort to interpret natural law and divine positive law (that is, revelation) as it related to the moral dimensions of medicine. The book contained the following declaration on the reverse side of the title page: "The '*nihil obstat*' and '*imprimatur*' are official declarations that a book or pamphlet is free from doctrinal or moral error. No implication is contained therein that those who have granted the '*nihil obstat*' and '*imprimatur*' agree with the contents, opinions, or statements expressed." This declaration, with its perplexing disclaimer, placed Father McFadden's efforts both within and beyond the church. The clear implication was that both natural law and divine positive law stood above specifically Catholic doctrine and were intended to be instructive to and binding upon all medical practitioners regardless of their specific religious beliefs.

The tradition of natural law has not served Catholic thinking alone. In 1955, the Protestant theologian Paul Tillich characterized the differences in doctrines of natural law between Catholicism and Protestantism:

> Catholicism believes that the natural law has definite contents, which are unchangeable and are authoritatively stated by the Church

(cf. the fight of the Roman Church against birth control). Protestantism, on the other hand, determines, at least today and in this country, the contents of the natural law largely by ethical traditions and conventions; but this is done without a supporting theory, and therefore Protestantism has the possibility of a dynamic concept of natural law. It can protest against each moral content which claims unconditional character.[18]

The inheritance of bioethics, then, as an emerging tradition in its own right, began with Catholic questions that pertained to "definite contents" but challenged the "unconditional character" of prevailing Catholic answers.

One line of criticism of bioethical thinking has been made about its seemingly relentless focus on autonomy and rights, among other distinctly American preoccupations. A different tack might take into account the intellectual framework in which bioethical deliberations have generally been conducted. As a largely normative, as distinct from empirical, enterprise, bioethics has long gained notice by its appeal to a kind of enlightenment casuistry in which Immanuel Kant and David Hume substitute for and supersede Saint Augustine and Thomas Aquinas. But this transition from the teachings of the Church Fathers to the teachings of the Enlightenment fathers conceals something of the methodological implications of appealing to any authority, whether religious or secular. When Stephen Toulmin observed in 1982 how philosophy was saved by the ethical conundrums of medicine, he appreciated better than most what was at stake institutionally in the longer run.[19] It would be the modern hospital in conjunction with the modern university (and its behavioral scientists and applied humanists) rather than the contemporary church that would serve as central sources of a new contemplative ideal out of which some semblance of authority over ethical questions in medicine in particular would develop. From this have flowed three forms of "managed" care in America: governmental, corporate, and bioethical. The last of these is by far the most trusted, as compared to the other two. Some in bioethics attribute this trust to their alleged disinterest, itself a form of guidance and authority.[20]

During the second half of the nineteenth century, physicians equated medical morality with the material and organizational interests of their professional practice. At the same time, more narrowly Catholic deliberations on medical morality, in the form of pastoral medicine, went virtually unnoticed by the mainstream medical profession. The decisive matters for Catholic physicians and moralists of the late nineteenth century (such as abortion, sexual sterilization, and specific operations such as craniotomy and Cesarean section—covered in chapter 2) would become far more decisive and divisive issues for American medicine and politics during the last quarter of the twentieth century. Specific kinds of medical practices that were in large part peripheral to the practices of most physicians would be catapulted to the center of normative conflict beyond the control of professional interests, pulling the profession along the way, often unwillingly, into the fray.

Intrigued by the role of pastoral medicine in the history of medical ethics, the well-known bioethicist Robert Veatch published an essay in 1995 entitled "Diverging Traditions: Professional and Religious Medical Ethics of the Nineteenth Century."[21] Veatch proposed several important arguments for understanding the relative influence of religious traditions on medical morality. He pointed out that the first Code of Ethics of the American Medical Association, adopted in 1847, must be seen as distinct from the Catholic tradition of pastoral medicine with its deliberations on specific medical-moral matters. Those physicians who formulated the 1847 code took no interest in the Catholic moralizers, and vice versa. In Veatch's rendition, they were two ships passing in the night.

Veatch's argument depends on the assumption that "Protestant thought in the mid-nineteenth century showed no concern about the ethics activities of the AMA."[22] Protestantism, Veatch argued, was central in the phenomenon of religious revival and the work of temperance, abolition, and charitable work (especially during and after the Civil War). This is an entirely straightforward and accurate depiction of the social movements within Protestantism, which led to the range of public political debates that define much of nineteenth-century American history. But Veatch did not mention the key social characteristic of American professional medicine during the same period. The American Medical Association was the embodiment of American Protestant concerns. It was, first of all, demographically a Protestant professional association. The code it promulgated addressed matters now called medical etiquette, while Catholic thinkers, by virtue of a different intellectual inheritance more central to very long-standing church preoccupations, were already addressing matters that now come under the rubric of medical ethics or bioethics.

By the middle of the twentieth century, the Protestant character of medical etiquette was lampooned by the Episcopal priest Joseph Fletcher in his *Morals and Medicine:*

> The extant literature on it [medical ethics] consists for the most part in homilies on the bedside manner and such calculated questions of propriety and prudence as shined shoes, pressed trousers, tobacco odors, whether to drink Madeira, and the avoidance of split infinitives! It is composed, in a phrase, of manuals or exhortations on competitive success.[23]

Fletcher was correct, in his time, to observe that the decorum of physicians was, in their opinion, crucial to the preservation of professional authority.

This was a consummately Protestant professionalism that appeared to bring little to bear, at least publicly, in the way of reflection and analysis on those matters addressed in the Catholic traditions of pastoral medicine.[24] In its endorsement and elaboration of such ideas as vocation and professionalism, Protestantism made individual conscience, rather than any church, the locus of decision-making about complex cases. Abortion is the central example. It does not figure in the AMA code but was nevertheless of great concern to Catholic moralists in Europe and to Protestant physicians who taught in the elite American medical schools of the time.[25]

Veatch's analysis did not address the fact that the same Protestant profession that remained silent in its code about abortion also led the "crusade," as James Mohr described it, to outlaw abortion in the United States in the latter half of the nineteenth century.[26] Mohr, too, had a difficult time reconciling the fact that elite Protestant doctors were leaders *against* abortion, while Protestant clergymen appeared all but silent on the matter. About abortion, then, there was a silent code, an indifferent Protestant clergy, an outspoken Catholic casuistry, and an activist Protestant medical profession, which formed the seemingly contradictory aspects of a growing public consensus.

Abortion was not a matter of public debate in 1850 (any more than it was in 1950), but the historiography, with few exceptions, of nineteenth-century abortion anachronistically seeks to find twenty-first-century (post–*Roe v. Wade*) validations for liberalized abortion practice. A seemingly indifferent Protestant clergy served as a good illustration of Protestant indifference generally. Yet abortion was, at that time, practiced in ways that came to be viewed as threatening not simply to the authority of physicians but to the safe and effective practice of medicine. Rather than citing clerical indifference as the key to Protestant acceptance of abortion, the question Mohr and others should have asked is why the Protestant clergy did not actively *resist* the criminalization of abortion led by Protestant doctors. The reason is because the societal or normative consensus was already clear—abortion was understood in Christian terms as a sin. In contrast to a Protestant, civil society approach to defining public morality about abortion, the Catholic tradition allowed for a framework of debate about exceptions to the general prohibition against it, given certain conditions. By the middle of the twentieth century, for the vast majority of Protestant physicians, abortion's illegality mattered more than any disputations from natural law about the approach to specific cases, unless specific medical or surgical indications could be found. The Catholic framework inspired Daniel Callahan's earliest efforts in bioethics, regardless of where he came out personally or politically on the matter of abortion.

Insiders and Outsiders

Like the term "sociology," bioethics is a neologism, that is, a new word coined for the purpose of crystallizing a new way of thinking, often about old problems. Comte's vision of positivism, a philosophy and science that would guide the administration of society, finds parallels in the normative approaches in bioethics. That no comparable efflorescence of intellectual oversight has developed for other professions and occupations other than medicine suggests a deeper connection between sociology and bioethics than is revealed at first sight by the broadness and abstractness of the former and the relatively narrow and concrete focus of the latter.[27]

The first use of the term "bioethics" is generally credited to a biochemist, Van Rensselaer Potter, whose *Bioethics: Bridge to the Future*, first published in 1971, is an instructive reminder of how the ambitions of one individual may inspire (but not direct) an emerging movement that has gone on to define the public situation of medicine during the past quarter century.[28] Potter's own agenda for bioethics, including "A Bioethical Creed for Individuals," has been summarized as "the enterprise of utilizing the biological sciences for improving the quality of life."[29]

Closer scrutiny of Potter's "Bioethical Creed" (and its subsequent elaboration in other writings) reveals diverging arguments about the future of medicine and the role of physicians in that future, whether in Potter's mostly marginalized vision or in the mainstream vision that now dominates public understanding and interest in bioethics. Potter's creed consisted of five beliefs and respective "commitments," beginning with, "I accept the need for prompt remedial action in a world beset with crises."[30] The commitment following this belief called for an effort to create a worldwide movement "that will make possible the survival and improved development of the human species in harmony with the natural environment." The second belief called for the acceptance of "the fact that the future survival and development of mankind" depends on present "activities and plans." Potter's Comtean inheritance is plainly stated in his third belief that each individual has an "instinctive need to contribute to the betterment of some larger unit of society in a way that is compatible with the long-range needs of society." Comte coined the term "altruism," which in its application to biological understanding remains one of the most powerful links between biological observations and social policy.

Potter's final two beliefs, which acknowledged the inevitability of human suffering and death, called for a commitment to "work toward the goal of eliminating needless suffering among mankind as a whole." As innocuous and reassuring as his creed may have been, Potter was more forthright about what he had in mind with respect to the role of physicians in the emerging gap between what medicine was promising and what it could always deliver, including sustaining life longer than ever before: "But what is to be the fate of the aging invalid? What is to be done while medical science tries to live up to the rising expectations of a society that breathes smoke-filled air frequently by choice, that consistently overeats and underexercises, and that places its faith in treatment rather than prevention? . . . Is it moral to prolong life when the chances for a return to sentient life are vanishingly small?"[31] Such questions, raised in 1971, were prescient in ways that helped to direct the public temperament toward calls for greater patient autonomy from the demands of medical research and hospital oversight in particular. But the success of bioethics was first and foremost its ability to appear without, or even beyond, a creed, that is, without an explicit agenda about how to resolve such questions, except to subject them to greater analysis.

The institutional success of bioethics cannot be underestimated. Already several attempts at canonical-like histories of the field have been written, including David J. Rothman's *Strangers at the Bedside*, Albert R. Jonsen's *The Birth of Bioethics*, and M. L. Tina Stevens's *Bioethics in America: Origins and Cultural Politics*.[32] Rothman's book, published in 1991, defined bioethics as "outside" medicine. In the book's epilogue, he concluded that "Outsiders to medicine, more conspicuously and successfully than physicians, now define the social and ethical questions facing the profession and set forth the norms that should govern it."[33] Rothman assumed, as most contemporary observers of medicine do, that physicians were once principally responsible for defining the social and ethical questions facing the profession and that a wary and disenchanted public took control of medical decision-making from them. This might be called the "civil rights" view of recent medical history, and in that sense is true insofar as physicians have become answerable to a host of outsiders, including courts and legislatures, clinical epidemiologists, women's health advocates, and bioethicists.

In another sense, outsiders in previous times were not so much excluded from the processes of medical deliberation, as they were insistent that physicians embody their cultural expectations about trust and duty. The doctor who in 1950 was anxious about tobacco odors or the shine on his shoes was not exemplifying behavior absent in the population—on the contrary, these Protestant preoccupations were decisive because they fused motive with action in the public mind. Rothman's portrayal of the recent history of the profession confirms that there was once a much greater correspondence between the motives of outsiders and insiders. Representative outsiders, far from being hostile to medicine, were intent upon finding ways to ride the wave of enthusiasm that was created by medical-scientific discoveries and treatments.

What is different today is how the critique of medical professionalism is understood. The problems that sociologists uncovered, for example in the work of Eliot Freidson and others, rarely proceed to litigation in the courts.[34] Sociologists reported empirical findings about the organization of medical practice, about the nature of the physician-patient relationship, and about the socialization of doctors into their profession often with the hope of achieving normative, that is to say, public policy, transformations in these areas. These empirical approaches had little to do with the interests of individual patients or physicians, and this is important to remember when examining how bioethics succeeded to public notice far beyond sociology in the past few decades. On the other hand, sociologists did have a strong sense of advocacy about the seeming indifference of medical professionals to patients' needs, about inequities in health care delivery, and about the corporate power of professionals generally. The remarkable force of change inspired also by new concerns about women's health is impossible to understand apart from the fusion of such advocacy with anecdotal "horror" stories in medicine.

Bioethicists, as they emerged with a distinct identity, may have shared much of the "civil rights" enthusiasm with comrade sociologists, at least initially. But to achieve institutional effectiveness, they had to take up old subjects in new ways, something that Albert Jonsen, among others, understood as well as anyone. The empirical study of abortion in 1969 started from the reality of its criminal character,[35] but the normative study of it in 1970 by Daniel Callahan began on a much different premise. Rather than assume, as many sociologists did, that the pursuit of women's rights around abortion was primarily a matter of advocating for and furthering the interests of a social movement, those humanists and theologians who examined the question sought a change in how to *think* about the problem. Callahan's singular achievement was to lead the way in changing the intellectual and disciplinary contexts in which life and death issues were raised. These contexts were much easier to change than the entrenched social, professional, or institutional ones, and in any case, redefining the ideas and values at stake reduced the importance of empirical description. Sociologists, by seeking first to describe empirical realities, were expected to explain how the norms emerged in relation to those realities as well. Calling for a change in what was empirically given was itself a form of advocacy for changing norms as well.

What developed is now a legacy of institutional transformation, so profound, and so systemic, that all debates about life and death matters in American society are indebted to the formulations made by the best-known bioethicists, and others with regular access to mass media. These are formulations that enable *other* professions, most conspicuously law and medicine (but also journalism), to propose strategies of transformation and normalization, according to each emerging dilemma. In the law, the historic confluence of Protestant medical opposition to abortion along with Catholic moral reasoning against it ended decisively when the Supreme Court no longer regarded professional interests as paramount. The Court did not completely disestablish those professional interests, and it left the question of access to be a perennially empirical matter, requiring continuing (and partisan) assessment of its relative availability. At the same time, each changed normative context has opened the way for the possible study of new empirical contexts, though it appears such developments as stem-cell research and human cloning will be more normatively than empirically important in public debates for some time to come. In other words, the unintended empirical consequences of permitting or forbidding this or that innovation will be observed as opportunities to propose new normative contexts in which to reassess them, leaving courts, and possibly legislatures, to respond to challenges from all sides.

Bioethicists possess no special institutional authority to claim jurisdiction over how such challenges are resolved, indeed they have until quite recently avoided appearing either too expert or too partisan as a matter of professional pride, thus conveying a broad, indeed, catholic sense of what Max Weber wished for sociology: value neutrality. This kind of disinterest, when ascribed correctly to the empirical world, means that advocacy can be separated from observation. On the other hand, disinterestedness about values themselves is something unique to democratic societies in which so many questions once deemed by consensus to be moral matters have been transformed by consensus to be matters of rights. In the process, the simplification of principles that are said to be in conflict has made for the rapid and effective communication of otherwise complex and often confusing issues. As Paul Tillich foresaw in the case of Protestant natural law, and as Joseph Fletcher recognized in filling the old bottles of Catholic casuistry with the new wine of liberal Protestant indeterminacy (what used to be known as antinomianism),[36] the professional success of bioethics has come in a sleight of hand that gives guidance about the questions that should be asked without claiming authority over, much less responsibility for, the answers that should be given.

This phenomenon of moving from the normative to the empirical (e.g., the method of bioethics), as distinct from the empirical to the normative (e.g., the method of sociology), illustrates the limits of both philosophical ethics and social-scientific research. Neither can provide definitive answers to the problems of human existence, and each has, in its own way, been associated with many types of false promises along that line. Bioethics is at the beachhead of modern mass communication about the dilemmas of scientific and medical innovation, with only residues of resistance remaining in the older fronts in this cultural struggle to define the purposes and limits of human life. Social science has a different mission than philosophical ethics, yet each has some reason to look back in time for sources that may help provide such purposes and limits. That these sources were historically defined as religious should not be viewed in hindsight as merely sectarian debates that have been superseded by the advocacy of social movements (in the case of sociology) or the refinement of enlightenment thinking (in the case of philosophical ethics). On the contrary, resistance to innovation, whatever its source, is an able guide to a research agenda in empirical sociology, just as the appearance of doctrine from church sources and the arguments from antisecular bioethicists should be a good guide to the evolution of mainstream bioethics.[37]

CHAPTER 7

Anxiety in the Age of Epidemiology

It will no longer be as it once was, that individuals could look to
the nearest eminence for orientation when things got somewhat
hazy before their eyes. That time is now past.
—Søren Kierkegaard, "The Present Age"

Death is another milestone on their way.
With laughter on their lips and with winds blowing round them
They record simply
How this one excelled all others in making driving belts.

This is festivity, it is the time of statistics
When they record what one unit contributed:
They are glad as they lay him back in the earth
And thank him for what he gave them.
—Stephen Spender, "The Funeral"

Stephen Spender's poem "The Funeral" goes on to speak of "straining red
flags" in the hands of those who "speak of world state" and who are no
longer "haunted by the individual grief / Nor the crocodile tears of European
genius."[1] As an ode to communist revolution, Spender's poem offers also a
testament to the failure of intellectuals to understand history. But as an ode to
"the time of statistics," the poem says more today about the ubiquity of census
than about particular historical or political destinies. Even though Spender may
have intended an elegy to one type of Western utopianism, his metaphorical
choice identified another type in which the tragedy of one death understood
correctly might sometimes become the key to the prevention of many others.[2]

Public anxieties about human progress have been expressed in many
ways. What is significant about the second half of the twentieth century is
how these anxieties grew dramatically among elites rather than among the
masses.[3] Certainly, in the aftermath of the use of atomic weapons, even with

the stabilization of international peace, fresh anxieties emerged among various elites about their role in the making and controlling of the nuclear age. These broad political anxieties existed alongside an unprecedented prosperity following World War II. Medical progress continued unabated, including antibiotic treatment for infections and public immunization programs against polio, which reduced the more immediate and palpable fears about late summer, swimming, and childhood disease. Anxieties associated with wide-scale nuclear war disappeared as the Cold War waned, while a real concern remains about the actions of rogue states and terrorists.[4] But the nuclear bombs already exploded have left a different legacy in the form of the study of long-term health effects on those exposed to the fallout released. National survival in the nuclear age has less public urgency than the fate of individual health in the postnuclear age, and for good reason: as collective threats have subsided, the search for and attention to threats to individual health have both been given impetus. The result among certain segments of the better educated has been the development of relatively informed anxieties about avoiding illness, getting well, and staying well.

The fateful basis for these anxieties owes its origin to a transformative moment in the progress of medical understanding: the development of social epidemiology after World War II.[5] Just as a constitutional democracy cannot fully function without a census that supplies the numerical basis for political representation, so modern medicine, and especially that part of medicine informed by public health, requires continuous epidemiological research to justify its numerous recommendations about health policy. The "art" of medicine was a practice born of intuition and experience, both powerful and important dimensions of the clinical encounter. But with the growth in scientific understanding of disease, the clinical encounter could no longer be isolated from what was being learned from the analysis of thousands and hundreds of thousands of similar encounters. A broadly based intervention of science and government into the lives of citizens has been taking place for more than two centuries, making real, for example, the legal compulsions that all children must be immunized against contagious diseases and that all minors must be treated for life-threatening illnesses regardless of their parents' religious convictions. As obvious and humane as these legal requirements have become to the vast majority of people, they have been established upon the scientific foundations of epidemiological understanding.

New Perspectives about the Evolution of Medicine

In his book first published in 1976, *The Role of Medicine: Dream, Mirage, or Nemesis?* Thomas McKeown challenged a central piety of the medical profession, namely, its historical role in the overall improvement of health. McKeown asked what determinants or measures ought to count toward establishing the comparative influences of medicine and other factors in this improvement. In accounting for the decline in mortality rates over the past several centuries in Western societies in particular, he pointed to the extraordinary transformation in factors that had once contributed to the cause and spread of such contagious diseases as plague, typhus, and malaria. These factors had little to do with the developments of medical science, still in its modern infancy, and more to do with widespread changes brought about by the rise of the industrial state that introduced improvements in housing, sanitation, nutrition, and the safety of food.[6]

Two things happened in rapid order: the size of populations increased and the numbers of people subject to fatal, contagious diseases declined. In fact, what he termed the "diseases of poverty" that had dominated the world's population for millennia were brought under control in the "advanced" or industrialized nations in less than a century, before the appearance of antibiotics and before the general use of antisepsis by physicians. Immunization, for smallpox for example, played its part, but McKeown's strong argument favored changes in the environment that improved the chances of ever larger numbers of people to survive past infancy and childhood.[7]

McKeown's thesis did not have to be entirely original in order to confirm that since the nineteenth century a developing medical common sense was coming to rely on increasingly global information about the effects of collective action in the control of contagious diseases.[8] Rather than diminish the significance of widely heralded and "heroic" achievements of medicine, the advocates of sanitary science or public health championed utilitarian and progressive theories of social improvement. Diseases of poverty were the result of *social*, rather than scientific, ignorance, and it was the duty of all citizens to recognize how changes in municipal policies could improve the health of all people, not just poor people. In fact, it was unnecessary to understand *medically* what caused these contagious diseases, if it could be established what was necessary *environmentally* to control and prevent them. Although the motivation to understand diseases' causation has its ultimate roots in the treatment and cure of sick individuals, the improvement of the public's health required acceptance of the ideal of prevention, thus reducing the need for treatment. The inference that such changes would reduce the need for physicians was characteristic of both utilitarian and progressive optimism rather than motivated by hostility toward physicians. In one of numerous books published on sanitation in the last quarter of the nineteenth century, Mrs. H. M. Plunkett's *Women, Plumbers, and Doctors; or, Household Sanitation* offered the following epigraph: "Showing that, if women and plumbers do their whole sanitary duty, there will be comparatively little occasion for the services of the doctors."[9]

The success of modern public health owes much to the logic of utilitarianism, where the simple formulation of the greatest good for the greatest number provided an impetus for collective improvements that helped to secure close ties between the modern state and public health authorities, leaving to patients and their physicians the control of those health problems seemingly unaffected by these policies. McKeown argued that what he termed "diseases of affluence" became the subject of greater public concern as a result of the success in reducing the mortality associated with diseases of poverty. In the language of epidemiology, a decline in the rate of infectious diseases was followed first by an awareness of a rise in the rate of chronic illnesses, the most common of which remain cancer and heart disease. As ever larger numbers of people lived longer, having either been spared or survived exposure to the diseases of poverty, these chronic illnesses would receive greater medical and public attention. The prevention of the diseases of affluence now poses the greatest challenge to those public health bureaucracies and movements that are allied with government and universities. The tactics pursued in the prevention of these diseases have clearly extended earlier ideas about the role of public health, but they have also given rise to new public controversies along the way.[10]

The "Worried Well"

It is a truism among physicians that they know far too much for their own good about the possible kinds of diseases that can be contracted, whether by heredity, environment, or contact with other human beings. Dr. Henry E. Sigerist (1891–1957), writing in retirement about his own cardiovascular disease, observed in 1952: "Physicians, as a rule, are poor patients; they know too much, and therefore never fully accept the guidance of a doctor as other sick people do."[11] A half century later, what was once true about an elite profession is widespread among college-educated and affluent citizens generally, those sometimes referred to as "the worried well."[12] Guidance about illness is no longer mediated by any single individual. On the contrary, as the sociologist Jonathan R. Cole found in his study of the role of scientists and the mass media in reporting links between dietary cholesterol and heart disease, a complex network now exists that informs the public, however tentatively or inaccurately, about the health consequences of the behavior of individuals.[13]

It is the focus on behavior as a medical problem, as distinct from, and sometimes in direct contrast to, a moral problem, that marks a significant shift in the ultimate task of medicine, whose relevance to an individual patient's health has grown correspondingly greater as more evidence has been collected about the relationship between behavior and disease. McKeown recognized that the intensity of this focus on behavior had unintended consequences, including the appearance of many more opportunities to diagnose diseases for which there were no, or no widely accepted, forms of treatment. Where physicians could do little or nothing for patients with terminal illness, for example, McKeown lamented the practitioner's loss of interest in such cases, making their diagnosis an end in itself and thus emphasizing their strictly medical aspects. He called for a revitalization of a "pastoral role" in medical education.[14]

Yet diagnosis has become an end in itself for patients as well in a collaborative medical strategy that reassures the "worried well" that they are not ill and that indemnifies physicians from being easily held responsible for not doing all that is possible to diagnose illness. As numerous economists have pointed out, this dynamic of medical reassurance, also known as "defensive" medicine, has added significantly to the costs of medical care.[15] The physician regarded as only interested in knowing what is wrong medically in the case of terminal illness is held responsible for not knowing what is wrong medically in situations where diagnosis of any serious illness is by most probabilities least likely. What at first may be seen as paradoxical is also understandable from the viewpoint of the development of medical understanding.

McKeown's observation about the overexpending of resources in the pursuit of diagnostic understanding of acute but untreatable illnesses was intended to explain why medical education devoted to such work is not sufficient. Physicians also have responsibilities to the majority of patients whose medical needs may be less medically interesting but far more common. Since the 1970s, when McKeown noted these developments, the rise of hospice care and the focus on the massive expense incurred in the last months of life by patients and families literally caught in the acute care complex of specialists and hospitals have diminished the public's enthusiasm for "medical heroics" at the end of life. But this does not mean that such expenses or such efforts are likely to be reduced dramatically in the near future, even with strong economic incentives to do so. Another collaborative medical strategy exists between physicians and a patient's family in which the family demands that everything be done for the care of their loved one. Anything less would be not only uncaring, but unloving.

The anxieties created by the absence of illness or in the pursuit of the preservation of health are not new. One therapeutic aspect of trusting doctors is that this trust offers an emotional buffer against the sheer randomness of living with the prospect of disease and death. Nevertheless, the incentives to be less trusting and more assertive in one's self-care have given us "alternative medicine," and most recently, "enhancement medicine," for example, in the form of cosmetic surgery, all assuming something of the status of an American "right."[16] Mark Twain's remarks about Aunt Polly's anxieties in *The Adventures of Tom Sawyer* are worth recalling:

> She was one of those people who are infatuated with patent medi-cines and all new-fangled methods of producing health or mending it. She was an inveterate experimenter in these things. When some-thing fresh in this line came out she was in a fever, right away, to try it; not on herself, for she was never ailing, but on anybody else that came handy. She was a subscriber for all the "Health" periodi-cals and phrenological frauds; and the solemn ignorance they were inflated with was breath to her nostrils. All the "rot" they contained about ventilation, and how to go to bed, and how to get up, and what to eat, and what to drink, and how much exercise to take, and what frame of mind to keep one's self in, and what sort of cloth-ing to wear, was all gospel to her, and she never observed that her health-journals of the current month customarily upset everything they had recommended the month before.[17]

Such "fever" is recognizable in the many pursuits of health that lead to the anxious search for ways to avoid illness as the means by which the anxiety is both maintained and relieved. The relief, however brief, is always achieved against a background of an impending return of symptoms that suggest otherwise.[18] Diagnostic testing may not be only an end in itself, as economists and others prefer to argue when calls are made to reduce their availability and frequency. The problem of supply and demand in this regard is complicated by a powerful psychological motivation to be reassured, not by probabilities, but by evidence that is specific to each individual. Something more than the garden varieties of hypochondria is at stake in the anxieties awakened by the explosion of information about the risks of illness and the relatively easy access to such information made possible by computers.[19]

As the diseases of affluence become causally associated with behavior (though, in certain important instances, with genetics or the larger environ-ment), the interest in wanting to be individually reassured increased as well, and more so among those with more education and awareness about health. Yet the identification of causal factors in the onset of such illnesses as cancer and heart disease pits the desire to be individually reassured against the kinds of knowledge routinely gathered about "risk factors" in the cause of illness. The recognizable anxieties that excited Aunt Polly have been complemented in the past half century by what might be called "epidemiological anxiety," which is defined by an awareness that some percentage of the population becomes ill because it engages in certain behavior, while some other per-centage of the population does not become ill despite the fact that it engages in the same behavior. In addition, the hesitation to engage in behavior that may be life threatening, whether immediately or in the longer term, cannot be separated from how common sense itself is informed by the findings of science. That these findings may at one moment reinforce moral convictions and at another moment undermine them has contributed directly to the diminishing authority that physicians have over patients, where "risk" estimation has superseded the "wages of sin." Advising patients how to live has never been the sole purview of medicine, but with greater public (and corporate) emphasis placed on prevention, the conflict between high-tech and low-tech interventions has put the physician in the unenviable position of having to be infallible, on the one hand, while sympathetic to and nonjudgmental about the patient's fallibilities, on the other. It should not be surprising, then, that in the past quarter century, physicians are relied upon more but listened to less.

The Case against Tobacco

Contemporary understanding of health ironically owes a great deal to the widespread resistance that existed throughout the 1940s and 1950s to the charge that cigarette smoking (or other uses of tobacco) caused disease. In light of present legal strategies to hold cigarette manufacturers accountable for the disease their product causes, it is difficult to accept such resistance at face value, since recounting it presently would appear to favor an industry about which there is no shortage of vilification.[20] The present financial stakes, if not the historical controversy itself, has also raised fascinating questions about the use of historians' opinions in such litigation, leading to sharp debate among historians themselves.[21]

The development of medical understanding reveals a conflict between observation at the individual level and generalization at a more collective level, that is, a level in which concrete diagnosis is replaced by probabilistic prognosis. Among cigarette smokers, only about 10 percent develop cancer of the lung from their habit. Other smokers, who do not develop lung or other cancers, certainly contract other illnesses, in particular, cardiovascular diseases and emphysema.[22] To claim that cigarette smoking is a cause of lung cancer is to say that it causes it in a certain percentage of those who smoke cigarettes, not in all people who smoke them. And further, for smoking to be a cause, it must be assumed that if these same people had not smoked, they would have been far less likely to develop lung cancer. This is an epidemiological generalization that was, in some quarters, fiercely resisted at first in the 1950s. Its acceptance required a new appreciation for the powers of statistical reasoning as a basis for the prediction about illness in particular. Poor prognostic skill in the treatment of disease, especially chronic, noninfectious disease, was sufficiently daunting for practitioners who were being told that behavior that seemed to have no immediate health effects could be decisive in the creation of disease years later.

The remarkable and tenacious campaign to persuade the American public of the dangers of cigarettes has been recounted in various ways.[23] The purpose here is to describe how a product, which was once praised for its stress-reducing effects and which was consumed at the height of its popularity in mid-twentieth-century America by 70 percent of white men, became the primary example of how to think (and worry) about potential illness as far off as twenty to forty years in the future. Cigarettes have been described as central to American culture and its values of independence and commercialism,[24] but the concern about their danger has led also to intense debates about liberty, consumer protection, and the responsibilities of industry.[25] In one respect, cigarettes are an ideological and moral bellwether, revealing whether the greater weight of responsibility should be placed on individuals who use them or on those who sell them. Either way, the mission of public health would appear to be the same (i.e., to reduce the incidence of disease), although the strategies to achieve that mission are considerably different from one another.[26]

Among the types of accounts that were intended to provide evidence of a relation between smoking and lung cancer, one was based on clinical observation of tissues determined to be cancerous; another on experiments conducted to produce cancer in laboratory mice (i.e., experimental carcinogenesis); and a third on medical records of patients who were diagnosed with cancer (i.e., retrospective studies), and later on records that followed patients who had not yet developed any disease (i.e., prospective studies). Taken together, these three types of investigation formed the foundation of postwar epidemiology, and they united in purpose and focus the work of surgeons, pathologists, government officials, voluntary associations such as the American Cancer Society, and numerous statisticians. So extensive was the interest in proving or disproving the dangers of smoking that with each new set of incriminating findings throughout the 1950s, the stakes for some kind of national consensus grew, culminating in the first surgeon general's report, *Smoking and Health*, in 1964.[27]

The clinical observation of lung cancer was the immediate responsibility of surgeons who operated on patients with pulmonary diseases. One of the first American physicians to acquire a reputation for associating cigarettes with carcinoma of the lung was Alton Ochsner (1896–1981), who had observed such tumors in situ and who was struck by the fact that these patients had also smoked cigarettes. In 1939, he outlined a number of problems about making the association:

> Although it is controversial whether the increase in pulmonary carcinoma in recent years is apparent or real, the German autopsy statistics would indicate that the increase is actual and not only apparent. There are several explanations for the actual increase in the incidence of pulmonary malignancies, most of which have not been satisfactory. A number of theories have been suggested. Winterniz, Wason, and McNamara, because of the presence of metaplasia in the bronchial mucosa of persons dying from influenza, suggested that this change is a precancerous lesion. The inhalation of irritating gases such as war gas or gas originating from the increased use of motor cars has been proposed as an etiological factor. In our opinion the increase in smoking with the universal custom of inhaling is probably a responsible factor, as the inhaled smoke, constantly repeated over a long period of time, undoubtedly is a source of chronic irritation to the bronchial mucosa. In addition to the actual increase in pulmonary malignancy, there is unquestionably a relative increase in those localities where routine postmortem examinations previously have not been made. This is due probably to the fact that the condition has not been suspected in many cases and adequate diagnostic procedures have not been employed. The recent development of thoracic surgery has stimulated interest in intrathoracic lesions. This, with the development of specialized methods of diagnosis, has facilitated the recognition of pulmonary malignancies.[28]

Ochsner's observation about whether the increase in pulmonary carcinoma was "apparent" or "real" referred to the fact that the medical records kept about "intrathoracic lesions" were not yet very well developed, considering that the first successful surgical removal of a lung had only taken place in 1935. Diagnostic accuracy was by no means well developed either. The question was whether surgeons and pathologists were stumbling on a more or less unchanged occurrence that had not been well observed and recorded previously (e.g., an apparent increase) or were observing something occurring more often than had been seen before (e.g., a real increase).[29] Part of the incentive to pay closer to attention to the appearance of lung tumors was due to improved surgical techniques and outcomes. Ochsner noted pathology reports from Germany, which he presumed were more reliable than what was yet available in the United States.[30]

In a second report on another series of cases in 1941, Ochsner and his associate Michael DeBakey (who would go on to become a famous heart surgeon) moved well beyond their clinical observations and claimed a "parallelism" between smoking and cancer of the lung:

> It is our definite conviction that the increase in the incidence of pulmonary carcinoma is due largely to the increase in smoking, particularly cigaret smoking, which is universally associated with inhalation. Every one of our patients, with the exception of 2 women, was an excessive smoker. Of particular interest in this connection is the comparison of the death rate per hundred thousand of population from cancer of the lung with the production of tobacco and automobiles in the United States during the seventeen year period 1920 to 1936 inclusive. It may be observed from a graphic representation of these incidences that, whereas there is no significant relation between the production of automobiles and cancer of the lung, there is an obvious parallelism between the increased production of tobacco and carcinoma of the lung.[31]

The authors presented a graph representing the death rates associated with the production of tobacco and automobile production in the United States between 1920 and 1936. They attributed the parallel between a steady rise in tobacco production and lung cancer, with a dramatic decline in automobile production during the same period, to be evidence of both more smoking and less car exhaust. These stark comparisons had persuaded Ochsner, at least, that to ignore the possibility of some association was a disservice to patients and the profession.

Ochsner's biographers acknowledged that such claims about tobacco use made in these reports on surgical cases were unfounded: "By strict scientific standards, they went off half-cocked. The cautious approach would have been to go into the laboratory, do experiments proving beyond reasonable doubt that cancer could be induced in the lung by the presence of tobacco smoke, and then—and only then—report their findings."[32] This observation invoked what in medical-scientific terms would be considered a very high standard of proof to establish cause and effect. Ochsner was a surgeon, not a laboratory researcher or a statistician.[33] In the 2000 surgeon general's report on tobacco, Ochsner's claims about the perils of smoking are attributed to his association with moralists and religious crusaders against tobacco:

> The Puritan temperament that had fueled anticigarette activity early in the century was on the defensive. Antipathy to Puritan moralism was strong enough to weaken faith in any research tainted by it. For example, Alton Ochsner's suggestions in the 1930s and 1940s of a connection between cigarette smoking and lung cancer were

discounted by his colleagues because he was known to be an "anti-smoking enthusiast."[34]

Ochsner's advice to patients may have been motivated primarily by religious belief, but it also suggests how scientific uncertainty played an important part in prolonging the debates between the defenders and detractors of tobacco. That tobacco was also a commercial behemoth and an immensely popular pastime during the same period explains why the search for scientific certainty was both less visible and less decisive to public sensibilities at first. Ochsner's opposition, grounded in religious conviction and verified to his satisfaction in clinical observation, limited the extent to which practicing physicians could be persuasive on such a matter as tobacco. A similar lack of effectiveness had defined the physician's role in the decades leading up to Prohibition.[35]

The fact that Ochsner's beliefs about smoking entangled religious conviction with scientific evidence should not necessarily diminish the significance of that evidence any more than it should diminish the depth of that conviction. What did motivate physicians historically to act in the best interests of their patients was rooted in more than evidence about physical harm. Even in the aftermath of Prohibition, smoking was associated with a judgment about character, and to that extent, *any* evidence that would suggest its harmfulness to health corresponded with a judgment about the moral implications of the behavior as well. Ochsner's passionate objection to smoking did not persuade a medical profession that by 1950 counted not only many among its own as smokers but also saw its "professional" role as distinct from the moralizing tendencies of clergymen.

The point made by Ochsner's biographers about the superiority of experimental evidence as proof of causation was addressed by others, in particular Ernst Wynder (1922–1999), who played a long and influential part in the controversy over the dangers of tobacco. Wynder's contributions were in two distinct areas of investigation, epidemiological and experimental.[36] In 1950, as a young medical researcher, he published, along with the distinguished pulmonary surgeon Evarts Graham (1883–1957), the first of what would be numerous studies by him and others showing an association between smoking and cancer. This new front in the study of the effects of tobacco on health was given added credibility by the research findings of two British researchers, Richard Doll and Austin Bradford Hill, whose extensive contributions to the epidemiology of smoking were central to legitimating the statistical approach to correlating behavior with disease.[37] Of greatest importance in the multitude of these findings was the existence of a "dose-response" relationship, which showed that the more cigarettes consumed, the higher the risk of an individual's developing lung cancer.[38]

Wynder's more eclectic style and independent spirit led him to investigate not only the correlation between patients with lung cancer and their smoking habits but also the direct and deleterious effects of tobacco on living tissue.[39] In 1953, he published his first findings on "Experimental Production of Carcinoma with Cigarette Tar," which demonstrated how the application of tobacco tar to the shaved backs of mice resulted in the formation of tumors.[40] It was Wynder's hope that whatever carcinogenic substances might be contained in that tar could eventually be isolated and removed. His experimentalist view of the causation of disease influenced how he thought about tobacco. Although he did not smoke himself and discouraged others from smoking, the establishing of cause and effect meant also isolating particular substances in tobacco that were thought to be carcinogenic. The possibility and pursuit of a "safer" cigarette for him was not a disingenuous endeavor.[41] Unlike others who emphasized prevention, Wynder's embrace of an experimental approach was consistent with a medical as distinct from a public health commitment to reducing the morbidity and mortality caused by tobacco.

In hindsight, Wynder's early methods in both epidemiology and experimental carcinogenesis may have been neither sophisticated nor definitive relative to later research, but he should be remembered for directing two principal approaches to the study of harm, both of which have led over time to greater scientific appreciation for and public anxiety about the dangers associated with long-term behaviors (such as smoking and excessive alcohol consumption) and with exposure to various substances in the environment. The public health strategies that emerged from these two approaches now contribute to both media sensationalism and medical investigation, each anxiously reinforcing the other.

The Physician and Tobacco

Thomas McKeown's thesis about the "role" of medicine argues that the overall improvement of health, as measured by morbidity and mortality rates, was never the primary approach of medical education or practice, and it also provides insight into why physicians have become less influential precisely on matters that appear to affect the largest numbers of patients. To advocates of public health, such matters center on the prevention of disease beyond direct patient intervention, thus diminishing, by definition, the role of physicians. But one of the unintended consequences of the discovery of the ways in which a chronic, noninfectious illness may develop over a long period of time has been to involve physicians more directly in the monitoring of health than ever before. The case of tobacco illustrates a central aspect of the physician's declining authority insofar as the determination of a link between tobacco and illness helped to undermine the effectiveness of persuasion in the clinical encounter itself.

When the first statistical studies began to appear in the early 1950s linking smoking with lung cancer, they were met in some quarters with enthusiasm, and in others with skepticism. The reactions among researchers of cancer were divided between those who found the statistical approaches novel but not persuasive, given the much greater investment already made in other types of research, and those who brought a new vision to cancer prevention as distinct from cancer cure. This divide is roughly illustrated by the different approaches and reactions of leaders and researchers at the National Cancer Institute (NCI) and those at the American Cancer Society (ACS).[42] For both organizations at the time, lung cancer was only one of many "sites" under investigation and for which there were numerous theories about their cause. NCI's government-supported research made it more deferential to well-established political interests, including tobacco growers and manufacturers and the senators and congressmen from their respective states. This does not mean that NCI was simply manhandled by such interests, but it does mean that government response to the growing awareness of the dangers of tobacco was pragmatic rather than alarmist.

On the other hand, the fortunes and prospects of the American Cancer Society depended from the start on two essential public features: first was the importance of demonstrating to the public that cancer could be detected and prevented, and second was the necessity of having broad publicity about what it did accomplish with cancer prevention. Unlike NCI, which was required to answer to Congress, ACS needed to justify itself to the public at large. Tobacco and tobacco interests posed different kinds of challenges to both organizations, with NCI pursuing research for the sake of curing specific cancers and ACS for the sake of detection and prevention. This obviously oversimplifies their mandates and understates their political differences and difficulties over time, but it gives an indication of the complexity of responses to the "dread disease."[43]

One way to illustrate how the American Cancer Society publicized its efforts can be found in its bimonthly report, *CA, A Bulletin of Cancer Progress*, which began publishing in November 1950 and which was intended primarily for physicians. (See table 1.)

Among the first and most enduring triumphs of the American Cancer Society was its support for research into the prevention of cervical and uterine cancer, which led to the general recommendation of the annual Pap smear as part of routine medical examination. Because early detection was so decisive in treating the disease, the strategy of screening secured a prominent place among the physician's responsibilities. Over a fifteen-year period, from 1950 to 1965, the topics of cytology (although not exclusively

Table 1

Topics of articles in *CA, A Bulletin of Cancer Progress*, 1950–65

Bone cancer	1	Leukemia	10
Brain tumors	1	Lung cancer	11
Breast cancer	19	Smoking	10
Cancer detection and diagnosis	13	Lymphoma	3
Cancer management	11	Occupational cancer	2
Cancer research	2	Oral (laryngeal)	14
Cervical-uterine cancer	16	Pancreas, liver cancer	2
Chemotherapy	4	Prostate cancer	7
Childhood cancer	5	Radiation therapy	7
Colostomy	4	Rectum and colon cancer	9
Cytology	22	Skin cancer (melanoma)	9
Gastrointestinal cancer	5	Stomach cancer	8
Genetics and cancer	1	Testicular cancer	1
Gerontology and cancer	1	Thyroid cancer	1
Head and neck cancer	1	Tumors	13

Note: The total number of issues between 1950 and 1965 was ninety. The total number of topics in the same articles covered more than one type of cancer.

devoted to cervical and uterine cancer) and cervical cancer ranked high in frequency in the pages of *CA*. In 1952, at its annual dinner, ACS honored George N. Papanicolaou, who had reported on his new method less than a decade earlier.

The first reports in *CA* about tobacco and lung cancer appeared in 1952, two years after the initial retrospective studies had been reported in the United States and England. ACS took the lead in pursuing the prospective or "follow-up" method, led by E. Cuyler Hammond, director of statistical research at ACS and a professor of biometry at Yale. Hammond, along with his associate Daniel Horn, recognized the deficiencies of the retrospective method, the most important of which was that among the several retrospective studies published up until that time, the *degree* of association between smoking and lung cancer varied widely enough to call into question the statistical methods used to establish any association at all.[44] What was required was an approach that could look at a large sample of the population without the disease in order to see what kinds of factors might contribute to its creation over time. By 1954, well into his prospective study, Hammond was still reticent about claiming a definitive association between smoking and lung cancer:

> In my opinion, the full facts are not yet known about any of these
> possible factors [listed in previous paragraph, cigarette smoking,

exhaust fumes from automobiles, and air pollution from coal and oil furnaces]. Some investigators have expressed the opinion that, while cigarette smoking may not be the only cause of lung cancer, it is at least by far the most important cause and accounts for the increase in the death rate. If this view is now accepted as fact, it inevitably will have the result of reducing research in respect to other possible causes. After all, you cannot expect the public to put up millions of dollars for investigation of other possibilities if everyone thinks the answer has been found. For this reason, if for no other, I should want very strong proof indeed before I would be willing to state as an absolute fact that I know cigarettes to be responsible.[45]

Hammond's reasoning was also influenced by his acknowledgment of the American experience with Prohibition, which was still very much a part of the American sensibility about the different strategies available to regulate behavior:

> I think you will agree with me that the American public has demonstrated a strong aversion to prohibition, so passing a law is not a likely solution. Persuasion through education (once the facts are known) is certainly more palatable and more likely to succeed. However, it is by no means easy for heavy smokers to give up the habit or even to cut their consumption down to a moderate level. Furthermore, it is amazing to see how little effect danger sometimes has as a deterrent to people doing what they want to do. The 39,000 preventable deaths and untold injuries last year from automobile accidents is sufficient to attest to this fact.[46]

The comparison with automobile accidents confirmed what scientific proof about the cause of lung cancer could not: whatever the evidence, if the risk is not assumed to create imminent danger, and even more, if the risk is stated in terms of probabilities, then the logic of personal decision-making will always depend on factors other than this kind of rational proof.[47]

The dilemma for physicians with regard to the emerging evidence of the harmfulness of tobacco was compounded by greater public controversy. By 1957, the progress of Hammond's and others' research on their prospective studies had reached the front page of the New York Times: "Cigarette Smoking Linked to Cancer in High Degree, American Society Makes Final Report on Study of 187,783 Men—Industry Disputes Statistical Studies." The article began: "A report to the American Medical Association yesterday showed a high degree of association between cigarette smoking and total death rates.

It added that there was an 'extremely high' association between cigarette smoking and death from lung cancer."[48]

The same *Times* article, as if to reinforce a broader cultural impression that *how* tobacco was used, rather than *if* it was used, was the source of health problems, reported that "Dr. E. Cuyler Hammond and Dr. Daniel Horn puffed on pipes yesterday as they submitted evidence on the relationship between lung cancer and smoking." And further, the report noted about the two researchers that "In some circles—medical and non-medical—their views are regarded with some reservation because neither is a Doctor of Medicine."[49] Such skepticism was not without reason, and the dissonance created by the claims of statistical research and the widespread use of tobacco lent a defense to experience that no amount of evidence of the sort obtained by such research could easily undermine.[50]

By the end of the 1950s, the American Cancer Society was promoting a much more direct message to medical practitioners about their responsibilities with respect to smoking. Dr. David Spain, a pathologist at Columbia University, insisted that "With every other advance in medicine the physician has made it his duty to inform himself of its value and use (poliomyelitis vaccine, diphtheria antitoxin, penicillin, etc.). So must he now accept the responsibility of adequately informing himself of the facts and their proper utilization as regards the effect of cigarette smoking on health."[51] And in 1960, in an editorial in *CA*, the prevention of lung cancer was finally heralded in more familiar scientific language as a "breakthrough":

Lung Cancer Prevention and the Physician: A "Breakthrough"—Lung Cancer Preventable! It has been estimated that 75 per cent or more of all lung cancer cases could be prevented if the knowledge now available about this disease was fully exploited. The uncovering of this information represents a "breakthrough" in cancer control. It was so described by Dr. Howard C. Taylor, Jr., Chairman of the American Cancer Society's Committee on Tobacco and Cancer, in an address to the Society's Board of Directors in June, 1959. At that time, the Board passed a resolution calling for a more intensified educational program on smoking and lung cancer for both physicians and the general public. It was recommended that particular emphasis be placed on bringing the facts on smoking and lung cancer to the attention of teen-agers before their smoking habits are formed. . . . This educational attack on lung cancer is long-range in prospectus and will encounter difficulties and obstacles. Its effectiveness will depend on the support of the entire community, particularly of parents, teachers and, most of all, physicians. . . . It is desirable that this be a voluntary noncoercive effort which involves both the public and the medical profession in a joint educational project. It must be conducted skillfully and persistently on a continuing basis. The American Cancer Society, with its lay and professional membership, located in every community throughout the United States, has this capability.[52]

Although having no real similarity with scientific breakthroughs of the diagnostic sort, such as the Pap smear, the claim that lung cancer could largely be prevented was a "breakthrough" of a new kind, both in terms of the acceptance of statistical evidence as "proof" and of the need for a widespread public campaign of information in the form of a "voluntary noncoercive effort."[53] In the former case, acceptance meant persuading professionals who were then obliged to speak out. In the latter case, the campaign against smoking required *mass* persuasion through information, an endeavor that would bring the worlds of advertising and public-health policy together and redefine the responsibilities of government and business along the way.

The support of physicians to accomplish these new ambitions required special attention, prompting the admonition that "Now, even though the M.D. may not himself be convinced of the bad effects of cigarettes, he is duty bound to inform his patients that there is mounting evidence of the harmful effects of cigarette smoking. How can he in good conscience do otherwise?"[54] The appeal to conscience, even rhetorically, was indicative of the nature of the problem itself, where certain doubts lingered about the whole matter. Nevertheless, the physician's ethical duty was to present patients with the potentially bad news, laying open the way for the now canonical admonitions produced by contemporary epidemiology about diet, exercise, and rest. Eventually, the physician who smoked at all would be judged by some as unsuitable to practice medicine.[55]

The expectation and drama associated with the issuance of the surgeon general's 1964 report *Smoking and Health*, which summarized and presented the research findings about smoking over several decades, should not be underestimated.[56] The ten-member Advisory Committee to the Surgeon General (then Dr. Luther Terry) was selected on the basis not only of their expertise but also because of their absence from the public controversy over smoking. None of these members had taken a public stand on the issue. This use of disinterest to assess a publicly and scientifically controversial issue was exemplary, and it helped to codify important advances in epidemiological thinking, leaving the postulates of Robert Koch to the era of infectious disease and opening the era of the study of chronic disease with new authority to influence public policy based on what the report called a "coherence of association" between smoking and disease.[57]

By introducing the idea that a disease could be caused by one of several factors and that those factors in different combinations could determine how slowly or rapidly such disease might develop, epidemiologists challenged stricter interpretations of biological causation that had dominated thinking in medicine for more than fifty years. Epidemiology's scientific authority did not rest on a single study or experiment, and its most influential findings were not so much directed toward medical practice as they were toward health-related behavior.[58] In that transition, the physician's authority to oversee both diagnosis and treatment was tempered by the challenges of chronic illness, which the vast majority of patients experienced in varying degrees. Doctors became superfluous in a new way: they now had to respond to their patients' conditions with the realization that each and every action on the physician's part could also potentially contribute to a collective, that is, epidemiological, understanding, which, in turn, would be recycled back as a form of probable guidance in the conduct of the physician-patient relationship. Rather than increasing certainty, the grounds for an increased tentativeness, even about smoking, were ironically secured.

This is not to claim that the number of physicians who were persuaded against smoking did not increase as a matter of course. But those most persuaded at first were more likely to be most familiar, in detail, with the potential dangers.[59] As *Medical Economics* reported in 1965: "With men who know lung tissue best, it's no smoking 5 to 1: A new survey of Florida M.D.s shows that only 18.5% of pathologists smoke, compared to 40% of urologists, 30% of all M.D.s."[60] Physicians, like most Americans, tended to require more immediate evidence, something that might translate to experience, in order to be persuaded that what they or their patients were doing was harmful.

Joseph Gusfield recognized that the process by which persuasion about long-term health risks was accomplished would require acceptance of new types of evidence and of new ways in which that evidence was communicated. The surgeon general's report of 1964 was more than a culmination and summary of research; it was the first symbolic authority to pronounce on smoking with the consent of all interested parties.[61] The few challenges, other than those directly mounted by the tobacco industry, to the report's findings remained in the realm of debates about statistical reasoning, far removed from the public's view.[62] The authority of the report was also a new species of authority, demanding new methods of achieving compliance. Whatever moral compulsion may have previously existed to discourage smoking, it was transformed into a judgment about the consequences such behavior had on a person's body, as distinct from a person's moral character. The achievement of epidemiology, in part, was to draw distinct lines between the new health behavior and the old morality.[63]

Questions for the Epidemiologist

The overview here of a significant chapter in the history of public health is intended to raise several questions about how physicians today manage the complexities of their profession in the larger marketplace of health care. The political economy of those complexities regularly gains the most public attention among the various experts now expected to lead the debates about what needs to be done. All of this proceeds on numerous assumptions about the transformative nature of technology, which often is cited as the reason for the problems of limited access and high expense. But the assumptions themselves, including two related claims, (1) that technology seems always to advance before it can be ethically evaluated and (2) that diagnosis outstrips the capacity to provide effective treatments, are built on a view of human nature that is rarely made explicit, even by those most critical of it. Both claims assume a certain idea about the perfectibility of human beings, and the stronger the belief is in such perfectibility, the greater the anxiety grows about achieving it.

The idea of human perfectibility, as John Passmore shows in his definitive study, *The Perfectibility of Man*, leads more often in the direction of despair rather than hope. Passmore notes that John Stuart Mill, in his *Autobiography*, lamented

> that since musical combinations are limited in number, music would sooner or later come to a standstill. . . . But once it is admitted that whole spheres of human life, by their very nature, can permit only limited prospects for improvement, the suspicion is naturally aroused that this might be true more generally—that human activity, in virtue of its very finiteness, is bound eventually to exhaust its capacity for improvement.[64]

Anxiety arises at this prospect, but so too does a search for its alleviation. Not surprisingly, Passmore illustrates this dilemma with a medical example:

> Men might be free of pain and frustration in a society in which liberty is lost, art and science are dead, and love is abolished. The possibility of creating such a society has become less remote as medical science has proved itself able to relieve anxiety and depression by drugs. . . . By now, it seems, men can be relieved of anxiety and depression not only without in the process becoming freer men but, in the sharpest possible contrast, by becoming drug-dependent.[65]

But the question is how this process actually proceeds, and why should the cigarette—perhaps the most effective drug-delivery device ever invented—be not only the central but the ur-villain in the rise of modern epidemiology? The epidemiological approach to health has exposed myriad failures in the "progress" of medicine, many of which have directly affected the health of women.[66] Among the most legendary by now, for example, was the use of diethyl-stilbestrol (DES) to enhance pregnancy and prevent miscarriage.[67] At the same time, the epidemiological approach has been successfully challenged in courts of law, where the anxieties unleashed by the meeting of probabilities with actualities, exemplified by and experienced in the physician-patient relation, become clashes between different interpretations and standards of proof in the courtroom.[68] Nothing, it seems, has prepared the modern patient for the transition from feeling anxiously hopeful about what medicine might achieve to demanding compensation for what medicine fails to deliver. Modern epidemiology has assured that no such preparation or easy transition is likely any time soon. This is because, quite apart from who may or may not be blameworthy in particular situations, neither the demand for perfectibility nor the search for ways to satisfy it is likely to diminish any time soon as well.

The cigarette, which stands at the top of the pyramid of sacrifice of human habits no longer tolerated among civilized people, is only the tip of the iceberg. Beneath it are legions of successors, waiting to take its place.[69] The way that assessments have been made of this meritocracy of harm is illustrated in two sets of exchanges that appeared in the pages of *Science* in 1988–89 and 1995, each one offering a glimpse of otherwise publicly unnoticed controversies in a field that continues to argue strenuously about both its methods and its missions.

Alvan R. Feinstein, who was professor of medicine and epidemiology and director of the Clinical Epidemiology Unit at Yale, offered a scathing indictment of the methodological shortcomings of epidemiology, as evidenced in the work of some of its most distinguished representatives, in his article "Scientific Standards in Epidemiologic Studies of the Menace of Daily Life." The "menace" consisted of "common entit[ies] of daily life," including nonmedical substances such as coffee, water, sugar, saccharin, and alcohol "that people eat and drink on their own" and pharmaceutical agents such as those prescribed for high blood pressure. Feinstein observed how the conclusions of scientific reports of such menace received "wide publicity by newspapers, television, and other media," but his criticism avoided any judgment of the process of communication, arguing rather the problem was with how studies, especially of noninfectious diseases, were conducted by epidemiological researchers. He praised the research by epidemiologists on infectious diseases, citing their use of "high-quality scientific methods," and directed his attention specifically to claims about cause-effect relationships between reserpine (a drug used for hypertension) and breast cancer; coffee and pancreatic cancer; and alcohol and breast cancer.[70]

In all three cases, Feinstein noted deficiencies in both the research design and the execution of the studies. Wary of the studies' conclusions, he wished to be persuaded by scientific method rather than by their design and statistical analyses. He thus carried forward the spirit, if not the substance, of criticisms offered by a variety of researchers who resisted the conclusions about tobacco and health for the same reasons that Feinstein questioned the conclusions of other epidemiological studies. He attributed rushed conclusions to the "underdeveloped state of epidemiologic science in noninfectious diseases," but described this state as "an entirely reasonable phenomenon":

> Because individual people are much more difficult to study than molecules or animals, and because groups of people are even more difficult to study than individuals, it is entirely reasonable for scientific methods to be less well developed in epidemiology than in other fields.[71]

Calling for the equivalent of a "paradigm shift" in such methods, Feinstein was also endorsing his own approach to what he and others called "clinical epidemiology," an effort to apply as well as possible the same standards of methodological sophistication used in randomized clinical-control, double-blind protocols.[72] In this way, he saw himself as contributing to the instigation of this shift.

His provocation had an effect. In letters to *Science* in March 1989, two leading researchers offered defenses of their work and the work of their colleagues. Edward H. Kass of the Harvard Medical School defended his colleagues ("epidemiologists of major stature") from charges that their research did not "satisfy the most rigorous criteria of scientific accuracy." Kass acknowledged that "large epidemiologic studies are difficult to conduct, and it is easy to become concerned about potential flaws that are quantitatively unimportant."[73] He suggested that Feinstein and his colleagues may have doubted conclusions of earlier studies because they were *too* focused on methodology without presumably seeing the larger picture. Samuel Shapiro of Boston University Medical School provided a synopsis of the confusions that arise between a "cause-effect" relation being established and an "association" being confirmed. In the jargon of epidemiology, the strength of an association had a great deal to do with whether or not a consensus could be formed about cause and effect. Shapiro took Feinstein to task for "distortion" and "selective citation." Smoking proved to be the lodestar that gave order to every other disagreement: "The reader should note that, while he [Feinstein] now says that the association between smoking and lung cancer is a 'splendid achievement' of epidemiologic research, he at one time wrote that it should be regarded with suspicion and suggested that it might be accounted for by cough leading to preferential diagnosis among smokers or by psychic stress."[74]

Feinstein's response on the same page displayed something of the deeply held emotions that were invariably a part of scientific disagreement despite a premium placed on disinterest and collegiality. He compared himself to Ignaz Semmelweis, the nineteenth-century obstetrician who endured strong criticisms from fellow practitioners over whether they were spreading disease as a result of not washing their hands before attending childbirth. "The defenders of the status quo attacked Semmelweis for not emphasizing all the successful harm-free deliveries and denounced his scholarship as untrustworthy and perhaps mentally deranged; but they made no acknowledgment of the dirty-hand problem and of his plea for cleanliness."[75] Similarly, Feinstein argued that the two published letters demonstrated a lack of acknowledgment of the deficiencies inherent in noninfectious disease epidemiology, and he accused members of the field of complacency in the face of a constant cycle of reporting about yet another "menace" of daily life where no such menace may exist.

Six years later, the question of epidemiology's shortcomings was raised in another article in *Science* by science journalist Gary Taubes, who interviewed numerous epidemiologists across the country about the problems they faced as researchers in establishing credibility, in particular, public credibility for their findings.[76] Many agreed that serious limitations were always present in epidemiologic investigation, but they were also insistent that these limitations were not a reason to abandon such research. Alvan Feinstein is quoted in the article without mention of his earlier piece in *Science* or the fact that he had addressed specific claims about whether reserpine in one case and coffee consumption in another were associated with a higher risk of developing cancer. Taubes missed the opportunity to credit Feinstein with having pointed out six years earlier much of what Taubes went on to conclude from his interviews with other epidemiologists.[77]

Taubes pointed out that the market nature of competition for research funds among epidemiologists resulted in support for studies that showed some type of association, whatever its strength, between a specific agent and disease. Research that showed no association was by competitive definition not interesting. This competition internal to the scientific enterprise was rooted in public anxieties that were stirred with each succeeding claim and counterclaim.[78] As another researcher concluded in a discussion about the relative costs of proving that something was either hazardous or safe, safety was always much more costly to confirm, even as the public's interest in possible hazards was always greater, and therefore this second kind of research would receive greater investment.[79] Not only was the reliability of scientific method at stake but also the relationship between the internal oversight of science and its public funding. The anxieties created by a general uncertainty about what scientific investigation can establish as proof at one time or another are never likely to be fully allayed because they are bound up in a fateful alliance with expertise, once specific to the authority of the doctor and now generic to epidemiology and its endless search for and uncovering of weak and strong associations.[80]

Taubes's overview of the state of epidemiology prompted numerous responses from many of those epidemiologists whom he had interviewed and who wanted to set the record straight that the methodological shortcomings of epidemiology must be placed in the larger context of what post–World War II epidemiology had contributed to well-established warnings and assurances about "lifestyle and environmental risk factors." In a letter signed by eight leading figures in epidemiology, a common defense of sorts was evident, where internal differences were minimized and the mission and mandate of epidemiology itself emphasized.[81] Other writers noted the impossibility of conducting anything like ethical research that might require human subjects to be in experiments for decades or to be subject to stringent oversight of their eating and drinking behavior. In the absence of such controlled experiments, the researcher is required to work backwards from disease to possible causes or to follow people's lives in the least intrusive ways possible over many years. The resulting recommendations of preventive strategies always represent an approximation of what in particular cases might be a contributing factor to the onset of disease.

But it is precisely the absence of certainty in any individual case that sustains a background anxiety, the alleviation of which was once achieved by the balm of faith rather than inflamed by the peril of tentative fact. The modern warnings and assurances of fact that epidemiology heralds are not simply successors to the religious admonitions and exhortations of faith that religious traditions offered, they are all that modern science can give. Epidemiology is by far the most fatalistic arm of medicine in contemporary life, giving little consolation for the fact that destiny is a puzzling but ultimately confirmable combination of genetics and behavior.[82] Consolation, in the older, religious meanings of the idea, was the inevitable response to the failure of the promise of facts. In this way a reversal of fortunes for fact and faith is completed in the project of epidemiology, which may, on occasion, call for a greater equality of suffering among those better and less better off,[83] but which offers no corresponding elements of consolation other than the facts of fate.

CHAPTER 8

Trust and Mortality

Trusting doctors has never been obvious or simple. Callicter (who may have lived at the time of Nero) came decisively down on the side of distrust:

> The physician, who killed me,
> Neither bled, purged, nor pilled me,
> Nor counted my pulse; but it comes to the same:
> In the height of my fever, I died of his name.[1]

In 1794 Matthew Prior described the same result *with* treatment, thus confirming the professional, if not public, sensibility that physicians are often damned no matter what they do:

> *The Remedy, Worse Than the Disease*
>
> I.
> I sent for Radcliffe, was so ill
> That other Doctors gave me over,
> He felt my Pulse, prescribed his *Pill*
> And I was likely to recover.
>
> II.
> But when the *Wit* began to wheeze,
> And Wine had warmed the *Politician*,
> Cur'd yesterday of my Disease,
> I died last night of my *Physician*.[2]

It is worth remembering that all individual perceptions and opinions about doctors have specific cultural and historical contexts, and that even in times when many expressed skepticism about the character of the physician and the efficacy of the treatments he could offer, trust in individual practitioners and their skills was alive and well. This can be seen in letters that George Washington wrote in 1789, ten years before he died, about his own health during an era when medical knowledge was limited and physicians usually practiced alone. Washington wrote to Dr. James Craik, the physician who was to attend to him in his final illness,

> The want of regular exercise, with the care of office, will, I have no doubt hasten my departure for that country from whence no Traveller returns; but a faithful discharge of whatsoever trust I accept, as it ever has, so it always will be the primary consideration in every transaction of my life be the consequences what they may.[3]

Several months earlier, Washington had received a letter from James McHenry, his secretary of war, expressing concern about Washington's medical treatment (for a tumor on his thigh) and recommending Dr. Craik, to which Washington replied that he was already one of Craik's patients:

> I thank you, my dear Sir, for the anxiety which you express that I should have some person about me, who is well acquainted with my constitution, and who has been accustomed to my confidence. The habits of intimacy and friendship, in which I have long lived with Dr. Craik, and the opinion I have of his professional knowledge, would most certainly point him out as the man of my choice in all cases of sickness. I am convinced of his sincere attachment to me, and I should with cheerfulness trust my life in his hands.[4]

In many ways, this depiction of attachment and mutual commitment between doctor and patient is as much a prefiguring of the nineteenth century's discussion of character as it is a reflection of professional realities—which included the fact that no matter how dedicated and caring a doctor was, the treatments he offered might fail. Washington's letters reveal the importance of caring and trust in the relationship between patient and doctor, an acceptance of the limitations of medical treatment, and the inevitable reality of mortality.

Although skepticism about physicians and medicine in general—which has always existed alongside trust in doctors—has a long and well-documented history, the question that remains intriguing for the sociologist is not why this distrust persisted over the centuries, but rather why it seemed to subside almost entirely in the United States for a period described by the historian John C. Burnham as "American Medicine's Golden Age," roughly from the end of the nineteenth century until the 1960s.[5]

Why, in one era, should trust be given to individual practitioners but not necessarily to their corporate identity as a profession, and in another, the "golden age," originate in that corporate identity and extend outward with few exceptions to all physicians practicing safely within that sphere? In the United States, trust in doctors never coincided completely with trust in medicine, but during the "golden age" the same (greatly expanded) corporate enterprise that identified itself as the medical profession seemed to offer guarantees that new techniques and treatments were available, or would be soon, to conquer disease and traumas of all kinds. In addition, by the early twentieth century the legal and scientific foundations affirming the institutional autonomy of medicine were either being developed or firmly in place, and after that autonomy was achieved, something like a vast collective amnesia ensued, making the "golden age" as much a cherished ideal as it was an ostensibly objective indicator of the physician's rising social status. For a brief time, as the hope for cure outweighed the importance of care in the public mind, the authority of the physician was embodied in the continually touted expansion of the powers of medicine. But as skepticism began to rise about medicine's actual powers, while the hope for cure did not subside, trust in the profession's "delivery system" and in those who delivered within it began to wane.

Evidence of challenge and decline are never precisely fixed in time. Writing in 1982, Burnham approached the growing public criticisms of physicians by referring to four distinct forces that had led, by the end of the 1960s, to the widespread undermining of public trust in the medical profession and its practitioners. First, chronic, as opposed to acute, diseases increasingly occupied the physician's attention over the course of the twentieth century. Second, medical care to patients was more routinely provided in large and impersonal hospitals, thus associating the delivery of medical care with uncaring bureaucracies. Third, the growth of consumer consciousness, a result of the shift from a manufacturing to a consumer society, intensified public scrutiny of all claims to expertise, not simply by individual consumers but also by the legions of new social movements and publications devoted to helping educate consumers to discriminate in more sophisticated ways about everything from music to vacations. This consumer consciousness was informed by a host of new onlookers of medicine, including journalists and social scientists, who exposed the medical-professional secrets that sometimes medicine could do more harm than good (i.e., iatrogenesis), and that often pretending to do something was believed to be more helpful than the dispensing of actual medicines (i.e., placebo effect). Finally, Burnham noted that increased attention to the psychosomatic aspects of illness—a clear consequence of the greater preponderance of chronic versus acute illnesses—left doctors with unwieldy and less tidy encounters with many of their patients.[6]

Before these forces began to undermine the physician's authority, that authority was not a subject of widespread debate. The focus, in the public mind, was less on the politics of professionalism and more on the routine enactment of the physician's oversight of all matters pertaining to illness and death, including profound questions about end-of-life care and the always contentious topic of abortion.

Yet from early on, public trust in the corporate enterprise of medicine was seen within the profession as dependent upon an institutional separation between the education of the medical professional and public awareness of the central place of mortality within that education. This view, in sociological terms, was founded in the belief that such separation was necessary and appropriate, and that the new and continually evolving content of medical-scientific education would ultimately require the physician to confront in a new way the public's fear of death (by identifying with the corporate, that is, professional, promise to find ways to forestall it) and to rise above that fear (by honoring that promise as best as possible).

William Osler and Death's Inevitability

A physician's opinion about death, in the face of a corporate enterprise devoted to forestalling it, reveals something about the way in which physicians historically achieved an ambivalent trust from those who sought them out. Until very recent times, except in the case of physician-assisted suicide (which may in fact have happened quietly, without notice, throughout the centuries), the medical profession has avoided as much as possible any perception about playing an active role in hastening death or accepting it or advocating for it "before its time." So too at the opposite end of the arc of life: although the Hippocratic oath specifically forbade it, we know that many doctors over the course of history performed abortions, sometimes even with the sanction of religious doctrine. But until the rise of the women's rights movement this issue remained largely unaddressed.

Part of the medical profession's efforts during the "golden age," then, was to maintain a clear demarcation in the public mind between death and its gatekeepers. It was thus a rare occasion, indeed, that some form of public ridicule of physicians and their connection to death in particular reached the front page of the newspaper. A spectacular, and thus revealing, instance occurred upon the occasion of William Osler's departure from the Johns Hopkins University in 1905.

Osler (1849–1919) is regarded as the doctor's doctor, and his name remains synonymous with humanistic medicine in the early days of its golden age. He was in every sense an iconic figure, larger than life, and an embodiment of vocation and dedication.[7] Osler's appointment at Hopkins as professor of medicine began in 1889, and he remained there for sixteen years. He was instrumental in the founding and subsequent fame of the medical school at Hopkins (which opened in 1893), and it was during this same time that his reputation and fame increased greatly. In 1904, he accepted the Regius Professorship of Medicine at Oxford, and left for England on May 15, 1905.[8]

How and why was it, then, that for a brief period he was widely regarded as an advocate of forced retirement and euthanasia? Various analyses of the specific incident that led to the ridiculing of Osler's reputation have been written defensively. They blame journalists but take little notice of what the widespread upset may have revealed about the public's perception of doctors. The canonical account is given by Harvey Cushing in *The Life of Sir William Osler*.[9] In preparing for his final address to his Hopkins colleagues in February 1905, Osler selected the title "The Fixed Period," after Anthony Trollope's novel of the same name.

The novel, published in 1882 at the end of Trollope's life, is set in 1980 and recounts the imaginary country of Britannula, where the citizens pass a law whose purpose is to rid themselves of the infirmities of old age—and the societal burden of caring for the infirm elderly—by fixing an exact age when all people should be euthanized. In his biography of Trollope, N. John Hall indicates that the author had based his story on the seventeenth-century play *The Old Law*, by Philip Massinger, Thomas Middleton, and William Rowley, "which he read in July 1876. The 'old law' would have men at 80 and women at 60 executed—'cut off as fruitless to the republic, and law shall finish what nature linger'd at.' "[10]

Trollope's novel is narrated by the president of Britannula, John Neverbend, who writes his account while returning to England after his efforts to carry out the plans for a fixed period are prevented by British authorities. Neverbend's sincerity never wavers about the merit of fixing a time when a person, by virtue of age (in Britannula, sixty-seven), should give up his life, in effect, for the good of all. It would also be a death with dignity: "I had felt it to be essentially necessary so to maintain the dignity of the ceremony as to make it appear as unlike an execution as possible."[11] The first candidate for "deposition" in a "college" where, after a year, he would be put to death, is Neverbend's "almost dearest" friend, Gabriel Crasweller. In the novel, the naming of the college Necropolis is a source of some debate, with Neverbend preferring Aditus, while another proposes Cremation Hall. Neverbend also imagines "a smiling hamlet might grow up at the gate, inhabited by those who would administer to the wants of the deposited; but I forgot that the deposited must come first."[12]

At the time it was published, literary critics described the novel as a *jeu d'esprit*. The American Robert Tracy, writing in 1978, concludes that it "is not a satire on Victorian England. It is instead—as the President's name suggests—a satire on the narrow-mindedness and the lack of human sympathy that characterize abstract reformers."[13]

Although Trollope may have been satirizing the lack of human sympathy of the vast array of reformers of his day, he was not unsympathetic to many of the boldly stated goals of various advocates of new proposals to advance human progress, who throughout the 1870s had rattled the sensibilities of religious leaders in England. His biographer Hall writes,

> With one of the aspects of Neverbend's project, cremation, Trollope was firmly in accord. In January 1874, Trollope had been one of sixteen prominent people at the home of Sir Henry Thompson, a distinguished physician and surgeon to Queen Victoria, who signed a document that brought into existence the Cremation Society of England:
> "We . . . disapprove the present custom of burying the dead, and we desire to substitute some mode which shall rapidly resolve the body into its component elements, by a process which cannot offend the living, and shall render the remains perfectly innocuous. Until some better method is devised we desire to adopt that usually known as Cremation."[14]

The advocates of cremation succeeded in legalizing it in England in 1884 after the acquittal of Dr. William Price on the charge of cremating an infant.[15] The same Henry Thompson who led this cause was also regarded, along with John Tyndall, as having incited one of the last publicly noticed conflicts between the clergy and reformers, over the efficacy of prayer, two years earlier. Trollope's satire was not divorced from a late-Victorian impatience with religious authorities that were said to interfere with arguably better ways to deal with many things in life, including disposal of the dead. Just as the case of prayer's efficacy (the prayer-gauge debate) challenged whether the results of faith could be scientifically measured, so cremation required the faithful to accept a more limited view of the sacredness of the body. Trollope had joined forces with that element of British religious skepticism whose claims to authority were built on pointing out the limits of faith in public life.

The medical profession was culpable in the ensuing public anxieties raised about the problems of aging. When William Osler took Trollope's *jeu d'esprit* and tossed it merrily into American public notice in his farewell address at Johns Hopkins in 1905, it did not occur to him that Americans might take this bit of British satire literally. Here is Osler:

> It is a very serious matter in our young universities to have all of the professors growing old at the same time. In some places, only an epidemic, a time limit, or an age limit can save the situation. I have two fixed ideas well known to my friends, harmless obsessions with which I sometimes bore them, but which have a direct bearing on this important problem. The first is the comparative uselessness above forty years of age. This may seem shocking, and yet read aright the world's history bears out the statement. . . . The effective,

moving, vitalizing work of the world is done between the ages of twenty-five and forty—these fifteen golden years of plenty, the anabolic or constructive period, in which there is always a balance in the mental bank and the credit is still good. . . . To modify an old saying, a man is sane morally at thirty, rich mentally at forty, wise spiritually at fifty—or never. . . .

My second fixed idea is the uselessness of men above sixty years of age, and the incalculable benefit it would be in commercial, political and in professional life if, as a matter of course, men stopped work at this age. In his *Biathanatos* Donne tells us that by the laws of certain wise states sexagenarri were precipitated from a bridge, and in Rome men of that age were not admitted to the suffrage and they were called *Depontani* because the way to the senate was *per pontem*, and they from age were not permitted to come thither. In that charming novel, *The Fixed Period*, Anthony Trollope discusses the practical advantages in modern life of a return to this ancient usage, and the plot hinges upon the admirable scheme of a college into which at sixty men retired for a year of contemplation before a peaceful departure by chloroform.[16] That incalculable benefits might follow such a scheme is apparent to any one who, like myself, is nearing the limit, and who has made a careful study of the calamities which may befall men during the seventh and eighth decades. . . . Whether Anthony Trollope's suggestion of a college and chloroform should be carried out or not I have become a little dubious, as my own time is getting so short.[17]

The reactions in newspapers to Osler's address were thunderous, leading him to speak out in his own defense on the front page of the *New York Times*. Five days after his address, following numerous news reports with headlines such as "Useless at 40" and "Professor Osler Recommends all at 60 to be Chloroformed," Osler responded,

I have been so misquoted in the papers that I should like to make the following statement: "First—I did not say that men at sixty should be chloroformed; that was the point in the novel to which I referred, and on which the plot hinged. Second—Nothing in the criticisms have shaken my conviction that the telling work of the world has been done and is done by men under forty years of age. The exceptions which have been given only illustrate the rule. Thirdly—It would be for the general good if men at sixty were relieved from active work. We should miss the energies of some young-old men, but on the whole it would be of the greatest service to the sexagenarii themselves."[18]

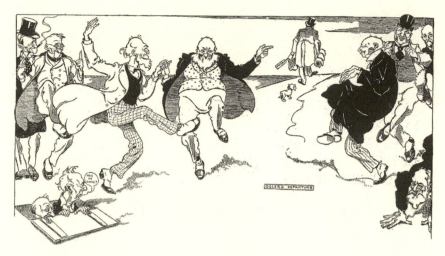

From *New York Times*, May 7, 1905, Part 3, First Magazine Section, p. 8.

Osler's insistence that he was primarily misunderstood and that Trollope's ideas were Trollope's and not his allowed him to distance himself from the more hyperbolic accusation that he himself endorsed the idea of literally disposing of the old. In the third edition of his deservedly famous book of essays, *Æquanimitas*, he wrote from England,

> To one who had all his life been devoted to old men, it was not a little distressing to be placarded in a world-wide way as their sworn enemy, and to every man over sixty whose spirit I may have thus unwittingly bruised, I tender my heartfelt regrets. Let me add, however, that the discussion which followed my remarks has not changed, but has rather strengthened my belief that the real work of life is done before the fortieth year and that after the sixtieth year it would be best for the world and best for themselves if men rested from their labors.[19]

It is impossible, from such a distance in time, to estimate the effects of Osler's remarks on the public, however much they may have been taken out of context. He rationalized, for example, that newspapers had been having their own fun at his expense. Twelve days before his departure from America, the *New York Times* published a cartoon depicting old men coming out from hiding as Osler walks off in the distance.

However, a few reports appeared of people committing suicide, their bodies found with news clippings about Osler's speech nearby.[20] His apology to "every man over sixty" and his continued insistence about the rightfulness of some of his own views about aging raise an interesting problem about the role of professional advice—individual and corporate—especially in light of the association of reports of suicides with his remarks. It is entirely possible that a few older people did take his words to heart, that is, they recognized the diminution of their own powers along with their social standing, and chose to end their own lives. But of course, rather than being a form of individual counsel, Osler's remarks were intended to draw attention to a societal issue. He failed to recognize the powerful connection in some minds between his authority as a physician with patients in his care and the meaning of his words outside that context.

Another problem emerges from this cautionary tale, in terms of the meaning of anecdotes and statistics. Osler based his half-satirical, half-serious social pronouncements on a literary text, a flight from a social reality that itself was captured, distorted, and sometimes missed in Trollope's imaginary musings. The missing part was soon reiterated in the newspapers in the form of examples of old people still vital and productive. Osler dismissed these examples as being exceptions to the rule, thus proving it, and—favoring incentives for retirement—he never gave up his conviction that institutional mechanisms must be used to make room for the young and vigorous. The arguments he provoked have continued to inspire debates about both retirement (now an accepted concept) and euthanasia, two things that lately seem to have been separated in the public mind. But the retired physician Jack Kevorkian, whether or not he knows of Osler or Trollope, has called attention once again to the question of whose authority it is, in principle and in practice, to give or take away life.

The Issue of Trust and the Transformation of Corporate Medicine

Over the past several decades, sociologists have formulated roughly three general explanations about the results of the transformation of American medicine after the golden age of nearly universal trust—explanations that have addressed organizational realities as paramount in prevailing definitions of efficiency and justice: (1) physicians became professionally dominant during the course of the twentieth century, which is to say that they achieved an autonomy over their work that became a model for every other form of professional dominance;[21] (2) they then became proletarianized, which is to say that many more of them worked for salaries than ever before;[22] and (3) they were then corporatized, which is to say that as individuals they had less and less autonomy, even though their incomes were still hardly proletarian. The critique of the medical profession by sociology illustrates the aspiration of others besides physicians to influence the organization and practice of medicine. That kind aspiration is not unique to sociologists.[23]

The struggle for the institutional establishment of scientific medicine toward the end of the nineteenth century was about competing visions and practices of therapeutic intervention. What else really mattered at the dawn of a new and promising era? But when former Supreme Court justice Sandra Day O'Connor appeared before the National Cancer Survivors Network decades later, in 1994, she spoke for millions of Americans frustrated not only about the difficulty of accessing information about cancer therapies, but also about the incredible lack of coordination among surgeons, radiologists, and others about the treatment plans for individual patients. Justice O'Connor's survival of breast cancer was not achieved easily; medicine obviously helped, but its corporate organization also interfered sufficiently to inspire her to speak about her struggles as a patient and specifically as a woman.[24]

Other explanations that have been offered for why trust in physicians has declined in recent decades involve the issue of character and caring. In 1960, the American Medical Association still honored a General Practitioner of the Year. In the same year, in their book *The Christian as a Doctor*, James T. Stephens and Edward LeRoy Long, Jr., quoted from the *Journal of the American Medical Association*, which described the award as "given each year to the physician who typifies the thousands of general practitioners throughout the country who have dedicated their lives to the practice of medicine, and who have given exceptional service to their communities."[25] Stephens and Long praised the idea of service but also stated, "Today it is important to cast the practice of medicine in a different light. The service motif by itself will not suffice." They quoted from a 1958 *New York Times* report about a survey of public attitudes toward the medical profession by the Chicago National Opinion Research Center, which concluded that "the vast majority of Americans believe that the best trait a doctor can have is to be up-to-date."[26]

In 1960, the professional balance between generalists and specialists still tilted decisively toward the generalists. The "G.P. of the Year Award" acknowledged this balance of power, even as a growing number of specialists began to influence the public's perceptions of medical competence. It is important to recognize the extent to which the perceptions of "service" (caring) and "competence" (medical knowledge and expertise) were now shaped in part by the relative balance between generalists and specialists. Thirty-five years later, Marilyn Chase's "Health Journal" in the *Wall Street Journal* spoke regularly about how much the old perceptions persisted in the radically transformed environment of star doctors (i.e., specialists) and primary-care physicians (i.e., generalists). Writing in 1996 about the marketing strategies that promote "best doctor" lists, Chase noted that

> seeking care from the most prominent practitioners can set people
> up for disappointment if their star specialist is elegant with a scalpel

but deficient in bedside manner. It's worse when the venerable physician who radiates the wisdom of the ages proves to have outdated medical knowledge.[27]

Chase reiterated many of the concerns of patients who continue to suffer the anxiety of experiencing the gap between elegance with a scalpel and a reassuring bedside manner. The separation of trust in competence and trust in the person has intensified a more visible range of anxieties about what consumers believe they are receiving in medical care. Some complain that they do not receive enough attention from their specialists (e.g., poor bedside manner). Patients are advised about finding out from their famous and busy surgeons who will actually be performing the surgery: "If you get your doctor to promise to do the surgery, he or she will feel legally bound to do it." This advice is given in recognition of the fact that many medical procedures are performed by teams of physicians and that the attending physician (the star) may not even be present. The division of labor to achieve a record of "competence" may thus undermine, if not defeat, the initial effort on the part of the patient to get "the best." At the same time, some patients are perfectly content with no bedside manner at all. Samuel Le Baron, an instructor in the family practice program of the Stanford University Medical School, acknowledged that a star "isn't going to be able to sit and ponder." Furthermore, a star often imparts "more technical [expertise] than care." Patients are advised to keep their primary care physician "in the loop."[28]

That loop is the web of trust without which the contemporary patient cannot be assured of knowing how to find out about what kinds of care are available and how such care is administered. Yet, as Charles Bosk noted thirty years ago in his now classic study of the training of surgeons, "At present, a physician's conscience is not only his guide but the patient's only protection."[29] Calls for reforming the health care system have proceeded unabated under the prevailing assumption that improving the structural, fiscal, and other management aspects of medicine will restore trust and equity in medical care. But the conscience of the physician precedes and is not necessarily consistent with such bureaucratic reformation. In this sense, "managed care" is a metaphor for the present time, and is deeply indebted to the extraordinary web of surveillance techniques established by modern epidemiology. The shaping of public expectations about the role of medicine and the education of physicians is played out among competing images of managed care, whether governmental, scientific, corporate, or bioethical.

If it were sufficient to argue that these images of managed care and the public role they play now summarize the political, and therefore the most important, realities of doctoring, then little more would need to be said about the vocation of medicine and trust in it. But the social and scientific conditions for another kind of reformation in medicine may nevertheless be beginning to appear.

The End-of-Life Debate

Among the questions facing physicians and public alike today is the one raised by William Osler—whether and under what circumstances society can officially permit physician-assisted suicide. Within the history of medicine, this is, like the problem of abortion, an ancient question, and such questions do not press upon the public in visible if conflicting ways unless something considerable is at stake for future generations, physicians and patients alike. In an assessment of the problem of death in medicine, Peter Sloterdijk, who has been described as a writer on the postmodern condition, observed:

> Part of today's crisis in medicine comes from the fact that, and the way that, it has surrendered its once functional connection with the priesthood and since then entered into a convoluted, ambivalent relationship with death. In the "struggle between life and death," priests and doctors are now in opposing camps. Only the priest, without becoming cynical, can take the side of death . . . because, in living religions and cosmologies, death is held to be the self-evident price for life and one phase in the grand designs with which the knowledge of priests once knew itself to be . . . connected. . . . For the doctor things are different. Doctors define themselves through having to take the side of life . . . thus the doctor comes into a mediating position: on the one hand, an "absolute" supporter of life; on the other, a partaker in the power of hegemonic powers over life.[30]

Max Weber had similarly concluded in 1918 that the physician was not called upon to define the meaning of life, but he stated the problem of the scientific attitude in medicine as a kind of neutrality over and against nature rather than as the font of "hegemonic powers":

> By his means the medical man preserves the life of the mortally ill man, even if the patient implores us to relieve him of life, even if his relatives, to whom his life is worthless and to whom the costs of maintaining his worthless life grow unbearable, grant his redemption from suffering. Perhaps a poor lunatic is involved, whose relatives, whether they admit it or not, wish and must wish for his death. Yet the presuppositions of medicine, and the penal code, prevent the physician from relinquishing his therapeutic efforts. Whether life is worth while living and when—this question is not asked by medicine.[31]

Weber insisted that this question about whether life is worthwhile living and when, cannot, and therefore ought not, be asked by medicine, even though the autonomous, professional status of the physician appeared to give the physician new license to act. The function of the penal code in this regard is evident, but because contemporary efforts on behalf of physician-assisted suicide are directed against such laws, Weber's more obscure characterization of the "presuppositions" of medicine requires further elaboration.

For Weber, scientific knowledge was a cultural astringent applied to ancient enchantments of the world, but it was only the latest in such astringents intended to pinpoint with greater exactness the causal relations between one fact and another. This "disenchantment of the world," as he described it, had been occurring for millennia, and medicine, to the extent that it was modern, was only lately reaching the recognition that its powers over life and death had achieved some new expression, one that could from then on be viewed as an indifference of two kinds. About one kind, Sloterdijk and many other "postmodern" critics have remarked, namely, the indifference that a fully modern, technical medicine has to the problem of human pain. In this case, the indifference is both personal and bureaucratic, allegedly inscribed in the hearts of medical students and enacted in hospital protocols.

Yet a second kind of indifference, perhaps even more cynical than any noted by postmodernists in search of pervasive yet elusive hegemonies, has defined the edges of life—before birth and in the last twilight of life—as useful for medicine itself, that is, for its progress. The imperative to help or save others at someone else's expense is not new. The Utilitarians of the nineteenth century and communitarians of the twentieth have given positive expression to policies that endorse collective improvement, often at the expense of whole classes of the most vulnerable, in areas of medicine from stem-cell research to standards for maintaining, or not, the lives of the comatose. This is not to argue that those vulnerable to new uses by medical science are or should be in every case absolutely off-limits, but the question of the meaning of vulnerability itself is also at stake over time. So it is in medicine that the greatest challenges in forestalling death have been met by a broader public acceptance of the usefulness of the death of one living being when it can save, or improve, the lives of many others. In this context, an automobile accident has an entirely new meaning. Indeed, what is potentially salvageable from any wreckage is more life for others. It is unlikely, and no doubt unseemly, that the death of Diana Princess of Wales might have also raised the question of the possible uses of her organs, as one final testament to her publicly celebrated benefactions, but the deaths of so many other lesser-known people surely are providing the material benefactions of an important and growing part of modern medicine.[32]

In another example, the death of Mickey Mantle in 1995, after an unsuccessful liver transplant, led to more calls that the public be persuaded to consider organ donation, but it was also a moment when the limits as well as the ambitions of medicine were put on public display. Mickey Mantle's death was the occasion for soul-searching about the distribution of scarce medical resources such as human organs as well as frustration about their acquisition. Not only were complaints made about the availability of organs for transplantation, but criticisms were also voiced about Mantle's celebrity being used as a criterion for his selection as a transplant recipient. The focus on his personal life and his use of alcohol also diminished the alliance between medicine's ambitions and the heroic appeal of a sports legend.[33]

Resistance among less educated citizens to organ transplantation requires a response not unlike those of efforts to combat smoking and obesity.[34] In all these cases, the progress of medical innovation, based on clinical and epidemiological research as well as ethical deliberation, depends on how useful others may be to purposes not specifically beneficial to those being used. Karen Ann Quinlan, whose case illustrated multiple dilemmas about the meaning of autonomy, the role of physicians and courts, and the uses of medical technology, did not die the way that many thought she would after she was removed from a respirator. The irony was more than implicit, since the meaning of her autonomy had as much to do with her quick death as with her freedom from the apparatus itself, and the role that doctors and courts played subsequent to the most publicized part of the drama quickly faded as she lived on for nine more years. Indeed, as time went on, the motivation to attend to issues about the "sanctity of life" was replaced by the insistence that autonomy should be absolute.[35] The clamor over her "case" had many justifications over time, all of which amounted to publicity for motives and arguments unrelated to her case specifically.

The Late-Twentieth-Century Transformations in Moral Sensibilities

Trust in doctors and the medical profession as a whole cannot be measured in any simple or decisive way. In the view of one thoughtful critic, the relationship between the physician and patient has evolved from one of mutual dependency to one that includes both the larger society's control of the profession and assertions by patients about their own rights.[36] Gilbert Meilander addressed the related problem of social expectations about what trust promises in a review of Eric J. Cassell's *The Nature of Suffering and the Goals of Medicine*:

> Despite all its appeal and importance, however, I think it claims too much and misidentifies the true healer. "The doctor-patient relationship is the vehicle through which the relief of suffering is

achieved." If that is the ground of our hope in the face of suffering, we are greatly to be pitied. And if we ask that of our physicians, we ask of them more than is within their power. Between a purely technical and contractual understanding of medicine, against which Cassell rebels, and the redemptive, salvific alternative he advocates, there ought to be some middle ground.[37]

The middle ground is never a secure ground, but it is maintained and transmitted in the still vital tradition of the physician's vocation, although this no longer provides either a definitive recipe for action or a blind trust in the person of the physician. In the Western world this vocation must find its new place among larger and healthier populations than have been seen in all of human history. Many in these populations live quiet lives in a modest pursuit of happiness, whether that happiness involves a decent and disease-free life or immortality itself, which is now a powerful part of the clinical goal of medicine as it seeks to create "prosthetic gods."[38]

It was Sigmund Freud's lamentation about happiness in *Civilization and Its Discontents* that introduced the idea of a prosthetic god:

> Man has, as it were, become a kind of prosthetic God. When he puts on all his auxiliary organs he is truly magnificent; but those organs have not grown on to him and they still give him much trouble at times. Nevertheless, he is entitled to console himself with the thought that this development will not come to an end precisely with the year 1930 A.D. Future ages will bring with them new and probably unimaginably great advances in this field of civilization and will increase man's likeness to God still more. But in the interests of our investigations, we will not forget that present-day man does not feel happy in his Godlike character.[39]

The unhappiness to which Freud refers may be for many the acknowledgment of mortality itself, but it may also be about how extensively the "Godlike character" of human beings is associated with those material circumstances that rightly account for much of what is meant by happiness. The material progress of medicine has given rise to two types of ethical debate: one has to do with the limits of such progress, the other with the autonomy of those subject to it.

These two debates are, in reality, reflections of one enduring problem about the nature of trust in individual persons (practicing professionals) and trust in "corporate" medicine (the profession as an organized entity with a decisive influence on individual doctors and the delivery of care). The significance of technology in relation to such problems of trust arises not so much in the nature of technology itself but in its application to those problems that arise as a result of confrontations with disease and death. These are not simply "technical" problems but ones finally taken up at many levels throughout the course of life, with and without the assistance of others. And in recent decades, as I have sought to make clearer in this book, the role of various social and intellectual movements, from feminism to bioethics, has transformed the nature of public trust in medicine and doctors in decisive ways.

The Issue of Patient Autonomy

Surely the reflections of Friedrich Nietzsche, famous (or infamous) as a champion of the power of individual will, establish one basis for understanding the new cultural meaning of autonomy as it has come to take its place in modern life:

> *A Moral Code for Physicians.*—The invalid is a parasite on society. In a certain state it is indecent to go on living. To vegetate on in cowardly dependence on physicians and medicaments after the meaning of life, the *right* to life has been lost ought to entail the profound contempt of society. Physicians, in their turn, ought to be the communicators of this contempt—not prescriptions, but everyday a fresh dose of *disgust* with their patients. . . . To create a new responsibility, that of the physician, in all cases in which the highest interest of life, of *ascending* of life, demands the most ruthless suppression and sequestration of degenerating life—for example in determining the right to reproduce, the right to be born, the right to live. . . .To die proudly when it is no longer possible to live proudly. Death of one's own free choice, death at the proper time, with a clear head and with joyfulness, consummated in the midst of children and witnesses: so that an actual leave taking is possible while he who is still living *is still there*, likewise an actual evaluation of what has been desired and what achieved in life, an *adding-up* of life—all of this is in contrast to the pitiable and horrible comedy Christianity has made of the hour of death.[40]

Nietzsche did not advocate a private dying; on the contrary he regarded the deliberate choice to end one's life as something to be "consummated in the midst of children and witnesses." Why children? One reason may have been to impress upon them from an early age a contempt for decrepitude that for Nietzsche was a small but significant part of his philosophy. Children do not easily and readily pay attention to adults; they are more often today served by adult attention. It is entirely better in Nietzsche's view that they learn early on to forget about needing to attend to those who cannot serve their attention. What better way than to witness suicide, perhaps regularly, and even better that kind of suicide now called "assisted" by the skilled hand of a physician? Such autonomy requires a corporate assent that includes family, friends, and earnest physicians. It is a socially and culturally defined autonomy of a particular kind.

Nietzsche's idea of autonomy found resonance, of course, among Nazi ideologues. But the idea of having some sort of control over one's departure from life does not condone murder. William Edward Hartpole Lecky (1838–1903), the Irish historian whose two works, *History of Rationalism* (1865) and *History of European Morals* (1869), established him as one of the major mediators between natural theology and modern rationalism in the nineteenth century, stated the dilemma less polemically than Nietzsche did:

> But the time must come when all the alternatives of life are sad, and the least sad is a speedy and painless end. When the eye has ceased to see and the ear to hear, when the mind has failed and all the friends of youth are gone, and the old man's life becomes a burden not only to himself but to those about him, it is far better that he should quit the scene. If a natural clinging to life, or a natural shrinking from death, prevents him from clearly realizing this, it is at least fully seen by all others.[41]

Others who wrote for the public (at least the well-educated public) came down on either side of the divide over euthanasia for those with terminal illnesses, those experiencing the indignities of decrepitude, and those facing a life of intractable pain, which William James remarked on in his chapter on "Saintliness" in *The Varieties of Religious Experience*:

> A strange moral transformation has within the past century swept over our Western world. We no longer think that we are called on to face physical pain with equanimity. It is not expected of a man that he should either endure it or inflict much of it, and to listen to the recital of cases of it makes our flesh creep morally as well as physically. The way in which our ancestors looked upon pain as an eternal ingredient of the world's order, and both caused and suffered it as a matter-of-course portion of their day's work, fills us with amazement.[42]

James's observations should not be taken as equivocations but more as evidence of perplexity about what to do in the face of such a clear and obvious transformation about what must or even should be endured as a matter of course.

The "strange moral transformation" that James described paved the way to the present circumstances in which the endurance of pain is unacceptable except as one may choose to endure it. The ever louder cultural protest has been, for at least a hundred years, against the blind acceptance of any inevitability regarding the human condition, including how we depart this life. What has happened in the course of truly great achievements in the history of public health and of modern medicine is that larger numbers of our fellow human beings are conscious that only one thing yet remains unavoidable—the certainty of one's death, that final relieving of the anxiety that our worries about health obviously anticipate. This is why James's remark about the strange moral transformation marks a cultural turning point in what the quest for health and well-being means in an era when only death, if not disease, seems defiant of rational apprehension. Genetic determinants of illness will be viewed in public opinion for some time to come as something akin to bad luck. But even this will change, perhaps in some series of dramatic breakthroughs, leaving in their wake the following sense of fate: neither the accident of consciousness (or what was once put philosophically and sociologically as the "accident of birth")[43] or accidents themselves (now high on the list of causes of mortality in those under fifty years of age) will yield to medical intervention or public health campaigns regarding prevention.

In the era of the wide spread of infectious diseases, discovery of how to control them led to the broad application of certain principles of professional and corporate conduct, including the requirements of purification and sterilization, which mark distinct, objective advances. Infection may not always be controllable, but more is known than ever before about when, how, where, and why it occurs. By virtue of their training and practice, public health professionals are deeply committed to environmental views of the causation of disease. Changing how people live has meant—under the dispensations of science and technology and the rise of epidemiology— changing first the environment in which people live and, more recently, changing their behavior, first through education then through regulation, and, only as a last resort, some form of direct coercion. Environmental changes have been accomplished largely outside the democratic process because no one would have thought to argue that any aspect of political rights was at stake in having access to, for example, cholera-contaminated water. Changing behavior through education and regulation has succeeded in many instances, but the democratic process has been implicated and challenged as the scope and mandate of such education and regulation has broadened. The idea that gun control can be viewed as a public health issue is not so incredible, but the resistance to a regulatory culture that defines the use of alcohol, tobacco, and firearms in epidemiological rather than commercial terms has cast the idea of liberty in a new light. It seems now probable that the public safety campaigns that began more than a hundred years ago as efforts to protect the public from various contaminants in water, food, and air will, down the road, focus relentlessly on behaviors that contribute to ill health and negative consequences both for the individual and for society.

What demographers have pointed out for some time is that with the decline in birthrates, despite the decline in infant mortality, and with the steady increase in longevity, due to a steady improvement in public health measures and medicine over the same time period, a world has been created in some places—but certainly not all—in which individual health and wellness are not only indirect benefits of centuries-long scientific and technological progress but have also become intense sources of investment, both emotional and financial.

In recent years, expenditures on health care in the United States have reached around 15 percent of the gross domestic product, or approximately $6,400 per capita. The percentage of GDP spent on health care in the United Kingdom is about half that in the United States. The significant point of comparison, however, is that the United States and England have comparable figures with respect to morbidity and mortality rates, longevity, and other principal measures of health and well-being.

For most analysts of public health, and in particular, economists, such a comparison is the equivalent of exposing not only inefficiency but immorality. Otherwise insistent about the imperatives of the rational actor, more than a few economists over much of the past century have never been entirely persuaded that the medical profession is anything other than it was portrayed in George Bernard Shaw's memorable remark, as "a conspiracy against the laity." Of course, Shaw was condemning the medical profession's concealment of malpractice, but he meant to convey that all professions, including the profession of economics, are conspiracies against the laity. It would be better to look beyond this remark, which Shaw made in the preface to his play *The Doctor's Dilemma*, to the even more powerful observations recorded in a series of articles that he wrote for *The English Review* toward the end of World War I: "Invited to contribute a series of articles in a Manchester paper in reply to the question, 'Have We Lost Faith?' Mr George Bernard Shaw gives his answer in this single sentence: 'Certainly not; but we have transferred it from God to the General Medical Council.'"[44]

Shaw's humor, the truth of which is recognized more clearly today perhaps than by readers of a century ago, had more to say about doctors than about patients, who are equally deserving of being reminded that when physicians profitably acquiesce to requests for more examinations and tests, the road to wellness has been paved with better intentions than either astute economists or complaining patients are necessarily ready to acknowledge. The fact that the United States leads the world in the consumption of health care resources may have less to do with the nature of medical practice than with the remarkable convergence of science, technology, faith, and affluence that also serves to inspire American complaints about everything to a finer degree than is possible anywhere else. For people (mostly of the upper classes, but also including anyone who is exposed to the media) to be exquisitely anxious about one's own health is a kind of cultural resignation to the absence of more immediate and momentous problems that have beset so much of humanity for so long.

The unintended consequence of living longer has been that it is expected, indeed demanded, that less happen in terms of adversity along the way. Such yearning for clear sailing is nothing new, and one should be hesitant to call this being selfish or spoiled in some new way. It represents a problem that was just as familiar to Plato in his *Dialogues* as it was to John Wesley and Cardinal Newman in their respective sermons on "The Danger of Riches." This problem for modern life is that health and well-being, although quite understandably conceived of as material things that once were conceived of as blessings, are now sought after as rights. Newman, for example, knew that having such riches and putting trust in them were two different things entirely. The trust, as he and many others after him have observed, is misplaced, a sight lower, as it were, than where such trust should be placed. But this is our modern fate after the backdrop of heaven and hell has fallen away and in its place such high expectations are placed on physicians and their science and technologies. The intensity of distrust in doctors is evidence of the demand for trust in things that are believed will sustain life longer, if not forever.

Ted Williams and Terri Schiavo: Counterpoints in the End-of-Life Debate

In light of a significant transformation in moral sensibilities about "quality of life" and its prolongation, two cases in recent years may seem at first to have little in common even though both served as public markers on the continuum that presently defines to what lengths some will go to maintain and sustain human life. And along with advances in cloning and the development of artificial intelligence, an extraordinary convergence may be at hand in establishing what previous generations, with utopian hopefulness, called a "new humanity."

After Ted Williams, the legendary Boston Red Sox player, died at the age of eighty-three in July 2002, public interest in his death took a bizarre turn when his son, John Henry, had his father's body transported to a "cryonics" facility—the Alcor Life Extension Foundation, in Scottsdale, Arizona. Various media reports noted that not only was Williams's body preserved in liquid nitrogen but it had also been decapitated. Williams's son was not purchasing a guarantee of immortality for his father, but was instead speculating on a hope that someday medical and technical science would be advanced sufficiently to bring Ted Williams (and John Henry himself, who died in 2004 and whose body was also sent to the cryonics facility in Arizona) back to life in the same bodies in which they had lived, or at least with the same consciousness they had possessed, during their "natural" lives. Ted Williams's eldest daughter, Bobby-Jo, fought in court to stop her brother and sister, Claudia, from keeping their father frozen in a nine-foot tall cylindrical steel tank but did not succeed.[45]

According to information provided by Alcor Life Extension Foundation and by a similar but unrelated facility, the Cryonics Institute, located outside of Detroit, there are approximately 140 "cryopatients" being "cryopreserved" at present, with well over a thousand people (between the two facilities) who have "completed their financial and legal arrangement for cryopreservation."[46] In an update of news about the Cryonics Institute on its website, an account is given of the "deanimation" and the cryopreservation of a seventy-nine-year old woman:

> May 16, 2006. The Cryonics Institute's 74th patient is a 79-year-old woman who was a victim of breast cancer—who was cryopreserved by her son. She deanimated (was pronounced dead) on Sunday, May 14th (Mother's Day). Of the most recent seven patients, five are mothers cryopreserved by their sons.
>
> This case typifies the popular conception of cryonics as something that is not arranged until time of death. Although the family had agreed upon cryonics in February, formal arrangements with the Cryonics Institute were initiated only a few days before deanimation, which occurred sooner than had been expected. Preparations were therefore not as good as they could have been. There was no use of heparin and shipment was briefly delayed because funding had to be wired. Under the circumstances, it went surprisingly quickly and smoothly, but more advanced preparation would have made a big difference.[47]

The *Wall Street Journal* reported on its front page about the emerging cryonics movement and the various financial implications in estate planning that attend to it. According to the *Journal*, cryonic hopefuls are planning to leave the bulk of their estates in trust to themselves in what are being called "personal revival trusts," which have something in common with what were previously called "dynasty trusts," once prohibited but now permitted by more than twenty states.[48]

The *Journal* also reported that a casino owner in Nevada who plans on being cryopreserved "opted against allowing a clone to get his money. He insisted that whoever gets the funds should have "my memories." This kind of insistence on preservation can be compared to the much more widely publicized family disagreement about the fate of Terri Schiavo, whose case became a referendum on the right to end life that was otherwise being maintained, or preserved, in what many argued was already a lifeless state except in the most minimal biological sense. The family quarrel over the disposition of Ted Williams, declared legally dead, tipped in favor (by a court's judgment) of an admittedly bizarre form of life preservation even as Terri Schiavo, legally alive, was allowed to die (also by a court's judgment).

The ink spilled and political capital squandered over Terri Schiavo's case illustrates one end of a continuum of anxiety about living for perhaps many years, as Karen Ann Quinlan did, in a state of completely irreversible coma. In Schiavo's case, this anxiety is of broad public significance. It is first most generally about the use of public, as distinct from private, funds to keep people alive who seem hopelessly destined to remain in a permanent vegetative state until they naturally expire. Those in such a state, as Terri Schiavo surely was, constitute a relatively small drain on the national economy in comparison to the vast sums of money that are spent each day on people in hospitals during the final weeks of their lives. And even larger numbers of the infirm and elderly require some forms of assistance that are bound to increase public expenses, even dramatically, in the years to come.[49] Yet the Schiavo case received extraordinary attention because it raised in some people's minds the specter of being maintained or preserved in some indefinite state with little or no promise of recovery to a "normal quality of life."

The principal difference between Ted Williams and Terri Schiavo seems to be that Williams *wanted* his body to be preserved (even though there was clearly a dispute within his family over his true final wishes), while Schiavo, according to her husband, did not want to be maintained in the state she was in (though there was also considerable dispute over whether this was, in fact, her expressed wish), and the issue of who should make the final decision, her husband or her parents, left doctors mostly on the periphery. Williams died and was immediately prepped for preservation; Schiavo had to be taken off all essential forms of sustenance, water in particular, and not too many days later she died and was eventually cremated. Williams's hope to defeat death and Schiavo's death despite her parents' hope for some degree of recovery are counterpoints in a strange alliance that gives expression to the extraordinary social complications that follow from both the overuse of medical technologies and the new demand for ever more sophisticated technologies to maintain life indefinitely. Williams's death was, after all, probably a more decisive fact than any speculative consideration about reanimation a hundred years from now. Schiavo's vegetative state presented a much more complicated calculus of emotional responses.

Here again, the case of Karen Ann Quinlan marks an important turning point. Thirty years ago seems almost an imponderable period of time to consider how profoundly different professional and legal attitudes were then about efforts to preserve life. At that time, hospital and state officials fought to keep Karen technically alive, arguing that they were ethically and legally responsible to guard her welfare, which meant, in fact, keeping her breathing on a ventilator. In a ruling that shifted the balance of power away from the professionals and the state, the New Jersey State Supreme Court decided that Karen's parents should have the final say in her welfare, and in this case, that final say could extend to whether or not she should be maintained on what was then widely considered to be "artificial" life support.

The legacy of the Quinlan decision remains a powerful influence in public attitudes about death and dying. What began as an argument about "artificial" and "extraordinary" care was eventually taken up by the Supreme Court in subsequent cases with the final result that the withdrawal of food and water could also be legally protected if a court could be persuaded that this was or had been the patient's wishes. The question of whether or not such decisions were in the patient's "best interest," in such matters of passive and active euthanasia, became less compelling as a matter of public policy. The anxieties stirred by Schiavo's case had to do with the very different ways in which people identified with her and her situation, not only the heartbreaking struggle among loved ones but also her specific medical condition. The intrusion of politics in the form of a (perhaps ill-informed) medical diagnosis when physician and Senator William Frist intervened publicly to offer his own assessment, exacerbated an already overpublicized struggle in which physicians were ritually expected to defer to court determinations about how to proceed.

Ted Williams and Terri Schiavo have more in common than may be obvious at first thought. Schiavo's parents sought to keep her alive, of course not indefinitely, but like Karen Ann Quinlan's parents, they enacted the same sense of obligation to her that once came with making a distinction between turning off a ventilator or starving and dehydrating someone to death. This may now be for many a distinction without much of a difference if the overriding intention is to hasten a death more of an "organism" rather than that of a "person." In Williams's case, another kind of ambition has taken root, which views the end of a natural life as a limitation of medical science and technology rather than one of the nature of life itself. Those who sought to keep Schiavo alive appear as the macabre ones, while those who endorsed what is regularly called a "death with dignity" seemingly have gained the upper hand in public debates about the "right to die." The anxiety conjured up by the image of a person in a long-term vegetative state and in need of constant care—it has been estimated that their numbers in this country may be between fourteen thousand and thirty-five thousand, adults and children combined—may someday evoke a much improved sense of hope as such people are joined with those already dead awaiting reanimation in a vast new enterprise to revive them all with their consciousness and memories intact.

Science Fiction and the Hope for Immortality

The prospect of immortality, which as a matter of public fascination remains a distant competitor to the pursuit of the "fountain of youth,"[50] has begun nevertheless to make a mark on how we think about what makes us human. For medical practitioners in the clinical trenches, such a mark may already be manifested by how much more the entire medical enterprise relies first on tests of all kinds and the information they produce, leaving the physical patient as an artifact of test "results" rather than the being at the center of sustained and coordinated medical attention by individual practitioners. In this process of displacement, the "digital age" as it is now known, has contributed a vocabulary of alliances between human beings and their technologies, the latter of which are seen to develop as substitutes for various components of the former. These are substitutions intended to enhance and promote human powers through new and imagined integrations of machine, body, and mind in the laboratory, in the surgical theater, and in the world of commerce.

In digital parlance and in the developing science of robotics, the stages of advancement are defined by the creation of bionic humans, cyborgs, and androids.[51] The underlying impetus for research into these technologies is the preservation of consciousness. The creation of bionic humans is the safest bet for the preservation of consciousness and memories, though they are the riskiest vessel in terms of long-term viability. To reduce the risk of a permanent loss of unique consciousness, the cyborg, with its replacement of all bodily mass with machine parts, conjures images of some new form of invulnerability. It is in the very nature of our lived-in bodies that we know not only consciousness but also vulnerability. Because of this, the perception of danger is a natural thing, even if common sense is not. Some believe that "off-loading" a unique consciousness and its memories into a machine of some kind may finally create a world in which no one would ever be permanently destroyed.

The androids present an alternative to natural consciousness. The film *A.I. (Artificial Intelligence)* gave popular expression to a world in which technology (a blessing and a curse) separates humans and androids into a new version of the haves and have-nots. Based on the short story "Supertoys Last

All Summer Long," by Brian Aldiss, first published in 1969, the film is about an android boy, David, who cannot please his mother but whose only wish is to become a "real" boy and thus win her affection.[52] This most Freudian and tragic sense of life exploits the idea that no robot/android could ever completely substitute for the unique consciousness that each human being is presumed to possess as a birthright. David is obsessed with being accepted. He is jealous of his human brother, who at the film's opening is in a cryogenically maintained state as doctors seek to cure him and bring him back to consciousness. Cast from the Garden of Eden of his mother's care, he embarks on a journey that introduces him to the pathetic android underworld and the immoral human overworld. At one point he finds himself again among his creator-inventors, who discuss what consciousness and awareness really mean.

By the close of the film, David has lived on for millions of years and the only thing different about the earth besides its being frozen over is that humanity is extinct. The film's director, Steven Spielberg, appears to bring back the same space creatures he used in *Close Encounters of the Third Kind*; they offer the poor android boy one final day with his mother, who has been reincarnated by a remarkable "memory extraction" technique. David enjoys his day and then goes to sleep forever next to his reimagined mother. In the end, *A.I.* cannot achieve a vision of hope for either androids or humans, because fate itself is a meaningless term except in a world where beginnings and endings are unique and unrepeatable. A paradise in which nothing ever changes and time never ends has no use for either hope or despair. The promise of eternal life by each of the world religions has only required the proof of faith to be fulfilled. But the determination to preserve one's active consciousness and memories in some permanent way joins technical progress with human vanity in a new and finally sinister way.[53]

Medicine's Power over Life and Death

There is something wonderful about the new forms of progress and also something wonderfully empty, as Freud lamented in his observations about "prosthetic Gods." The goal of complete prosthetic replacement parallels the obsessive avoidance of all that may imperil health and well-being. The logic of such developments, as sociologists and anthropologists long ago recognized, defines the nature of institutions in which those aspects of individuality, including the individual himself, are necessarily dispensable. No individual is an institution, at least not for long. Freud recognized that discontents were not principally based on the organization of the human environment—although the central dogma of public health would so contend—except for that vast internal environment within each individual, inaccessible to others and very often to oneself as well.

Of the several contemporary campaigns against psychoanalysis, two stand out: The first has been led by the psycho-biological study of the mind, producing a pharmacopoeia that has been aimed (whether its advocates admit it or not) at taming the will in the young and lessening the burden of existence in older age. The second is a campaign of suspicion about both the credibility and applicability of psychoanalytic insight. In both campaigns the question of trust has shifted focus from the authority of the practitioner to the power of his technique. Most pastoral counseling, of which Freud's "talking cure" was a secular manifestation, takes place outside of medicine proper, but technique is still very much tied to the effects produced in this realm. The therapeutic sphere has always required that concrete results be produced, and it has become now a matter of public indifference about what works as long as it does work and does not harm. Over the past quarter century, much has changed for physicians, who are no longer visibly in charge of their corporate fate as a profession. Yet there is something about the nature of their vocation that will not be reduced to the sum of their corporate identity at any given moment in time but will also not be sufficiently protective of their individual identity to ensure any lasting loyalty.

What is allowed to be done or not done is no longer consistently mediated by personal authority, and so looking for answers by looking for people to provide them misconstrues what is at stake in trust built on probabilities and fragmented oversight. But what is the alternative? Part of the absence of certainty about what is not to be done in particular arises from the hope of progress itself. Max Weber, in such formulations as "the disenchantment of the world" and "the rationalization of the world," envisioned a cold, brisk wind blowing across Occidental ideas about the connection between hope and progress. Progress proceeds, as it were, with neither a sense of divine intervention nor the certainty of some definitive success.

Among his most brilliant insights, C. S. Lewis observed that when the apostles preached to the pagans, the pagans had and feared their own gods, even as so many in the West today doubt the existence of even one universal God. The pagan fear was about a choice among divine powers, whereas the modern fear is that no power can be decisive, and if not decisive, then it must be arbitrary. The religious mission has become doubly difficult, as Lewis believed in the Christian case, because the laity has to be persuaded that they actually possesses a spiritual condition before that condition can be offered a cure, whatever it may be. Such was the older meaning of hope. Torn from any number of spiritual moorings, this hope might be seen now as a will to power, at which complaints have been directed for over a century. Unfortunately these complaints have not succeeded in changing the character of "progress." The Weberian imperative of a science and technology projecting onto the world a vision of control of that world gives no indication of any kind of mediating authority about *who* is in control.

Taking control of one's life, as the therapeutic prescription now requires, means trusting in others only to the extent absolutely necessary, and no more. Perhaps this shallowness of trust is inversely related to the intensity of many people's disappointments. At the center of this control, from opposite ends of the continuum of life, abortion and physician-assisted suicide, both employing relatively simple technologies, are manifestations of the shallowness of trust and the bitter heart of disappointment. But they are the preconditions for much of the prosthetic technologies and subsequent hopes that have followed for the individual. In a collectivist sense, the era of social engineering gave tyrants a license to imagine themselves as prosthetic gods. Perhaps the next utopian idea after the repudiation of collectivism will come to be seen as the complete exercise of "private" control over human beings in their removal from the world. Both abortion and physician-assisted suicide are the private abandonment of hope for and beyond this life. They are constantly heralded as public rights against which any resistance, however construed, is called infringement. But an enormous cultural inversion has taken place, since what is now perceived of as an infringement, at least in moral terms, was once regarded as protection based on a general prohibition against the taking of life.

Some years ago in one of the many iterations of debate over the "right" to die, the following three sentences appeared in a letter to the *New York Times*:

> I prefer to die without being able to ask for a doctor to help me kill myself. Come the time, I will not even want to think about that.
> I surely will not want the people around me thinking I should be thinking about that.[54]

Whether or not this observation, made by Mr. Julius B. Poppinga in 1994, represents a majority sentiment over time, it clearly does stand in stark contrast to the pronouncements of secular elites who are central to envisioning and thus promoting a world in which the pain of living may be as much a pain to others as it is to the person in pain. Mr. Poppinga, an attorney and an elder of Grace Presbyterian Church in Montclair, New Jersey, suggested a plausible alternative to Nietzsche's proposed solution of 1889: the *that* in his plea "I surely will not want the people around me thinking I should be thinking about *that*" is a form of double forgetting, a double not thinking about "that." Mr. Poppinga was asking not only that he not have to consider the subject of physician-assisted suicide "come the time" but also that he not have to think about such an "option" as something on the minds of others "around" him.

The Undoing of Cultural Repressions

The term "around," as in "I surely will not want the people around me thinking" defines the social context, that is, the role of the will of others, in this kind of double forgetting. In this context, what sociologists call cultural repression is a form of prohibition that exists prior to consciousness and its deliberations; in this case the idea of physician-assisted suicide would be something that one would have to acknowledge to oneself and that others might expect one to consider. Individual "autonomy" is presently credited as the source and arbiter of this particular view of the end of life. Yet such a widely debated expectation should also be seen as the failing of a cultural repression that was once sufficient in its capacity to judge the individual consideration of all suicide to be a kind of self-doubt, a failure on the part of the individual. The next step in a failing cultural repression is the replacement of that self-doubt with collective affirmation that it is instead a species of self-control.

In the case of assisted suicide, the failing cultural repression does not, by the fiction of autonomy or by the collective indifference to suffering, necessarily have to lead to a widespread practice of euthanasia. This would require a wholly different degree of public coercion.[55] Instead, an uneasy balance exists in the United States between those who are intent on hastening their own deaths by active intervention and those who acknowledge that pain, as William James observed, does not have to be endured for its own sake. This must be seen as a vast improvement, leading to more attentive hospice care, for example. In democratic societies especially, the resistance to shifting this balance too far in the direction of support for assisted suicide is likely to remain fairly strong, thus avoiding a broad transformation in the social patterns of how people die.

In the case of abortion, which also involves the question of who is to decide in matters life and death, that question is even more important but seemingly less urgent to the present priorities of women, couples, and medical researchers. Among all the distinctively Christian transformations in moral judgments about abortion is the near extinction of both the shame regarding resort to it and shame regarding the circumstances in which an unwanted pregnancy came about. A mere half century ago, women were subject to humiliations that seem remote, if not impossible to imagine, in more recent generations. Shame and humiliation have residual manifestations, including expressions of regret and other clinically defined psychological disorders. These residual expressions of anxiety about the "right" to abortion are adaptations to the extinction of a cultural repression whose provenance was once central not only to defining the distinctiveness of human life at its beginning as well as at its end, but also to an insistence that the sexual relations that bring about its creation must be more than the satisfaction of physical desire.

The right-to-life movement has adapted to the gradual undoing of this particular cultural repression by avoiding any association that makes it appear to be judgmental about sexual relations. This represents a decisive departure from earlier modalities of shame, in which the private and public significance of "getting a girl into trouble" was associated less with the potential child than with a family's dishonor in the context of those, who were, as Mr. Poppinga put it, "around." The shift in focus to a concern for the unborn child, regardless of the circumstances of its creation, released a powerful motivation to defend interests that up until the legalization of abortion seemed securely dedicated to the preservation of life. Sexual morality within all the major religious traditions had accomplished this end indirectly, if not always successfully. With the abolition of a highly judgmental view of sexual morality as it was once understood, in which the person was hedged in by shame and the avoidance of such shame through modesty, the "right to life" has become the expression of another, all but extinct, cultural repression.

What remains for those now dedicated to "a right to life," both at its beginning and at its end, is to untangle an even more difficult knot that ties the interests of the preservation of life outside the womb to the destruction of life within it. Were it not for the intensified interest in finding ways to treat some of the most debilitating diseases later in life (a function, demographically speaking, of the growing proportion of the aged within the population of the United States), the uses of fetal life—in the form of stem-cell research usually using extra embryos created in the process of artificial insemination that would otherwise be discarded—to save presently living adults might be condemned even more broadly than it appears to be from the clamor of political debate about this issue. The abortion right, it must be admitted, has made everything else possible. In this way, contrary to the prevailing myth that technological innovation creates unforeseen and new ethical dilemmas, such innovation would not have been imaginable, at least in some respects, had not the ethical crossroad been reached where abortion before the third trimester of pregnancy is now legally permitted without the stipulation that it involves the physical health of the pregnant woman. Quite apart from the resistance to wholesale approval for euthanasia, given alternatives for pain relief, for example, resistance to abortion is no longer rejected because it denies the evolution of a new sexual ethic, but rather because such resistance interferes with scientific and commercial advancement. As the social movements arising from both religious and secular bases organize to resist this advancement, it would behoove them both to revisit how sexual morality relates to abortion freedom rather than how that freedom relates to medical and technological innovation.[56]

In contemporary debates about the various corruptions and deficiencies of the medical profession, the harshest criticisms have been aimed at the entrepreneurs of managed care and for-profit medicine. They certainly have something to answer for, although it seems that patient satisfaction in general has not suffered as much as some critics would like to contend. On the other hand, various social and intellectual movements, in and around medicine, have diminished the status and importance of the individual practitioner in ways that have yet to be fully accounted for. Such practitioners operate, literally, in the twilight of many moral sensibilities about the meaning of human life. When he examined comparable problems of physician authority thirty years ago in *Ethics at the Edges of Life*, the theologian Paul Ramsey concluded, "Our children and our children's children will not even have been cognizant of the fact they have journeyed on into the setting sun of Western law and morality, not seeing the shadows. We may even now be living 'between the evenings' (a beautiful—and, I believe, Jewish—expression for 'twilight'). That's the sum of it."[57]

ACKNOWLEDGMENTS

Of the many personal and intellectual debts I owe to others in the matter of this book, the first are to the Reverend William E. Dubocq and the Reverend William Alexander Johnson, who directed my earliest intellectual considerations of religion. Reverend Dubocq was chaplain during my boarding school years at Governor Dummer Academy in Byfield, Massachusetts. I remember with great affection that he took me to hear Rabbi Abraham Heschel at Brandeis University and that we read Paul Tillich's *Dynamics of Faith* together. He impressed me with a lifelong interest in how religious conscience informs personal and institutional responsibility.

William Johnson affirmed my abiding faith in the experiment of American religious pluralism, a continuing source of strength and tension in American life. During my undergraduate years at Brandeis University, he introduced me to nineteenth-century American Protestantism, which remains, I believe, a starting point for understanding many things about American life and its anxieties in our own time.

Since we live only one life—if we live even one, as my graduate mentor, Philip Rieff, often remarked—I have never aspired to be a Protestant minister, though the calling of the ministry embodied in American Protestantism is by every cultural and historical measure the archetype for understanding the enduring meaning of the idea of vocation in all professions over the past two hundred years. As Rieff understood, a powerful consciousness of doubt now undermines many relations that by necessity operate on trust. Rieff taught in the true spirit of vocation, insisting that noble character was a principal element in establishing and maintaining trust over time.

Renée C. Fox continues to teach me the humility of the observer, who understands both the persistence of that which is ephemeral and that which endures. The work that she set out to accomplish a half century ago stood alone in its anticipation of the uncertainties about health and human progress that are today the subject of so much debate and controversy. She has remained a constant source of encouragement, friendship, and intellectual inspiration.

Several people took the time and effort to read manuscript in its stages of preparation. Charles Bosk, in particular, provided detailed comments and advice along the way. His wisdom and sagacity about many matters both scholarly and personal will always be appreciated. Others have offered encouragements and assistance of many kinds, and I am honored to name them here: Brigitte and Peter Berger, Irving Louis Horowitz and Mary Curtis, Steven Grosby, Alan Mittleman, Peter Skerry, Stephen Bates, Thomas Cushman, Guy MacLean Rogers, Elissa Koff, Dr. Robert Insoft, Daniel J. Mahoney, Tom Riley, Dennis Wrong, James T. Patterson, and Alex Zwerdling. Several Wellesley College students were particularly helpful, especially Akemi Joy Tanaka and LaShaune Patrice Johnson. Chris Kochansky and Richard Isomaki provided essential copy-editing and a fresh eye near the completion of this work, as did Nathan Carr and Clara Platter of Princeton University Press. Both Peter Conrad and Raymond De Vries acted as conscientious reviewers of the book, and I thank them for their time and effort. And my deepest thanks go to Peter Dougherty.

Initial support for the research and writing of this book came from the Woodrow Wilson International Center for Scholars, where I was a fellow. The generosity of the Wellesley College Class of 1949 in endowing a chair in ethics aided in research and preparation, and I wish to thank all of them for their interest and confidence in my work. Parts of this book were presented at various times and in various places as public lectures. I am grateful to the then Dean of the College, Nancy H. Kolodny, for inviting me to speak about my research in a Wellesley College faculty seminar; to the late James H. Cassedy of the National Library of Medicine for his invitation to address a seminar on the history of medicine; to James Davison Hunter for inviting me to present my work at the University of Virginia two times at the beginning of the research and at the end of the writing of this book. Several people helped specifically in securing materials, including Gail M. Pietrzyk, Public Service Archivist, University of Pennsylvania; Janice Braun, Assistant Historical Librarian, Yale University, Historical Library, Harvey Cushing/John Hay Whitney Medical Library; G. David Anderson, University Archivist, Gelman Library, George Washington University; Ida Cohen Selavan, Ph.D., Judaica Librarian, Hebrew Union College–Jewish Institute of Religion, Cincinnati, Ohio; Margaret Zeller, Tulane University Medical School, Rudolph Matas Medical Library, Special Collections; Susan J. Sullivan, Associate Librarian for Information Services, Presbyterian Church, Department of History, Philadelphia; Karen Jenson, Wellesley College; and Cynthia H. Krusell.

I have had the privilege over the past twenty-five years to advise and recommend many young women going on to medical school from Wellesley College. I have also taught many of these same students in one particular course on medical sociology and social epidemiology. Although they are too numerous to acknowledge here, I am indebted to all of them, including some with whom I have remained in correspondence as they give accounts of their life journeys in medicine and public health. I pray for younger physicians, as they grow older, that they may bequeath a legacy to their successors of higher hopes beyond any narrow, personal ambition and toward a better world.

Wellesley College
December 13, 2007

APPENDIX 1

Extant Addresses, Sermons, and Eulogies by Clergymen

This list consists only of separately published materials, including some that appeared in volumes of collected essays. Newspapers and medical periodicals of the period often provided excerpts from and accounts of addresses delivered by many other clergymen.

The denominational affiliation of the author, if known, is listed at the end of each entry.

1823   Bates, Joshua. Address Delivered in Castleton, December 2, 1823, at the Commencement of the Vermont Academy of Medicine: connected with Middlebury College. Smith & Shute Printers, Castleton, VT. 16 pages.

1825   Bailey, Rufus William. An Address, Delivered at the Annual Commencement of the Berkshire Medical Institution, Pittsfield, December 23, 1824. P. Allen, Pittsfield, MA. 24 pages. [Presbyterian]

1825   Marsh, John. The Beloved Physician. A Sermon Occasioned by the Death of Doct. Andrew F. Warner, of Haddam, June 23, 1825. Hartford: Goodwin. 20 pp. [Congregational]

1840   Hopkins, Mark. "Address, delivered before the Medical Class at Pittsfield, Nov. 4, 1840." *Miscellaneous Essays and Discourses* (Boston: T.R. Marvin, 1847), pp. 197–213.

1841   Crane, Silas Axtell. Christian truths and motives; the surest basis and best means of education. Address, graduating of first medical class of Kemper College. Chambers & Knapp, St. Louis. 18 pages.

1844   Boardman, Henry Augustus. The Claims of Religion Upon Medical Men. A Discourse Delivered in the Tenth Presbyterian Church, Philadelphia, November 24, 1844. Book and Job Printing Office, Philadelphia. 24 pages. [Presbyterian]

1845   Hope, M. B. A Discourse Designed to Show that Physiological Inquiries Are Not Unfriendly to Religious Sentiment. Delivered in the Tenth Presbyterian Church, Philadelphia, January 18, 1845. Barrett and Jones, Philadelphia. 16 pages. [Presbyterian]

1847   Barrows, Elijah Porter. The Harmony of Creation: and the Subordination of the Physical Part of it to the Moral. An Address Delivered before the

Trustees, Faculty, and Students of the Medical Department of the Western Reserve College, Cleveland, February 24, 1847. Hudson [Ohio] Observer Press, Cleveland. 22 pages. [Presbyterian]

Krebs, John Michael. The Reciprocal Relations of Physicians and Clergymen: A Speech. Delivered at the Anniversary Dinner of the New York Society for the Relief of Widows and Orphans of Medical Men, November 17, 1847. Henry Ludwig, New York. 10 pages. [Presbyterian]

1848   Berg, Joseph Frederick. The Faithful Physician; a Discourse Addressed to the Students of the Medical Colleges of Philadelphia, December 10, 1848. W. S. Young, Philadelphia. 16 pages.

Parker, Joel. A Sermon on the Moral Responsibility of Physicians. Addressed to the Medical Students of Philadelphia, February 6, 1848. A. Scott, Philadelphia. 22 pages. [Presbyterian]

1849   Day, Henry Noble. The Professions. An Address Delivered at the Commencement of the Medical Department of Western Reserve College. At Cleveland, February 21, 1849. Observer Office, Hudson, OH. 23 pages. [Congregational]

Mott, Lucretia Coffin. A Sermon to the Medical Students, Delivered by Lucretia Mott, at Cherry Street Meeting House, February 11, 1849. W. B. Zeiber, Philadelphia. [Quaker]

1850   Rogers, Ebenezer Platt. The Medical Profession and the Duties of its Members. A Sermon Delivered Before the Members of the Graduating Class of the Medical College of Georgia, March 3, 1850. J. & L. Metcalf, Northampton, MA. 20 pages. [Presbyterian]

1851   Quintard, Charles Todd. An Address Delivered Before the Graduating Class of the Medical College of Georgia, March 1851. McCafferty, Augusta, GA. 20 pages. [Episcopal]

Thompson, Matthew La Rue Perrine. A Sermon Preached by Request before the Medical Class of the University in the City of Buffalo, December 28, 1851. E. A. Maynard's Steam Power Press, Buffalo, NY. 28 pages. [Presbyterian]

1852   Chapin, Edwin Hubbell. The Post of Duty. A Discourse Occasioned by the Death of Dr. A. Sidney Doane, Delivered in the Murray Street Church, February 15, 1852. Press of Baker, Godwin & Co., New York.

Hall, Nathanial. A discourse delivered in the First Church, Dorchester, on the Sunday succeeding the funeral of Robert Thaxter, M.D. Ebenezer Clapp, Jr., Boston. 23 pages.

Quintard, Charles Todd. The True Physician: An Address to the Graduating Class of the Memphis Medical College, Session 1851–52. Appeal Book & Job Office Print, Memphis, TN. 15 pages. [Episcopal]

Smyth, Anson. The Beloved Physician: Sermon occasioned by the death of Calvin Smith, M.D. Preached at Toledo, Ohio, September 19, 1852. Hosmer, Andrews and Co., Toledo, OH. 16 pages.

Stevens, William Bacon. A Sermon Preached Before the Students of the Several Medical Colleges of the City of Philadelphia, December 5, 1852, in St. Andrew's Church. King & Baird, Philadelphia. [Episcopal]

1854   Bartol, C. A. The Relation of the Medical Profession to the Ministry: A Discourse Preached in the West Church, on the Occasion of the Death of Dr. George C. Shattuck. John Wilson and Son, Boston.

Newell, Frederick R. The beloved physician: a sermon in Littleton, funeral of Jacob Gault Elliot, M.D., November 26, 1854. Crosby, Nichols, and Co., Boston. 14 pages.

1855   Quintard, Charles Todd. Address to the Graduating Class of the Memphis Medical College, Session of 1854–55. n.p. 14 pages. [Episcopal]

1856   Bittinger, John Baugher. The True Mission of the Physician: An Address, Delivered at the Commencement of the Western Reserve Medical College, Cleveland, February 29, 1856. Cleveland, Cowles, Pinkerton & Co. [Presbyterian]

Parker, Joel. The Beloved Physician: A Tribute to the Memory of James C. Bliss, M.D., A Discourse on the Combined Influence of the Gospel and the Medical Profession in Forming the Character. Samuel S. & William Wood, New York. 29 pages. [Presbyterian]

Tappan, Henry Philip. The Mutual Responsibilities of Physicians and the Community, Being an Address to the Graduating Class of the Medical College of the University of Michigan, March 27, 1856. Free Print Press, Office of Peninsular Journal of Medicine, n.p.. 25 pages. [Congregational]

1857   Brown, Frederick Thomas. The "Physician Should Be a Christian"; An Address, Delivered at the Commencement of the Western Reserve Medical College, February 27, 1857. E. Cowles & Co., Cleveland. [Presbyterian]

1858   Kennedy, Duncan. A Clergyman's Idea of a Model Physician: An Address Delivered at the Commencement of the Albany Medical College, June 8, 1858. Munsell & Rowland, Albany, NY. 24 pages. [Presbyterian]

Stevens, William Bacon. The Religious Teachings of Medical Science. A Sermon Delivered before the Medical Students of the Several Colleges of Philadelphia in St. Andrew's Church, November 7, 1856 and Repeated by Request in the Same Place, December 6, 1857. C. Sherman, Philadelphia. 40 pages. [Episcopal]

1860   Rudder, William. The Complete Physician: An Address Pronounced Before the Graduates of the Albany Medical College, in the Assembly Chamber, Dec. 24, 1860. Frank H. Little, Albany. 30 pages. [Episcopal]

Stevens, William Bacon. Hospitals and the Church. An Address Delivered before the Convention of the Diocese of Pennsylvania in St. Andrew's Church, Philadelphia, May 24, 1860. Ashmead, Philadelphia. 31 pages. [Episcopal]

1861   Daggett, O. E. The beloved physician: a sermon preached in the First Congregational Church, Canandaigua, N.Y., at the funeral of Edson Carr, M.D., Sunday, December 1, 1861. J. J. Mattison, Canandaigua, NY. 24 pages. [Congregational]

1862   Clapp, A. Huntington. The Beloved Physician. A sermon occasioned by the death of Joseph Warren Fearing, M.D.: preached in the Beneficent Congregational Church, Providence, December 7, 1862. Knowles, Anthony & Co., Providence, RI. 20 pages. [Congregational]

Townsend, M.D., Rev. Stephen. Valedictory Sermon Preached in Saint Luke's (The Beloved Physician) Methodist E. Church, Philadelphia, March 10, 1862. Perkinpine & Higgins, Philadelphia.

Woods, Leonard. An address delivered on the opening of the New Hall of the Medical School of Maine, February 21, 1862. Telegraph Office, A. G. Tenney, Brunswick, ME. 24 pages.

1863   Clark, Rufus Wheelwright. The Sources of a Physician's Power. An Address Delivered at the Commencement of the Albany Medical College, May 28, 1863. Steam Press of C. Van Benthuysen, Albany, NY. 30 pages.

Townsend, M.D., Rev. Stephen. Sermon to the Students of Jefferson Medical College, Preached in Green Street M.E. Church, February 15, 1863. Perkinpine & Higgins, Philadelphia. 24 pp. [Methodist]

1864   Bacon, Leonard. The Beloved Physician: A discourse delivered in First Church in New Haven, at the internment of Jonathan Knight, M.D., Late Professor of Surgery in Yale College. Thomas J. Stafford, New Haven, CT. 28 pages.

Cobb, Oliver E. The Beloved Physician. Sermon Preached at the Funeral of Denis Wortman, M.D., in the Reformed Dutch Church, Hopewell, NY, May 5, 1864. N. Tibbals, Library Association, New York. 21 pages.

Haven, Erastus Otis. The Relations of the Medical Profession to Science. An Address Delivered before the Graduating Class of the Department of Medicine and Surgery of the University of Michigan, March 30, 1864. L. Davis, Ann Arbor, MI. 20 pages. [Methodist]

1865   Beadle, Elias Root. The Sacredness of the Medical Profession, A Sermon Delivered before the Students of Jefferson Medical College and the Medical Department of the University of Pennsylvania, November 19, 1865. James S. Claxton, Philadelphia. 16 pages. [Presbyterian]

Sprague, William B. A Sermon Addressed to the Second Presbyterian Congregation, Albany, Sunday Morning, April 2, 1865, on Occasion of the Death of Sylvester D. Willard, M.D., Surgeon-General of the State of

New-York. Van Benthuysen's Steam Printing House, Albany, NY. 32 pages. [Presbyterian]

1866   Kennedy, Duncan. A Sermon on the Occasion of the Death of Thomas W. Blatchford, M.D., delivered in the Second Street Presbyterian Church, Troy, on Sunday Morning, Jan. 28, 1866. Scribner, Troy, NY. 58 pages. [Presbyterian]

1867   Bellows, Henry Whitney. Address before the College of Physicians and Surgeons, at Their Annual Commencement, March 14, 1867. J. F. Trow & Co., New York. 12 pages. [Unitarian]

Clark, Rufus Wheelwright. A Discourse on the Life and Character of Howard Townsend, M.D., late professor of materia medica and physiology in the Albany Medical College: Preached in the North Dutch Church, Albany, Sunday Morning, Jan. 20, 1867. Albany: Gray. 18 pages.

Ludlow, James M. In Memoriam, Howard Townsend, M.D.: Died January 16, 1867. Munsell, Albany, NY. 41 pages. [Presbyterian]

Tucker, Henry Holcombe. "The True Physician." An Address Delivered before the Graduating Class of the Medical College of Georgia at its Annual Commencement, March 1, 1867. E. H. Pughe, Augusta, GA. 15 pages.

1868   Haven, Erastus Otis. Duties of the Medical Profession. An Address before the Class of 1868 of the Department of Medicine and Surgery of the University of Michigan. Dr. Chase's Steam Printing House, Ann Arbor, MI. 20 pages. [Methodist]

1869   Haven, Erastus Otis. The Medical Profession. Address Delivered to the Medical Class at the University of Michigan, March 31, 1869. Dr. Chase's Steam Printing House, Ann Arbor, MI. 16 pages. [Methodist]

1870   Peabody, Andrew Preston. What the Physician Should Be. An Address Delivered at the Commencement of the Medical School of Harvard University, at the Medical College in Boston, March 9, 1870. Welch, Bigelow, & Co., Cambridge, MA. 23 pages. [Unitarian]

1871   Lewis, Charlton Thomas. The Professional Spirit and Scientific Medicine. Address to the Class of the College of Physicians and Surgeons at the Annual Commencement, March 1, 1871. New York Printing Co., New York. 13 pages. [Methodist]

Palmer, Benjamin Morgan. The Pious Physician; or, The Claims of Religion Upon the Medical Profession. Presbyterian Committee of Publication, Richmond, VA. 31 pages. [Presbyterian]

1874   Beadle, Elias Root. The True Physician: A Sermon, Delivered before the Students of Jefferson Medical College and the Medical Department of the University of Pennsylvania, January 11, 1874. Philadelphia, Turner Hamilton. 16 pages. [Presbyterian]

1875   Crosby, Howard. The Ethics of Medical Men. An Introductory Lecture to
        the Medical Course of the University of the City of New York, September
        28, 1875. John F. Trow & Son, New York. 15 pages.

1877   Bartol, C. A. The Man and the Physician. A Sermon. Preached in the
        West Church, Boston, Sunday, Dec. 9, 1877. A. Williams & Co., Boston.
        26 pages.

        Lewis, Charlton Thomas. Ancient and Modern Hygiene Contrasted: the
        Influence of Civilization on the Duration of Life. A Discourse at the Annual
        Meeting, Boston, October, 1876. American Public Health Association. River-
        side Press, Cambridge, MA. 11 pages. [Methodist]

        West, Nathaniel. The Medical Science and Profession, Commencement
        Address before the Trustees, Faculty and Graduating Class of the Miami
        Medical College, February 27, 1877. Cincinnati Lancet Press, Cincinnati. 14
        pages. [Presbyterian]

1880   Clendening, Thomas C. Sermon, Preached Before the Students of Hahn-
        emann Medical College. Rand, McNally, Chicago. 16 pages.

        Thompson, Hugh Miller, Curative Value of High Character in the Physi-
        cian. Annual Addresses before the Louisiana State Medical Society.
        J. S. Rivers, Printer, New Orleans. 13 pages. [Episcopal]

1881   Palmer, Benjamin Morgan. Address at the Commencement Exercises of
        the Medical Department of the University of Louisiana, New Orleans,
        March 17, 1881. New Orleans, n.p. 12 pages. [Presbyterian]

1882   Burton, Nathaniel J. The Beloved Physician: In Memoriam (Lucian S. Wil-
        cox, M.D.) Case, Lockwood & Brainard, Hartford, CT. 18 pages.

        Ware, Loammi Goodenow. The Beloved Physician: A sermon preached in
        the First Congregational Church, Burlington, Vermont, Sunday, November
        19, 1882. Free Press Association, Burlington, VT. 19 pages. [Congregational]

1883   Chace, George Ide. Theism Viewed from the Physician's Standpoint. An
        Address Delivered before the Rhode Island Medical Society, June 19, 1883.
        Providence, RI, n.p. 17 pages. [Baptist]

        Mercer, Lewis Pyle. The Soul and the Body; a Sermon to Medical Students,
        with an Appendix on the Doctrine of Swedenborg. O. Clapp & Son, Bos-
        ton. 31 pages.

1884   Bartol, C. A. The Beloved Physician: A Sermon in West Church after the
        Decease of Dr. Calvin Ellis. Cupples, Upham, Boston. 19 pages.

        Lyman, Albert Josiah. "The Modern Physician the Mediator of Science. An
        Address Delivered at the Academy of Music, Brooklyn, May 21, 1884, before
        the Graduating Class of the Long Island College Hospital." New York Medi-
        cal Journal 39, June 21, 681–85. [Congregational]

Thompson, Hugh Miller. Address Presented at the 11th Annual Meeting of the American Public Health Association, Detroit, Michigan, November 13–15, 1883, on Nov. 15. In *Public Health Papers and Reports,* vol. 9, pp. 352–57. Republican Press Association, Concord, NH. [Episcopal]

1885　　Thwing, Edward Payson. The beloved physician: a tribute to the memory of the late Prof. Samuel G. Armour, M.D., LL.D., Dean of Long Island College Hospital, Brooklyn, NY, Memorial discourse delivered November 8, 1885 at St. Matthew's Evangelical Lutheran Church, Brooklyn, by E. P. Thwing, Minister in Charge. New York Academy of Anthropology, New York. 16 pages. [Lutheran]

1886　　Millen, Charles Watson. Address Delivered at the 25th Commencement of the Eclectic Medical College of the City of New York, Chickering Hall, March 25, 1886. The Day Star, New York. 8 pages. [Methodist]

1890　　Bonham, James William. The Looking Cure: A Sermon Preached to the Students of Jefferson Medical College. Thomas Whittaker, New York. 31 pages.

1891　　Ball, Wayland Dalrymple. "Valedictory Address, Delivered at the 84th Commencement of the University of Maryland Medical Department, April 1, 1891." *Maryland Medical Journal* 24 , April 11, pp. 507–17. [Presbyterian]

　　　　Brooks, Phillips. "The Beloved Physician." In *The Light of the World and Other Sermons* (New York: E. P. Dutton, 1891), pp. 216–33. [Episcopal]

1893　　Dandridge, Nathaniel Pendleton. Hospitals, their work and their obligations: the valedictory address delivered at the commencement exercises of the Miami Medical College, Cincinnati, March 30, 1893. Robert Clarke, Cincinnati, OH. 23 pages.

　　　　Palmer, Benjamin Morgan. The Representative Life and Character of Dr. Richardson. Faculty of the Medical Department of the Tulane University of Louisiana, New Orleans. 16 pages. [Presbyterian]

1895　　Purcell, J Bryan. "Medical Ethics, Being the Annual Oration Delivered Before the Alumni Association of the University of Maryland, Medical Department, April 16, 1895." *Maryland Medical Journal* 33, May 18, pp. 79–83.

1899　　Voorsanger, Jacob. "Overcrowding the Professions. An Address Delivered Before the Faculty and the Graduating Class (1899) of Cooper Medical College, San Francisco, August 22, 1899." In *Sermons and Addresses* (New York: Bloch, 1913), pp. 214–225. [Jewish]

APPENDIX 2

Philadelphia Medical Sermons

1844   Boardman, Henry Augustus. The Claims of Religion Upon Medical Men. A Discourse Delivered in the Tenth Presbyterian Church, Philadelphia, November 24, 1844. Book and Job Printing Office, Philadelphia. 24 pages.

1845   Hope, Matthew Boyd. A Discourse Designed to Show that Physiological Inquiries Are Not Unfriendly to Religious Sentiment. Delivered in the Tenth Presbyterian Church, Philadelphia, January 18, 1845. Barrett and Jones, Philadelphia. 16 pages.

1848   Parker, Joel. A Sermon on the Moral Responsibility of Physicians. Addressed to the Medical Students of Philadelphia, February 6, 1848. A. Scott, Philadelphia. 22 pages.

        Berg, Joseph Frederick. The Faithful Physician; a Discourse Addressed to the Students of the Medical Colleges of Philadelphia, December 10, 1848. W. S. Young, Philadelphia. 16 pages.

1849   Mott, Lucretia Coffin. A Sermon to the Medical Students, Delivered by Lucretia Mott, at Cherry Street Meeting House, February 11, 1849. W. B. Zeiber, Philadelphia.

1852   Stevens, William Bacon. A Sermon Preached Before the Students of the Several Medical Colleges of the City of Philadelphia, December 5, 1852, in St. Andrew's Church. King & Baird, Philadelphia. 34 pages.

1858   Stevens, William Bacon. The Religious Teachings of Medical Science. A Sermon Delivered before the Medical Students of the Several Colleges of Philadelphia in St. Andrew's Church, November 7, 1856 and Repeated by Request in the Same Place, December 6, 1857. C. Sherman, Philadelphia. 40 pages.

1860   Stevens, William Bacon. Hospitals and the Church. An Address Delivered before the Convention of the Diocese of Pennsylvania in St. Andrew's Church, Philadelphia, May 24, 1860. Ashmead, Philadelphia. 31 pages.

1862   Townsend, M.D., Rev. Stephen. Valedictory Sermon Preached in Saint Luke's (The Beloved Physician) Methodist E. Church, Philadelphia, March 10, 1862. Perkinpine & Higgins, Philadelphia. 20 pages.

1863   Townsend, M.D., Stephen. Sermon to the Students of Jefferson Medical College, Preached in Green Street M.E. Church, February 15, 1863. Perkinpine & Higgins, Philadelphia. 24 pages.

1865   Beadle, Elias Root. The Sacredness of the Medical Profession, A Sermon Delivered before the Students of Jefferson Medical College and the Medical Department of the University of Pennsylvania, November 19, 1865. Philadelphia, James S. Claxton. 16 pages.

1874   Beadle, Elias Root. The True Physician: A Sermon, Delivered before the Students of Jefferson Medical College and the Medical Department of the University of Pennsylvania, January 11, 1874. Philadelphia, Turner Hamilton. 16 pages.

1880   Clendening, Thomas C. Sermon, Preached Before the Students of Hahnemann Medical College. Rand, McNally, Chicago. 16 pages.

1890   Bonham, James William. The Looking Cure: A Sermon Preached to the Students of Jefferson Medical College. New York: Thomas Whittaker. 31 pages.

Long Island College Hospital Commencements, 1860–1899

In the following list, a physician delivered the commencement address in eleven years (27%), a minister in twenty years (49%; shown in boldface), a person other than a physician or minister in nine years (22%; shown in italics). In one case (2%) the profession of the speaker is unknown. Sources are the *New York Times*, the *Brooklyn Daily Eagle*, the *New York Medical Record*, the *Dictionary of American Biography* (*DAB*), and Joseph H. Raymond, *The L.I.C.H. and Its Graduates* (Brooklyn, NY: Association of the Alumni, 1899).

1860   Theodore L. Mason, M.D.

Austin Flint (*DAB*)

1861   De Witt Clinton Enos, M.D., July 16, 2nd Comm., Anatomy, Operative Surgery

1862   Edwin Nesbit Chapman, M.D.

Joseph Chrisman Hutchison, M.D., "An Address on the life and character of C. E. Isaacs, M.D."

1863   Austin Flint, M.D. (*DAB*)

1864   Joseph Chrisman Hutchison, M.D.

1865   Frank Hastings Hamilton, M.D. (*DAB*)

1866   Richard Salter Storrs, D.D. (*DAB*)

1867   Abram N. Littlejohn, D.D., LL.D., Episcopal Bishop of Long Island (*DAB*)

1868   Joseph Kimball, D.D.

1869   Edward Swift Dunster, M.D.

1870   Samuel G. Armor, M.D.

1871   Alpheus Benning Crosby, M.D.

1872   Ethelbert S. Mills, Esq.

1873   Richard Salter Storrs, D.D. (*DAB*)

1874   Henry Martyn Scudder, D.D., M.D.

1875   John Godfrey Saxe, LL.D. (*DAB*)

1876   Joshua Marsden Van Cott, "Legal and Ethical Standards of Professional Duty and Responsibility."

1877   Jesse B. Thomas, D.D., First Baptist Church, Pierrepont St. (*DAB*)

1878   Octavius B. Frothingham, D.D. (*DAB*)

1879   Snively, William A., D.D., Grace Church on the Heights

1880   James Monroe Buckley, D.D. (*DAB*), Hansen Place Methodist Episcopal Church

1881   Henry Ward Beecher, D.D.

1882   Joshua Marsden Van Cott

1883   Charles Henry Hall, D.D., S.T.D., Rector of Holy Trinity Church (*DAB*)

1884   Albert J. Lyman, D.D., "The modern physician the mediator of science." (*DAB*)

1885   St. Clair McKelway, LL.D., Editor-in-Chief, *Brooklyn Daily Eagle*

1886   Henry J. Van Dyke, D.D., 2nd Presbyterian Church in Brooklyn (*DAB*)

1887   John Humpstone, D.D., Emanuel Baptist Church

1888   T. De Witt Talmage, D.D. (*DAB*)

1889   Leander T. Chamberlain, D.D., Classon Ave. Presbyterian Church

1890   Truman Jay Backus, LL.D., President, Packer Collegiate Institute of Brooklyn (*DAB*)

1891   Theodore Gaillard Thomas, M.D., Columbia, emeritus (*DAB*)

1892   Robert R. Meredith, D.D., Tompkins Ave. Congregational Church

1893   Alexander Hutchins, M.D.

1894   Chauncy DePew, U.S. senator (1880 at Bellevue, 1884 at NYU) (*DAB*)

1895   Joseph C. Hendrix, Banker and Congressman (*DAB*)

1896   Willard Bartlett, Medical Jurisprudence

1897   Francis Landey Patton, D.D., President, Princeton University (*DAB*)

1898   Thomas B. McLeod, D.D.

1899   John D. Adam, D.D., Reformed Church on the Heights, Brooklyn

NOTES

PREFACE: A SOCIOLOGICAL PERSPECTIVE

1. See P. M. Ellwood, Jr. and G. D. Lundberg, "Managed Care: A Work in Progress," *JAMA* 276 (1996): 1083–86.

2. During this period, interest in the character of the physician has moved from a constructive elaboration of temperament and duty to a detailed, indeed clinical accounting of the "lost" physician. The most recent literature on the topic falls under the rubric of the "impaired" physician. A useful summary of views about the deviant practitioner is Paul Jesilow, Henry N. Pontell, and Gilbert Geis, *Prescription for Profit: How Doctors Defraud Medicaid* (Berkeley and Los Angeles: University of California Press, 1993).

3. See Jonathan B. Imber, *Abortion and the Private Practice of Medicine* (New Haven: Yale University Press, 1986), especially chap. 6, "Innovation and the Refuge of Private Practice."

4. Created in 2002, the council has issued numerous reports on a wide range of subjects, including *Human Cloning and Human Dignity: An Ethical Inquiry* (2002); *Beyond Therapy: Biotechnology and the Pursuit of Happiness* (2003); *Monitoring Stem Cell Research* (2004); *Reproduction and Responsibility: The Regulation of New Biotechnologies* (2004); and *Taking Care: Ethical Caregiving in Our Aging Society* (2005).

5. See Edward C. Halperin, "The Jewish Problem in U.S. Medical Education, 1920–1955," *Journal of the History of Medicine* 56 (2001): 140–67.

6. A poignant account is given by Wilbur H. Watson, *Against the Odds: Blacks in the Profession of Medicine in the United States* (New Brunswick, NJ: Transaction, 1999).

INTRODUCTION

1. In the past several years, numerous books that seek to bridge the gap between a compassionate profession and an incredulous public have appeared, all written by physicians. See Danielle Ofri, *Incidental Findings: Lessons from My Patients in the Art of Medicine* (Boston: Beacon Press, 2005); David Watts, *Bedside Manners: One Doctor's Reflections on the Oddly Intimate Encounters between Patient and Healer* (New York: Harmony Books, 2005); Atul Gawande, *Better: A Surgeon's Notes on Performance* (New York: Metropolitan Books, 2007); Jerome Groopman, *How Doctors Think* (Boston: Houghton Mifflin, 2007); and Perri Klass, *Treatment Kind and Fair: Letters to a Young Doctor* (New York: Perseus Book Group, 2007).

2. Such ethnographies include Charles L. Bosk, *Forgive and Remember: Managing Medical Failure*, 2nd ed. (Chicago: University of Chicago Press, 2003); Terry

Mizrahi, *Getting Rid of Patients: Contradictions in the Socialization of Physicians* (New Brunswick, NJ: Rutgers University Press, 1986); Robert A. Hahn, *Sickness and Healing: An Anthropological Perspective* (New Haven: Yale University Press, 1995); Nicholas A. Christakis, *Death Foretold: Prophecy and Prognosis in Medical Care* (Chicago: University of Chicago Press, 2000); Elizabeth M. Armstrong, *Conceiving Risk, Bearing Responsibility: Fetal Alcohol Syndrome and the Diagnosis of Moral Disorder* (Baltimore: Johns Hopkins University Press, 2003); and Adam Hedgecoe, *The Politics of Personalised Medicine: Pharmacogenetics in the Clinic* (New York: Cambridge University Press, 2005).

CHAPTER 1 Protestantism, Piety, and Professionalism

1. M. B. Etziony, *The Physician's Creed* (Springfield, IL: Charles C Thomas, 1973), p. 13. Despite a broad public expectation that the Hippocratic oath has some binding capacity upon the actions of physicians, few empirical studies exist of physicians' understanding of its relevance to their medical practice. In 1928, Eben J. Carey, acting dean of the Marquette University School of Medicine, conducted a survey of seventy-nine medical schools as to the use of the oath at commencement exercises. Carey received seventy-four responses and determined that only thirteen schools required medical students to take the oath. Eben James Carey, "The Formal Uses of the Hippocratic Oath for Medical Students at Commencement Exercises," *Bulletin of the Association of American Medical Colleges* 3 (1928): 159–66. See also Donald P. Irish and Daniel W. McMurray, "Professional Oaths and American Medical Colleges," *Journal of Chronic Diseases* 18 (May 1965): 276–90. The *Journal of the American Medical Association* in its "Medical News" section reported that at graduation exercises at Stanford University in 1969, "the 59 graduates . . . broke precedent by abandoning the time-honored oath," and that "For the first time in its 186-year history, students graduating from Harvard University took two pledges rather than the Hippocratic Oath alone." Students insisted at the time on the need for greater relevance of any oath to their lives. *JAMA* noted that the Declaration of Geneva, adopted in 1948 by the Second General Assembly of the World Medical Association, was being used as well. See "Hippocratic Oath Remains Most Used Pledge for New MD's," *JAMA* 209 (1969): 21–22. Less than thirty years later, the disputes about idealism were no longer salient, but the oath's relevance to medical practice was still cited, if only in terms of what it did not contain. Dr. Samuel Pallin, medical director of the Lear Eye Clinic in Phoenix defended his right to sue other ophthalmologists who used his patented method of surgery without paying him royalties: "The Hippocratic oath says nothing about intellectual property. It does say a doctor shall not participate in abortion, or be paid for passing on teachings to other doctors. But as we know, doctors are paid to do abortions, and to teach in medical schools." "Why Is This Surgeon Suing? A Split on Patents," *New York Times*, June 8, 1995, p. D5. I briefly examined the oath with respect to abortion in Imber, *Abortion and Private Practice*, pp. 115–16.

2. Ludwig Edelstein, *Hippocrates the Oath or the Hippocratic Oath* (Baltimore: Johns Hopkins University Press, 1943), p. 3.

3. http://www.pbs.org/wgbh/nova/doctors/oath_modern.html (accessed July 23, 2007).

4. See Owsei Temkin, *Hippocrates in a World of Pagans and Christians* (Baltimore: Johns Hopkins University Press, 1991). See also Leon R. Kass, "Is There a Medical Ethic? The Hippocratic Oath and the Sources of Ethical Medicine," in *Toward a More Natural Science: Biology and Human Affairs* (New York: Free Press, 1985), pp. 224–46.

5. See Chester R. Burns, "Reciprocity in the Development of Anglo-American Medical Ethics, 1765–1865," in *Proceedings of the XXIII International Congress of the History of Medicine* (London: Wellcome Institute of the History of Medicine, 1974), 1:813–19, reprinted in *Legacies in Ethics and Medicine*, ed. Chester R. Burns (New York: Science History Publications, 1977), pp. 300–306.

6. Burns, *Legacies*, p. 305. See also Donald E. Konold, *A History of American Medical Ethics, 1847–1912* (Madison: State Historical Society of Wisconsin, for the Dept. of History, University of Wisconsin, 1962). Worthington Hooker's work was entitled *Physician and the Patient or, a Practical View of the Mutual Duties, Relations, and Interests of the Medical Profession and the Community* (1849). See also Chester R. Burns, "Medical Ethics and Jurisprudence," in *The Education of American Physicians: Historical Essays*, ed. Ronald L. Numbers (Berkeley and Los Angeles: University of California Press, 1980), pp. 273–89.

7. John Harley Warner, *The Therapeutic Perspective: Medical Practice, Knowledge, and Identity in America, 1820–1885* (Cambridge: Harvard University Press, 1986), p. 11.

8. See John Harley Warner, "Science, Healing and the Physician's Identity: A Problem of Professional Character in Nineteenth-Century America," in *Essays in the History of Therapeutics*, ed. W. F. Bynum and Vivian Nutton (Atlanta: Rodopi, 1991), pp. 65–88.

9. Rev. Nathaniel West, D.D., *"The medical science and profession." Commencement address by the Rev. N. West, D.D., before the trustees, faculty and graduating class of the Miami medical college. Delivered in Pike's opera house, Cincinnati, Ohio, February 27th, 1877* (Cincinnati: Cincinnati Lancet Press, 1877). Warner does not appear to have inquired into who N. West was. Similarly, Lilian R. Furst cites West, by way of Warner, and uses the dichotomy between redemption and science to construct an argument about the balance of power in medicine itself. See Lilian R. Furst, *Between Doctors and Patients: The Changing Balance of Power* (Charlottesville: University Press of Virginia, 1998), pp. 86ff.

10. An obituary appears in *Minutes of the Synod of Minnesota*, vol. 4, no. 2 (St. Paul: Jackson and Smith, 1906), p. 173.

11. West, *Medical Science and Profession*, p. 3.

12. Oliver Wendell Holmes, "The Medical Profession in Massachusetts," in *Medical Essays* (Boston: Houghton Mifflin, 1911), p. 367.

13. West, *Medical Science and Profession*, pp. 10–11.

14. James H. Cassedy examined an early example of consumer consciousness, insofar as ministers were particularly sensitive to the perception among their flocks that homeopathy seemed a gentler means to the same ends sought more harshly by allopathic methods, including bloodletting and blistering. I examine in what follows the advice that ministers offered physicians in particular about the duties of their vocation, not about therapy. James H. Cassedy, "Biting the Hand: Medical Courtesy,

Quackery, and the Antebellum Clergy," *Second Opinion* 5 (1987): 100–119. See also Richard H. Shryock, "Public Relations of the Medical Profession in Great Britain and the United States: 1600–1870, a Chapter in the Social History of Medicine," in *Annals of Medical History*, n.s. 2, no. 3 (1930): 308–39.

15. Bruce Kimball, *The "True Professional Ideal" in America: A History* (Cambridge, MA: Blackwell, 1992), offers a sustained critique of the distrust implicit and explicit in the social-scientific analysis of professionalism, thus challenging contemporary (or what he calls "presentist") images of professional dominance. Commentary and advice—what Maximillian Graff Walten described as "character-writings"—about the role of professionals clearly formed the intellectual, and thus cultural, basis of what would emerge within Protestantism as doctrines of vocation. See Thomas Fuller's *The Holy State and the Profane State*, 2 vols., ed. Maximillian Graff Walten (New York: Columbia University Press, 1938), 1:119.

16. In chapter 4, I examine in more detail the medical school commencement and its symbolic importance for defining the role of future physicians.

17. A full-scale, historical reconstruction of the participation of clergymen in the admonitory instruction of physicians is beyond the scope of this book. In the decade between 1880 and 1890, the number of medical schools was estimated to be between 100 and 133 (due to openings, closings, and uncertain designations), and thus between 1,000 and 1,330 graduations could have occurred. Most medical schools have kept few easily accessible records of such events; some have preserved programs, and virtually none have retained copies of the addresses themselves. The tradition of clergy addresses to audiences outside of churches extends back to the beginnings of the Republic. The major genres of such sermons, including pulpit, funeral, election, and college chapel types, are reviewed in Nelson R. Burr, *A Critical Bibliography of Religion in America* (Princeton, NJ: Princeton University Press, 1961), pp. 943–51. See also A. W. Plumstead, *The Wall and the Garden: Selected Massachusetts Election Sermons, 1670–1775* (Minneapolis: University of Minnesota Press, 1968); and A. W. Plumstead, "The Election Sermons," chap. 5 in *Religion in American History: Interpretive Essays*, ed. John M. Mulder and John F. Wilson (Englewood Cliffs, NJ: Prentice-Hall, 1978), pp. 57–73. For further background to the profound influence of clergy on American life, see, among other works, David D. Hall, *The Faithful Shepherd: A History of the New England Ministry in the Seventeenth Century* (Chapel Hill: University of North Carolina Press, 1972); and H. Richard Niebuhr and Daniel D. Williams, eds., *The Ministry in Historical Perspectives* (New York: Harper, 1956), esp. chap. 8 by Sidney E. Mead, "The Rise of the Evangelical Conception of the Ministry in America: 1607–1850," pp. 207–49, and chap. 9 by Robert S. Michaelsen, "The Protestant Ministry in America: 1850 to the Present," pp. 250–87. I owe my discovery of a Protestant literature on medical vocation to James H. Smylie. See James H. Smylie, "The Reformed Tradition," in *Caring and Curing: Health and Medicine in the Western Religious Traditions*, ed. Ronald L. Numbers and Darrel W. Amundsen (New York: Macmillan, 1986), pp. 204–39, esp. 236 nn. 35 and 36.

18. At medical colleges established exclusively for women (e.g., Medical College of Pennsylvania), commencement addresses were sometimes delivered by women.

19. In at least two instances in the nineteenth century, a rabbi delivered such an address: at Wayne State University in 1897 and Cooper Medical College in 1899. I have found no evidence that a Catholic priest delivered such an address during this time.

20. For example, between 1850 and 1893, commencement speakers at the Medical Department of the University of Pennsylvania (which held ceremonies separate from the University) were, to a man, physicians. William Osler delivered the address in 1889. Many of these physicians brought to the commencement occasion an abiding sense of what John S. Haller, Jr. has called "a common nineteenth-century theme of a medical priesthood," whereby graduating physicians were exhorted to think of themselves as pursuing a ministry. This theme did not arise spontaneously among members of the medical profession; rather the theme itself was embedded in the distinctly Protestant idea of vocation, which designated the ministry as the highest embodiment of authority among the professions. See John S. Haller, Jr., *American Medicine in Transition, 1840–1910* (Urbana: University of Illinois Press, 1981), pp. 280–84.

21. Based on the reconstructed records of addresses at these schools (in the author's possession).

22. As late as 1890, the tradition of calling Philadelphia medical students into area churches was strongly pursued. The Reverend J. W. Bonham, M.D., church evangelist in St. Andrew's Church, described lectures on Sunday evenings by eminent Philadelphia physicians and ministers in various churches: "The congregations were very large, composed of students of the University of Pennsylvania, Jefferson Medical College, and other Medical Colleges of Philadelphia." *The Looking Cure: A Sermon Preached to the Students of Jefferson Medical College* (New York: Thomas Whittaker, 1890), p. vi.

23. John Kearsley Mitchell, M.D. (1793–1858), a member of the faculty of Jefferson Medical College, and Nathaniel Chapman (1780–1853), a member of the faculty of the University of Pennsylvania Medical School, served as liaisons between the students and Rev. Boardman. Dr. Mitchell served again in this capacity two months later when Matthew Boyd Hope, M.D., who was also a clergyman, preached in the Tenth Presbyterian Church. See M. B. Hope, *Discourse designed to show that physiological inquiries are not unfriendly to religious sentiment, delivered in the tenth Presbyterian church, Philadelphia, January 18, 1845* (Philadelphia: Barrett and Jones, 1845).

24. Henry A. Boardman, *The Claims of Religion upon Medical Men* (Philadelphia: Book and Job Printing Office, 1844), p. 6. Boardman also preached about other professions, including lawyering and business. See *The importance of religion to the legal profession: with some remarks on the character of the late Charles Chauncey, esq.* (Philadelphia: W. S. Martien, 1849); and *The Bible in the counting-house: a course of lectures to merchants* (Philadelphia: Lippincott, Grambo, 1853).

25. Boardman, *Claims of Religion*, p. 7.

26. Ibid., p. 10.

27. Ibid., pp. 12–13.

28. Ibid., p. 14.

29. Such studies include Joseph F. Kett, *The Formation of the American Medical Profession: The Role of Institutions, 1780–1860* (New Haven: Yale University Press, 1968); William G. Rothstein, *American Physicians in the Nineteenth Century: From*

Sects to Science (Baltimore: Johns Hopkins University Press, 1972); Martin Kaufman, *American Medical Education: The Formative Years, 1765–1910* (Westport, CT: Greenwood Press, 1976); James G. Burrow, *Organized Medicine in the Progressive Era: The Move toward Monopoly* (Baltimore: Johns Hopkins University Press, 1977); Haller, *American Medicine in Transition*; Paul Starr, *The Social Transformation of American Medicine* (New York: Basic Books, 1984); Kenneth M. Ludmerer, *Learning to Heal: The Development of American Medical Education* (New York: Basic Books, 1985); William G. Rothstein, *American Medical Schools and the Practice of Medicine: A History* (New York: Oxford University Press, 1987); James H. Cassedy, *Medicine in America: A Short History* (Baltimore: Johns Hopkins University Press, 1991); and John Duffy, *From Humors to Medical Science: A History of American Medicine*, 2nd ed. (Urbana: University of Illinois Press, 1993). See also Ronald L. Numbers, "The Fall and Rise of the American Medical Profession," in *The Professions in American History*, ed. Nathan O. Hatch (Notre Dame, IN: University of Notre Dame Press, 1988), pp. 51–72; and John Harley Warner, "Science in Medicine," in *Osiris*, 2nd ser., 1 (1985): 37–58.

30. In addition to Paul Starr, see Bernhard J. Stern, "The Income of Physicians," in *American Medical Practice: In the Perspectives of a Century* (New York: Commonwealth Fund, 1945), pp. 87–102; George Rosen, *Fees and Fee Bills: Some Economic Aspects of Medical Practice in Nineteenth-Century America* (Baltimore: Johns Hopkins Press, 1946); and William A. Glaser, *Paying the Doctor: Systems of Remuneration and Their Effects* (Baltimore: Johns Hopkins University Press, 1970).

31. Charles Quintard's life is described in the *Dictionary of American Biography*. Quintard was first a physician, a professor of physiology and pathological anatomy. He studied with Valentine Mott and in 1847 received the M.D. degree from NYU (University of the City of New York). He spent a year at Bellevue Hospital, then moved to Athens, Georgia, where he practiced until 1851, at which time he moved to Memphis Medical College. In 1854 he began his studies for the ministry, was ordained a priest in 1856, and in 1865 was elected the second Episcopal bishop of Tennessee. He spent the Civil War ministering and doctoring to Confederate troops. See Sam Davis Elliott, ed., *Doctor Quintard, Chaplain C.S.A. and Second Bishop of Tennessee: The Memoir and Civil War Diary of Charles Todd Quintard* (Baton Rouge: Louisiana State University Press, 2003). Quintard's aphorism, "Good men are not all physicians, nor are all physicians good men," was stated similarly by Francis Bacon in the early seventeenth century: "Physicians are some of them so pleasing and conformable to the humor of the patient, as they press not the true cure of the disease; and some other are so regular in proceeding according to art for the disease, as they respect not sufficiently the condition of the patient. Take one of a middle temper; or, if it may not be found in one man, combine two of either sort; and forget not to call as well the best acquainted with your body, as the best reputed of for his faculty." Francis Bacon, *Essays or Counsels, Civil and Moral* (London: Collins' Clear-Type Press, n.d.), p. 274.

32. *Ohio Medical and Surgical Journal*, May 1, 1853, 444–45.

33. *New-York Medical Press*, March 17, 1860, 189.

34. Troyen A. Brennan, *Just Doctoring: Medical Ethics in the Liberal State* (Berkeley and Los Angeles: University of California Press, 1991), p. 75.

35. See Burton J. Bledstein, *The Culture of Professionalism: The Middle Class and the Development of Higher Education in America* (New York: Norton, 1976).

36. Fabian Franklin, *The Life of Daniel Coit Gilman* (New York: Dodd, Mead, 1910), p. 29.

37. See A. McGehee Harvey, *Science at the Bedside: Clinical Research in American Medicine, 1905–1945* (Baltimore: Johns Hopkins University Press, 981). Johns Hopkins University did not escape entirely the public notice of its rapid withdrawal from religiously defined purposes of university education. See the account of the dedication of the statue of Christus Consolator at Hopkins in 1896. Nancy McCall, "The Statue of the Christus Consolator at the Johns Hopkins Hospital: Its Acquisition and Historic Origins," *Johns Hopkins Medical Journal* 151 (July 1982): 11–19.

38. Barbara Gutmann Rosenkrantz, "The Search for Professional Order in 19th Century American Medicine," in *Sickness and Health in America: Readings in the History of Medicine and Public Health*, ed. Judith Walzer Leavitt and Ronald L. Numbers, 2nd. ed. (Madison: University of Wisconsin Press, 1985), p. 225–26.

39. Ibid., p. 226.

40. Ibid., p. 229. See also an earlier version of Rosenkrantz's essay with the same title in *Proceedings of the XIVth International Congress of the History of Science* (Tokyo: Science Council of Japan, 1975), pp. 113–24. And see John Harley Warner, "Ideals of Science and Their Discontents in Late Nineteenth-Century American Medicine," *Isis* 82, no. 313 (1991): 454–78.

41. Roy Porter remarks, "The religious inputs in medical practice need much further study. Historians have been so concerned with questions such as the secularization of the medical-world view that they have neglected to study the continuing religious motivations for medical practice." "Thomas Gisborne: Physicians, Christians and Gentlemen," in *Doctors and Ethics: The Earlier Historical Setting of Professional Ethics*, ed. Andrew Wear, Johanna Geyer-Kordesch, and Roger French (Atlanta: Rodopi, 1993), p. 267. In one sense, Porter is correct if he means by "religious motivations" the lack of study of what today we mean by the character of the medical practitioner. But a substantial literature already exists about the relationship between religion and medicine, and in particular about the clerical physician, about the religious influences on approaches to healing, and about religion and mental health. On the clerical physician, see Walter R. Steiner, "The Reverend Gershom Bulkeley of Connecticut, An Eminent Clerical Physician," in *Medical Library and Historical Journal* 2, no. 2 (1904): 91–103; Otho T. Beall, Jr. and Richard H. Shryock, *Cotton Mather: First Significant Figure in American Medicine* (Baltimore: Johns Hopkins University Press, 1954); Henry M. Parrish, "Contributions of the Clergy to Early American Medicine," in *Journal of the Bowman Gray School of Medicine* 14, no. 4 (1956): 55–64, 67; Margaret Humphreys Warner, "Vindicating the Minister's Medical Role: Cotton Mather's Concept of the Nishmath-Chajim and the Spiritualization of Medicine," *Journal of the History of Medicine* 36 (1981): 278–95; and Patricia Ann Watson, *The Angelical Conjunction: The Preacher-Physicians of Colonial New England* (Knoxville: University of Tennessee Press, 1991). On religious approaches to healing, see Richard Thomas Barton, *Religious Doctrine and Medical Practice* (Springfield, IL: Charles C Thomas, 1958); Martin E. Marty and Kenneth L. Vaux, *Health/Medicine*

and the Faith Traditions: An Inquiry into Religion and Medicine (Philadelphia: Fortress Press, 1982); and Numbers and Amundsen, *Caring and Curing*. On religion and mental health, see Edward S. Cowles, *Religion and Medicine in the Church* (New York: Macmillan, 1925); and David Belgum, ed., *Religion and Medicine: Essays on Meaning, Values, and Health* (Ames: Iowa State University Press, 1967).

42. Boardman, *Claims of Religion*, p. 18. Boardman took his quote from Nathaniel Chapman. See Nathaniel Chapman, *An Introductory Lecture to a Course of Lectures on the Theory and Practice of Medicine, in the University of Pennsylvania: Delivered at the Opening of the Session of 1838–39* (Philadelphia: Bailey, 1838).

43. Boardman, *Claims of Religion*, , p. 19.

44. Joel Parker, *A Sermon on the Moral Responsibility of Physicians. Addressed to the Medical Students of Philadelphia, February 6, 1848* (Philadelphia: A. Scott, 1848), p. 5. Parker's biography is contained in the *Dictionary of American Biography*.

45. Ibid., p. 8.

46. Ibid., p. 12.

47. Ibid., p. 13.

48. Ibid., p. 18.

49. Ibid.

50. Ibid., p. 21.

51. Ibid.

52. Parker had at least one more occasion to reflect on the relations between ministry and medicine, after he returned to New York in 1852. See Joel Parker, *The Beloved Physician: A Tribute to the Memory of James C. Bliss, M.D., A Discourse on the Combined Influence of the Gospel and the Medical Profession in Forming the Character* (New York: Samuel S. and William Wood, 1856).

53. Joseph Frederick Berg, *The Faithful Physician; a Discourse Addressed to the Students of the Medical Colleges of Philadelphia, December 10, 1848* (Philadelphia: W. S. Young, 1849), p. 5.

54. Ibid., p. 8.

55. Ibid., p. 11.

56. Elias Root Beadle, *The Sacredness of the Medical Profession. A Sermon Delivered Before the Students of Jefferson Medical College and the Medical Department of the University of Pennsylvania, November 19, 1865* (Philadelphia: James S. Claxton, 1865), p. 9.

57. Ibid., p. 13.

58. Ibid., pp. 11–12.

59. Elias Root Beadle, *The True Physician: A Sermon, Delivered before the Students of Jefferson Medical College and the Medical Department of the University of Pennsylvania, January 11, 1874* (Philadelphia, Turner Hamilton), pp. 6–7.

60. Ibid., p. 9. Compare Beadle's view of the physician's special access to the lives of patients with the sociologist Georg Simmel's similar observations about the role of the priest: "To date, this is the greatest example in history of the formation of a social group which cuts across all other existing social groups. . . . The priesthood could establish a relationship to, and could communicate with, all existing social strata in a manner which was entirely unbiased, because the individual priest was

completely released from the ties with his social stratum; he was not even permitted to retain his name. Otherwise, those ties would have determined the personality of the priest together with those which he had newly gained in the priesthood." Simmel added that "celibacy is the most radical method by which the individual priest was put outside the network of group affiliations. Georg Simmel, "The Web of Group-Affiliations" (1922), in *Conflict and The Web of Group-Affiliations*, trans. Kurt H. Wolff and Reinhard Bendix (New York: Free Press, 1955), p. 144. The role of the physician partook of similar expectations, including the importance assigned to being called "Dr." as an instance of subordinating the person to the office. Contemporary publicity about charges of sexual indiscretions among all professionals points to the cultural dilemma of distrust in which "radical" methods (e.g., celibacy) are no longer defended as a means to ensure the reputation of office over and against the temptations (and sins) of individuals.

61. Stephen Townsend, M.D., *Sermon to the Students of Jefferson Medical College, Preached in Green Street M.E. Church, February 15, 1863* (Philadelphia: Perkinpine and Higgins, 1863), p. 19. Townsend continued that "Our judicial and legal institutions yield a revenue of influence and instrumentality, sustaining by their official decisions and holy life and example, the cause of piety." See also Rev. Stephen Townsend, M.D., *Valedictory Sermon Preached in Saint Luke's (The Beloved Physician) Methodist E. Church* (Philadelphia: Perkinpine and Higgins, 1862).

CHAPTER 2   The Influence of Catholic Perspectives

1. Medical exceptionalism is typically defined in therapeutic terms, as in the case of divergent therapies from the allopathic tradition such as homeopathy and eclecticism. My interest here is in the manners and morals of professional exceptionalism, illustrated in the case of Catholic approaches to medically complex problems.

2. The single best history of Catholic health care in the United States is Christopher J. Kauffman, *Ministry and Meaning: A Religious History of Catholic Health Care in the United States* (New York: Crossroad, 1995). See also Ursula Stepsis and Dolores Liptak, eds., *Pioneer Healers: The History of Women Religious in American Health Care* (New York: Crossroad, 1989).

3. See Bledstein, *The Culture of Professionalism*.

4. William Osler, "Vocation in Medicine and Nursing," in *Essays on Vocation, First Series*, ed. Basil Mathews (London: Oxford University Press, 1919), pp. 119–28. Osler notes, "This chapter reproduces material scattered through the author's books '*Aequanimitas*' and '*Counsels and Ideals*'," thus making it particularly appropriate as a summation of his thoughts on vocation. See also "Internal Medicine as a Vocation," in *Aequanimitas, With other Addresses to Medical Students, Nurses and Practitioners of Medicine*, 3rd ed. (Philadelphia: P. Blakiston's Son, 1932), pp. 131–45.

5. See Rev. John Blowick, *Priestly Vocation* (Dublin: M. H. Gill, 1932); and Rev. Berard M. Riegert, *The Obligation of Following a Religious Vocation: A Study of Theological Opinion from the Seventeenth to the Nineteenth Centuries* (Washington, DC: Catholic University of America Press, 1962).

6. See Jenny Franchot, *Roads to Rome: The Antebellum Protestant Encounter with Catholicism* (Berkeley and Los Angeles: University of California Press, 1994).

7. For a thorough study of nineteenth-century medical jurisprudence, see James C. Mohr, *Doctors and the Law: Medical Jurisprudence in Nineteenth-Century America* (New York: Oxford University Press, 1993).

8. See Konold, *History of American Medical Ethics.*

9. David F. Kelly, *The Emergence of Roman Catholic Medical Ethics in North America: An Historical-Methodological-Bibliographical Study* (New York: Edwin Mellen Press, 1979), p. 44. Kelly's book is a nearly definitive undertaking of the substantial literature produced on medical matters under Catholic auspices.

10. Ibid., p. 55.

11. Ibid., p. 56.

12. Ibid.

13. Ibid., pp. 58–59 n. 127.

14. See Immanuel Jakobovits, *Jewish Medical Ethics: A Comparative and Historical Study of the Jewish Religious Attitude to Medicine and Its Practice* (1959; New York: Bloch, 1975), and Fred Rosner and J. David Bleich, eds., *Jewish Bioethics* (New York: Sanhedrin Press, 1979). See also Menachem Elon, "Jewish Law and Modern Medicine" (1969), in *Jewish Law in Ancient and Modern Israel, Selected Essays with an Introduction by Haim H. Cohn* (Hoboken, NJ: Ktav Publishing, 1971), pp. 131–42.

15. Kelly cites one treatise by a Protestant physician, Ernst Joseph de Valenti (1798–1871), first published in 1831. See *Medicina clerica; oder, Handbuch der Pastoral-Medizin, für Seelsorger, Pädagogen und Aerzte, nebst einer Diätetik für Geistliche* (Leipzig: Kohler, 1831).

16. Carl Franz Nicolaus Capellmann, *Pastoral Medicine* (New York: F. Pustet, 1879). See also Joseph G. Ryan, "The Chapel and the Operating Room: The Struggle of Roman Catholic Clergy, Physicians, and Believers with the Dilemmas of Obstetric Surgery, 1800–1900," *Bulletin of the History of Medicine* 76 (2002): 473–78.

17. Carl Capellmann, *Pastoral Medicine*, trans. Rev. Wm. Dassel (New York: Fr. Pustet, 1882), p. iv. See Robert M. Veatch, "Diverging Traditions: Professional and Religious Medical Ethics of the Nineteenth Century," in *The Codification of Medical Morality: Historical and Philosophical Studies of the Formalization of Western Medical Morality in the Eighteenth and Nineteenth Centuries*, vol. 2: *Anglo-American Medical Ethics and Medical Jurisprudence in the Nineteenth Century*, ed. Robert Baker (Dordrecht: Kluwer, 1995), p. 128. Veatch's interesting essay notes the importance of Capellmann's work, contrasting pastoral medicine to the medical ethics of the AMA, with no mention of the distinctly Protestant character of the latter.

18. Capellmann, *Pastoral Medicine* (1882), p. v.

19. Ibid., p. 12.

20. Ibid., pp. 12–13.

21. The definitive discussion in English on the evolution in Catholic thinking on abortion is John Connery, S.J., *Abortion: The Development of the Roman Catholic Perspective* (Chicago: Loyola University Press, 1977); see, in particular, chaps. 12–15.

22. Capellmann, *Pastoral Medicine* (1882), p. 15.

23. Ibid., p. 16.

24. Ibid., p. 16n.

25. I have outlined this progress in Imber, *Abortion and Private Practice.*

26. Capellmann referred to various operations for inducing labor and delivery, including perforation (of the uterus), cephalotripsy (crushing of the fetal head to facilitate delivery), embryotomy (cutting up of the fetus to facilitate delivery), embryothlasy, and craniotomy (surgical cutting to pieces of the fetal skull to facilitate delivery). For a study of the ancient practice of craniotomy, see Louis Bakay, *An Early History of Craniotomy: From Antiquity to the Napoleonic Era* (Springfield, IL: Charles C Thomas, 1985).

27. See Carl Capellmann, *De occisione foetus: quam abortu provocato, perforatione, cephalotripsia medici audent: eine Studie fur Aetzte und Theologen* (Aachen: Rudolf Barth, 1875).

28. Capellmann, *Pastoral Medicine* (1882), p. 18.

29. Ibid., p. 19.

30. Martin S. Pernick, *A Calculus of Suffering: Pain, Professionalism, and Anesthesia in Nineteenth-Century America* (New York: Columbia University Press, 1985).

31. Capellmann, *Pastoral Medicine* (1882), p. 24.

32. Ibid., p. 26.

33. Ibid., pp. 26–28.

34. For an account of Busey's early life, see his *A Souvenir, with an Autobiographical Sketch of Early Life and Selected Miscellaneous Addresses and Communications* (Washington, DC: n.p., 1896). See also Samuel C. Busey, *Personal Reminiscences and Recollections of Forty-Six Years' Membership in the Medical Society of the District of Columbia and Residence in this City with Biographical Sketches of Many of the Deceased Members* (Washington, DC: Dornan, 1895). The latter book contains voluminous accounts of Busey's involvement in all the medical-political issues of his day. See also Ryan, "Chapel and Operating Room," 483 n. 104.

35. Busey, *Souvenir*, p. 10.

36. Ibid., p. 158.

37. John R. Bodo, *The Protestant Clergy and Public Issues, 1812–1848* (Princeton, NJ: Princeton University Press, 1954), pp. 24–25. For background on these and similar tensions, see Stow Persons, "Religion and Modernity, 1865–1914," in *The Shaping of American Religion*, ed. James Ward Smith and A. Leland Jamison (Princeton, NJ: Princeton University Press, 1961), pp. 369–401.

38. An important study of the evolution of alcohol policy in the welfare state is Dan E. Beauchamp, *Beyond Alcoholism: Alcohol and Public Health Policy* (Philadelphia: Temple University Press, 1980).

39. See Daniel Feller, *The Jacksonian Promise: America, 1815–1840* (Baltimore: Johns Hopkins University Press, 1995).

40. Busey, *Souvenir*, p. 21.

41. Ibid., p. 23.

42. Ibid., p. 26.

43. *"The Romish Intrigue: Frémont a Catholic!!"* (New York: Robert M. De Witt? 1856), p. 15. For background on Frémont's career and the issue of his religious affiliation in particular, see Ferol Egan, *Frémont: Explorer for a Restless Nation* (Garden City, NY: Doubleday, 1977), pp. 508–9; and Michael F. Holt, "Another Look at the Election of 1856," in *James Buchanan and the Political Crisis of the 1850s*, ed. Michael

J. Birkner (Selinsgrove, PA: Susquehannna University Press, 1996), pp. 37–67. See also Sally Denton, *Passion and Principle: John and Jessie Frémont, the Couple Whose Power, Politics, and Love Shaped Nineteenth-Century America* (New York: Bloomsbury, 2007).

44. Busey, *Souvenir*, p. 223.

45. Ibid., p. 226.

46. Ibid., pp. 226–27 n. 3.

47. Ibid., p. 242.

48. Ibid.

49. Ibid., p. 244.

50. Joseph T. Durkin, S.J., *Georgetown University: The Middle Years (1840–1900)* (Washington, DC: Georgetown University Press, 1963), p. 30.

51. Busey, *Souvenir*, p. 246.

52. Ibid., p. 247. See Christopher J. Kauffman, *Tradition and Transformation in Catholic Culture: The Priests of Saint Sulpice in the United States* (New York: Macmillan, 1988).

53. Ibid., p. 271. The address was also published as a separate pamphlet. Samuel C. Busey, *The Wrong of Craniotomy upon the Living Fetus: Sixth Annual Address of the President, Delivered before the Washington Obstetrical and Gynecological Society, October 19th, 1888* (New York: William Wood, 1889).

54. Ibid., p. 273.

55. Ibid., p. 280.

56. Ibid., p. 274n.

57. Ibid., p. 289.

58. Ibid., p. 288.

59. Ibid., pp. 288–89.

60. See Ellen Wilson Fielding, "The Good Doctor," *Human Life Review* 22, no. 3 (1996): 87–92.

61. Andrew Klarmann, *The Crux of Pastoral Medicine: The Perils of Embryonic Man*, 4th ed. (New York: Frederick Pustet, 1912), pp. vi, vii.

62. Stanislaus Woywod, *The Casuist: A Collection of Cases in Moral and Pastoral Theology* (New York: Joseph F. Wagner, 1924). Woywod was also the author of *Cura Infirmorium: Containing in Latin with English Translation all the Titles in the latest Edition of the Rituale Romanum on the Care of the Sick and the Dying* (New York: Joseph F. Wagner, 1934). Published in the form of a small manual, it could accompany the priest attending the sick and dying.

63. Ibid., p. 192.

64. Ibid., p. 224. In the four other volumes in this five-volume collection of cases, the question of responsibilities specific to the physician is taken up two times: "Does the Performance of Craniotomy Incur Excommunication" (3:178–81), and "A New Operation in Childbirth" (4:249–50). In both cases, the pieces are signed by physicians. On the other hand, the numerous dilemmas and contingencies attending to extreme unction, in particular, the duties of the priest, resulted in the subject being addressed nine times: "Extreme Unction" (2:81–85); "Repetition of Extreme Unction During the Same Illness" (2:306–9); "An Incomplete, Yet Valid Confession: Extreme

Unction Not Repeated After Invalid Reception" (3:156–59); "Rite of Extreme Unction, When Several Persons Are to Receive It at the Same Time" (3:247–49); "Does the Effect of Extreme Unction Revive?" (4:97–101); "Extreme Unction in Casu Necessitatis (4:184–87); "Conditional and Unconditional Administration of Extreme Unction in the Case of Unconsciousness" (5:228–32); and "Extreme Unction Neglected" (5:233–35).

CHAPTER 3   The Scientific Challenge to Faith

1. George Wood Bayless, *Some of the Rewards of Medicine: An Introductory Address Delivered in the Kentucky School of Medicine, October 30, 1858, at the Opening of the Session of 1858–9* (Louisville, Ky.: Morton and Griswold, 1858), p. 13.

2. Edwin Hubbell Chapman, *The Post of Duty. A Discourse Occasioned by the Death of Dr. A. Sidney Doane, Delivered in the Murray Street Church, February 15, 1852* (New York: Press of Baker, Godwin, 1852), p. 12. Sumner Ellis, Chapin's biographer, notes, "When some one asked him what he lectured for, he replied: 'For f-a-m-e, fifty and my expenses.' But this was in the long-ago, when lecturing was a more serious but less paying service than it has been in more recent years." *Life of Edwin H. Chapin, D.D.* (Boston: Universalist Publishing House, 1882), p. 252.

3. Editorial, *Medical Register* (Philadelphia), April 2, 1887, p. 258.

4. For scholarly attempts that assess the status of the professions relative to one another during the nineteenth century, see R. D. Gidney and W.P.J. Millar, *Professional Gentleman: The Professions in Nineteenth-Century Ontario* (Toronto: University of Toronto Press, 1994); Samuel Haber, *The Quest for Authority and Honor in the American Professions, 1750–1900* (Chicago: University of Chicago Press, 1991); Kimball, *True Professional Ideal*; William R. Johnson, "Education and Professional Life Styles: Law and Medicine in the Nineteenth Century," *History of Education Quarterly* 14 (1974): 185–207.

5. Holmes made the allusion to "medicated novel" in "A Second Preface," insisting that "The real aim of the story was to test the doctrine of 'original sin' and human responsibility for the disordered volition coming under that technical denomination." *Elsie Venner: A Romance of Destiny* (New York: New American Library, 1961), p. xii. For a review of Holmes's life and career, see Miriam Rossiter Small, *Oliver Wendell Holmes* (New York: Twayne, 1962). The best account of his reputation as a medical man remains Neille Shoemaker, "The Contemporaneous Medical Reputation of Oliver Wendell Holmes," *New England Quarterly* 26 (1953): 477–93. And see Thomas Franklin Currier, *A Bibliography of Oliver Wendell Holmes* (New York: New York University Press, 1953).

6. Holmes, *Elsie Venner*, p. 213.

7. See John Steadman Rice, *A Disease of One's Own: Psychotherapy, Addiction, and the Emergence of Co-Dependency* (New Brunswick, NJ: Transaction, 1996). See also Howard L. Kaye, "Why Freud Hated America," *Wilson Quarterly* 17, no. 2 (1993): 118–25.

8. The cultural implications of this transfer of authority are examined by Nathan G. Hale, Jr., *Freud and the Americans: The Beginnings of Psychoanalysis in the United States, 1876–1917* (New York: Oxford University Press, 1971); and Francis G.

Gosling, *Before Freud: Neurasthenia and the American Medical Community, 1870–1910* (Urbana: University of Illinois Press, 1987).

9. The Church of England as well as the Roman Catholic Church were equally vulnerable to the criticisms of freethinkers, given the generalized nature of the dissent. See John Mackinnon Robertson, *A History of Freethought in the Nineteenth Century* (New York: G. P. Putnam, 1930).

10. The orthodoxies that Tyndall challenged in the latter part of the nineteenth century were often described as superstitions; in this sense, the formulation of orthodoxy today and the challenges to it arise from even deeper disagreements about the nature of moral authority.

11. John Tyndall, "Presidential Address of the British Association for the Advancement of Science, 1874," in *Victorian Science: A Self-Portrait from the Presidential Addresses of the British Association for the Advancement of Science*, ed. George Basalla, William Coleman, and Robert H. Kargon (New York: Anchor, 1970), pp. 474–75. On Tyndall's life, see Arthur Stewart Eve and C. H. Creasey, *Life and Work of John Tyndall* (London: Macmillan, 1945). See also Joe D. Burchfield, "John Tyndall: A Biographical Sketch," in *John Tyndall: Essays on a Natural Philosopher*, ed. William Hodson Brock, Norman D. McMillan, and R. Charles Mollan (Dublin: Royal Dublin Society, 1981), pp. 1–13.

12. John Tyndall, "Apology for the Belfast Address" (1874), in *Fragments of Science* (New York: P. F. Collier and Son, 1902), p. 219.

13. Ibid., 220–21. For an early, somewhat hostile, summary of Tyndall's religious views, see Richard A. Armstrong, *Agnosticism and Theism in the Nineteenth Century: An Historical Study of Religious Thought* (London: Philip Green, 1905), chap. 4, "Materialism and Atheism: John Tyndall and Charles Bradlaugh," pp. 101–34.

14. Frank M. Turner, "The Victorian Conflict between Science and Religion: A Professional Dimension," *Isis*, 69, no. 248 (1978): 372. Consider Maurice Cowling's summary of Tyndall: "Whatever Tyndall may have thought he was doing, what he was also doing was to create a mentality for a new intelligentsia—a scientific intelligentsia which would have its own subject-matter to complement the subject-matter of classical scholarship and which, by involving itself in literature as well as science, would effect a modern synthesis and give permanent shape to the moral impulse through which, as Tyndall believed, Fichte, Emerson, and Carlyle had given him the strength to become a scientist in the first place." Maurice Cowling, *Religion and Public Doctrine in Modern England*, vol. 2: *Assaults* (Cambridge: Cambridge University Press, 1985), p. 148.

15. Wilfrid Ward, *Problems and Persons* (London: Longmans, Green, 1903), pp. 246–47.

16. See Edward A. White, *Science and Religion in American Thought: The Impact of Naturalism* (Stanford, CA: Stanford University Press, 1952); John C. Greene, "Science and Religion," in *The Rise of Adventism: Religion and Society in Mid-Nineteenth-Century America*, ed. Edwin S. Gaustad (New York: Harper and Row, 1974), pp. 50–69; James R. Moore, *The Post-Darwinian Controversies* (Cambridge: Cambridge University Press, 1978); Ronald L. Numbers, "Science and Religion," in *Historical Writing on American Science: Perspectives and Prospects*, ed. Sally Gregory Kohlstedt

and Margaret W. Rossiter (Baltimore: Johns Hopkins University Press, 1985), pp. 59–80; and David C. Lindberg and Ronald L. Numbers, eds., *God and Nature: Historical Essays on the Encounter between Christianity and Science* (Berkeley and Los Angeles: University of California Press, 1986). For a critical reflection on the revisionist "neo-harmonist" historiography of recent decades, see David A. Hollinger, "Justification by Verification: The Scientific Challenge to the Moral Authority of Christianity in Modern America," in *Religion and Twentieth-Century American Intellectual Life*, ed. Michael J. Lacey (Cambridge: Woodrow Wilson International Center for Scholars and Cambridge University Press, 1989), pp. 116–35.

17. See Philip Kitcher, *Abusing Science: The Case against Creationism* (Cambridge: MIT Press, 1982); Marcel Chotkowski La Follette, ed., *Creationism, Science, and the Law: The Arkansas Case* (Cambridge: MIT Press, 1983); Raymond A. Eve and Francis B. Harrold, *The Creationist Movement in Modern America* (Boston: Twayne, 1991); Ronald L. Numbers, *The Creationists: The Evolution of Scientific Creationism* (New York: Alfred A. Knopf, 1992); George E. Webb, *The Evolution Controversy in America* (Lexington: University Press of Kentucky, 1994); and Edward J. Larson, *Summer for the Gods: The Scopes Trial and America's Continuing Debate over Science and Religion* (Cambridge: Harvard University Press, 1998).

18. See James Davison Hunter, *Culture Wars: The Struggle to Define America* (New York: Basic Books, 1991); Philip Rieff, "The Newer Noises of War in the Second Culture Camp: Notes on Professor Burt's Legal Fictions," *Yale Journal of Law and the Humanities* 3 (1991): 315–88; and David Martin, *A General Theory of Secularization* (New York: Harper and Row, 1978). Creationism may be taught without sanction in private schools; the issue has remained of legal consequence in public schools.

19. Frank M. Turner, quoting Asa Briggs, concludes, "The conflict between science and religion petered out, giving way to new debates about the nature not of the Universe but of society." Turner, "Victorian Conflict," p. 376, quoting Asa Briggs, *The Age of Improvement, 1783–1867* (New York: David Mckay, 1964), p. 488.

20. Stephen S. Kim, *John Tyndall's Transcendental Materialism and the Conflict Between Religion and Science in Victorian Britain* (Lewiston, NY: Mellen University Press, 1996), p. 179. Others who have advanced an amelioristic thesis about Tyndall's intentions regarding the reconciliation of the realm of the spiritual with the world subject to scientific laws include Paul L. Sawyer, "Ruskin and Tyndall: The Poetry of Matter and the Poetry of Spirit," in *Victorian Science and Victorian Values: Literary Perspectives*, ed. James Paradis and Thomas Postlewait (New York: New York Academy of Sciences, 1981), pp. 217–46; and Gillian Beer, *Open Fields: Science in Cultural Encounter* (Oxford: Clarendon Press, 1996), who defends Tyndall's "transcendental edge" by which "he contrived to keep some dark space for an ordering, though not a pre-emptive, Intelligence" (p. 249).

21. See Frank M. Turner, "Rainfall, Plagues, and the Prince of Wales: A Chapter in the Conflict of Religion and Science," *Journal of British Studies* 8, no. 2 (1974): 48. See also Frank M. Turner, *Contesting Cultural Authority: Essays in Victorian Intellectual Life* (Cambridge: Cambridge University Press, 1993), in which a revised version of the same essay appears, pp. 151–70. My discussion in the following pages is indebted to Turner's work and draws from it conspicuously.

22. Charles Kingsley, "Lord Palmerston and the Presbytery of Edinburgh," *Fraser's Magazine* 49 (1854): 47, 51, quoted in Turner, "Rainfall, Plagues," p. 50.

23. Turner, "Rainfall, Plagues," p. 51.

24. Ibid., p. 54.

25. The finest account of the successive interpretations of the cause of cholera, from religious to scientific explanations, is Charles E. Rosenberg, *The Cholera Years: The United States in 1832, 1849, and 1866* (1962; Chicago: University of Chicago Press, 1987).

26. *Fortnightly Review*, December 1, 1865.

27. Quoted in Eve and Creasey, *Life of Tyndall*, p. 125. Stanley sought toleration in principle and in practice. See Rowland E. Prothero, ed., *The Life and Correspondence of Arthur Penrhyn Stanley*, vol. 2 (New York: Charles Scribner's, 1893), p. 348–49; and Frances J. Woodward, *The Doctor's Disciples: A Study of Four Pupils of Arnold of Rugby* (London: Oxford University Press, 1954), p. 58–59.

28. Quoted in Eve and Creasey, *Life of Tyndall*, p. 126. Although Tyndall would figure more prominently later in what would come to be known in England and America as the prayer-gauge debate, his first attempts in print at criticizing petitionary prayer did not go unnoticed, even as Dean Stanley, who would later preside at Tyndall's marriage, sought amelioration. See Rev. Thomas Groser, *On Prayer: With Special Reference to Professor Tyndall's Objections. A Sermon Preached in the Catholic Apostolic Church* (London: Thomas, Bosworth, 1866).

29. Turner, "Rainfall, Plagues," p. 62.

30. See also Allan Mazur, *The Dynamics of Technical Controversy* (Washington, DC: Communications Press, 1981), pp. 10–12; and Jon H. Roberts, *Darwinism and the Divine in America: Protestant Intellectuals and Organic Evolution, 1859–1900* (Madison: University of Wisconsin Press, 1988), pp. 72–75.

31. The best collection of primary materials on this controversy appeared in the United States ed. John O. Means, *The Prayer-Gauge Debate by Prof. Tyndall, Francis Galton, and Others, Against Dr. Littledale, President McCosh, The Duke of Argyll, Canon Liddon, and "The Spectator"* (Boston: Congregational Publishing Society, 1876). Sir Henry Thompson, although implicated in initiating this round of the "prayer-gauge debate," took direct part in helping to legalize cremation in England in 1884.

32. Ibid., pp. 11–12. Those supplications included spiritual improvement, moral superiority, intellectual power; national supremacy; preservation from pestilence, famine, battles; protection against murder and sudden death; and "the prayer for 'sick persons,' which is not precise in it requests on their behalf."

33. Ibid., p. 13. Thompson eliminated many other prayer tests because of the difficulty in establishing any systematic way of measuring such effects apart from other influences.

34. Ibid., p. 15.

35. It is striking how much Thompson's observation about this distinction between general and specific prayers reflects the deeply held perceptions about class distinctions in Britain, and later in industrial societies generally. Contemporary epidemiological studies still derive much of their political and moral salience in the studies of mortality and morbidity rates based upon social class, and more recently,

in Britain, upon more refined gradations among the employed. See, for example, M. G. Marmot, G. Rose, M. J. Shipley, and P.J.S. Hamilton, "Employment Grade and Coronary Heart Disease in British Civil Servants," *Journal of Epidemiology and Community Health* 32 (1979): 244–49.

36. Means, *The Prayer-Gauge Debate*, p. 16.

37. Ibid., p. 18.

38. Ibid., p. 19.

39. Originally in *The Spectator*, July 6, 1872, pp. 846, 847. Means, *The Prayer-Gauge Debate*, p. 24.

40. Ibid.

41. Ibid., p. 26.

42. Ibid., pp. 28–29.

43. Ibid., p. 30.

44. In his affectionate summary of the "ingenuity of his [Galton's] idiosyncratic methods," Stephen Jay Gould noted, "He even proposed and began to carry out a statistical inquiry into the efficacy of prayer!" *The Mismeasure of Man* (New York: Norton, 1981), p. 75. For studies of Galton, see among other works, D. W. Forrest, *Francis Galton: The Life and Work of a Victorian Genius* (New York: Taplinger, 1974); Ruth Schwartz Cowan, *Sir Francis Galton and the Study of Heredity in the Nineteenth Century* (New York: Garland, 1985); Nicholas Wright Gillham, *A Life of Sir Francis Galton: From African Exploration to the Birth of Eugenics* (New York: Oxford University Press, 2001); Michael Bulmer, *Francis Galton: Pioneer of Heredity and Biometry* (Baltimore: Johns Hopkins University Press, 2003); and Martin Brookes, *Extreme Measures: The Dark Visions and Bright Ideas of Francis Galton* (New York: Bloomsbury 2004). See also The Galton Institute, *Sir Francis Galton, FRS: The Legacy of His Ideas* (Houndsmills, Basingstoke, Hampshire, England: Macmillan in association with the Galton Institute, 1993).

45. Originally in *Fortnightly Review*, August 1872, pp. 125–35. Means, *The Prayer-Gauge Debate*, p. 88.

46. Ibid., p. 89.

47. See appendix A, "Mortality of Registered Physicians in England and Wales, 1920–22," in Frederick L. Hoffman, *Life and Death in the Medical Profession* (Newark, NJ: Prudential Press, 1932), pp. 25–26.

48. Means, *The Prayer-Gauge Debate*, pp. 93–94.

49. Ibid., p. 101.

50. *British Medical Journal*, February 7, 1874, p. 182. An interesting correspondence followed this announcement about various authorities on the Sabbath. See *BMJ*, March 7, 1874, p. 334; *BMJ*, March 14, 1874, p. 368; and *BMJ*, April 4, 1874, p. 470.

51. A Committee of Clergy, *The Medical Aspect of Fasting* (London: W. Knott, 1897). The authors proposed that "dispensations" or exemptions from various fast requirements might be given on the basis of health, but they maintained some semblance of religious authority, distinct from exemption, when they noted that "The Fast before Communion is really a separate question. The obligation of its observance is far greater than that for the ecclesiastical fasts and days of abstinence. Being the universal immemorial custom of the whole Church, there is no question of dispensation" (p. 6).

52. John H. Jellett, *The Efficacy of Prayer, Being the Donnellan Lectures for the Year 1877*, 3rd ed. (London: Macmillan, 1880). In the appendix to his lectures, Jellett describes the unreasonableness of both sides, those who think that statistics can and should play no role in the discussion (here he cites James Augustus Hessey, *Moral Difficulties Connected with the Bible, Being the Boyle Lectures for 1871, Preached in her Majesty's Chapel at Whitehall* [London: Society for Promoting Christian Knowledge, 1872]) and those who believe that statistics resolve the matter conclusively (here he cites Francis Galton). See p. 174.

53. Ibid., p. 60.

54. Ibid., pp. 63–64.

55. Ibid., p. 65.

56. Ibid., p. 187.

57. See Martha S. Vogeler, *Frederic Harrison: The Vocation of a Positivist* (Oxford: Clarendon Press, 1984).

58. Jellett, *The Efficacy of Prayer*, p. 182.

59. See Roberts, *Darwin and the Divine*, pp. 19–20. For further background, see also Herbert Hovenkamp, *Science and Religion in America: 1800–1860* (Philadelphia: University of Pennsylvania Press, 1978), and J. David Hoeveler, Jr., *James McCosh and the Scottish Intellectual Tradition from Glasgow to Princeton* (Princeton, NJ: Princeton University Press, 1981). See also William Milligan Sloane, ed., *The Life of James McCosh: A Record Chiefly Autobiographical* (New York: Charles Scribner's, 1896).

60. Means, *The Prayer-Gauge Debate*, p. 144.

61. Mark Hopkins, *Prayer and the Prayer Gauge* (New York: Dodd and Mead, 1874), p. 40. Hopkins originally delivered the text as a sermon. See Mark Hopkins, *Prayer and the Prayer Gauge: A Discourse Delivered in the First Presbyterian Church, Troy, NY, December 15, 1872* (Albany, NY: Weed, Parsons, 1873).

62. Hugh Miller Thompson, "The Christian Doctrine of Prayer," in *Christian Truth and Modern Opinion. Seven Sermons Preached in New York by Clergymen of the Protestant Episcopal Church* (New York: Thomas Whittaker, 1874), p. 64.

63. Quoted in Eve and Creasey, *Life of Tyndall*, p. 171. Eve and Creasey give an account of Tyndall's visit to America, in chapter 14.

64. Edward Lawrence Godkin, " Tyndall and the Theologians," in *Reflections and Comments, 1865–1895* (New York: Charles Scribner's Sons, 1895), p. 131. The editorial originally appeared in *The Nation*, September 17, 1874, pp. 181–82. A week earlier, September 10, 1874, pp. 171–72, an extended commentary on the text of Tyndall's address appeared.

65. Ibid., pp. 135–36.

66. *The Nation*, November 19, 1874, p. 327. Two weeks later, Godkin picked up the mantle again, pursuing in finer detail his disappointment in both Tyndall and Huxley: "Both these gentlemen have now had so many encounters with the clergy on scientific ground, and have so often come off victorious, that they have got to like fighting, and have at last been carried by their bellicose zeal into the one region which ought to be closed to all true scientists." *The Nation*, November 26, 1874, p. 343.

67. *The Nation*, December 24, 1874, p. 420.

68. William James, "The Mood of Science and the Mood of Faith" (1874), in *The Works of William James: Essays, Comments, and Reviews* (Cambridge: Harvard University Press, 1987), pp. 115–17. James cited Tyndall and Huxley in particular as deserving of rebuke when "they propound what is merely one out of several equally unverified conceptions as if it were an established truth and proceed to rally the faithful around them by pealing the slogan, and branding in advance all critics of this particular hypothesis as minions of 'Ecclesiasticism' . . ." (p. 116).

69. Rev. Dr. Frederick de Sola Mendes, *Tyndallism and Judaism: Substance of a Sermon Delivered Nov. 14, 1874, In the Synagogue, "Shaaray Tefila," 44th St., New York* (New York: Printed by Request, 1874), p. 9.

70. William James, *The Varieties of Religious Experience* (Cambridge: Harvard University Press, 1985), p. 365. The responses to Tyndall's challenges continued for decades. Several years after James dismissed the narrowing of purpose of prayer, a Brooklyn Presbyterian minister, Leander Chamberlain, concluded: "Prayer is, in itself, incapable of submission to preemptory tests. It comes to its place in the relations of cause and effect, only through an adoring appeal to the divine wisdom and love." *The True Doctrine of Prayer* (New York: Baker and Taylor, 1906), p. 144. W. B. Selbie, following James in his exploration of comparative religion, remarked on prayer as an essential element in all religion: "we are dealing here, not with something strained, forced, and artificial, but with the spontaneous outgrowth of man's elemental needs and the normal working of his higher consciousness." *The Psychology of Religion* (Oxford: Clarendon Press, 1924), pp. 218–19.

71. C. S. Lewis addressed the "efficacy" of prayer in *Atlantic Monthly* in 1959, recalling much of the debate reviewed here. C. S. Lewis, "The Efficacy of Prayer," in *The World's Last Night and Other Essays* (New York: Harcourt, Brace, 1960).

72. See C.R.B. Joyce and R.M.C. Weldon, "The Objective Efficacy of Prayer: A Double-Blind Clinical Trial," *Journal of Chronic Diseases* 18 (April 1965): 367–77; Platon J. Cullipp, "The Efficacy of Prayer: a Triple-Blind Study," *Medical Times* 97 (1969): 201–4; Stephen G. Brush, "The Prayer Test," *American Scientist* 62 (1974): 561–63; R. C. Byrd, "Positive Therapeutic Effects of Intercessory Prayer in a Coronary Care Unit Population," *Southern Medical Journal* 81 (1988): 826–29; William Kruskal, "Miracles and Statistics: The Casual Assumption of Independence," *Journal of the American Statistical Association* 83 (1988): 929–40; C. Marwick, "Should Physicians Prescribe Prayer for Health? Spiritual Aspects of Well-Being Considered," *JAMA* 273 (1995): 1561–62; and Herbert Benson et al., "Study of the Therapeutic Effects of Intercessory Prayer (STEP) in Cardiac Bypass Patients: A Multicenter Randomized Trial of Uncertainty and Certainty of Receiving Intercessory Prayer," *American Heart Journal* 151 (2006): 934–42. Press reports on this last study by Benson et al. received front-page attention in "Long-Awaited Medical Study Questions the Power of Prayer," *New York Times*, March 31, 2006.

73. For example, see Theodore J. Chamberlain and Christopher A. Hall, *Realized Religion: Research on the Relationship between Religion and Health* (West Conshohocken, PA: Templeton Foundation Press, 2000); and Harold G. Koenig and Harvey Jay Cohen, eds., *The Link between Religion and Health: Psychoneuroimmunology and the Faith Factor* (New York: Oxford University Press, 2002). Both of these

volumes were sponsored by the John Templeton Foundation, the leading supporter of such investigations in recent years.

CHAPTER 4   Public Health, Public Trust, and the Professionalization of Medicine

1. See John Duffy, *The Sanitarians: A History of American Public Health* (Urbana: University of Illinois Press, 1990). I do not intend to address in this chapter the history of public health, but in addition to the work of John Duffy, I am indebted for insight and context to the following: Barbara Rosenkrantz, "Cart Before Horse: Theory, Practice and Professional Image in American Public Health, 1870–1920," *Journal of the History of Medicine and Allied Sciences* 29 (1974): 55–73; and Charles E. Rosenberg and Carroll S. Rosenberg, "Pietism and the Origins of the American Public Health Movement," *Journal of the History of Medicine and Allied Sciences* 23 (1968):16–35.

2. Daniel J. Macgowan, *Claims of the Missionary Enterprise on the Medical Profession: An Address Delivered Before the Temperance Society of the College of Physicians and Surgeons of the University of the State of New-York, October 28, 1842* (New York: William Osborn, 1842), p. 13.

3. The best account of foreign missions is William R. Hutchison, *Errand to the World: American Protestant Thought and Foreign Missions* (Chicago: University of Chicago Press, 1987), in particular, pp. 163ff. See also A. F. Walls, " 'The Heavy Artillery of the Missionary Army': The Domestic Importance of the Nineteenth-Century Medical Missionary," in *The Church and Healing*, ed. W. J. Sheils (Oxford: Basil Blackwell, 1983), pp. 287–97; and Henry Warner Bowden, "An Overview of Cultural Factors in the American Protestant Missionary Enterprise," in *American Missions in Bicentennial Perspective*, ed. R. Pierce Beaver (South Pasadena, CA: William Carey Library, 1977), pp. 40–62. For a contemporaneous assessment of foreign missions in the first quarter of the twentieth century, see Archibald G. Baker, "Though Concerning Protestant Foreign Missions," in *Religious Thought in the Last Quarter-Century*, ed. Gerald Birney Smith (Chicago: University of Chicago Press, 1927), pp. 207–27.

4. James S. Dennis, *Christian Missions and Social Progress: A Sociological Study of Foreign Missions* (New York: Fleming H. Revell, 1899), 2:400–433. See also W. J. Wanless, M.D., *The Medical Mission: Its Place, Power and Appeal* (Philadelphia: Westminster Press, 1900).

5. For a Catholic account, see T.W.M. Marshall, *Christian Missions: Their Agents, and Their Results*, 5th ed., 2 vols. (New York: P. J. Kennedy, 1896).

6. Speaking before the Men's National Missionary Congress in 1910, Dr. Winfield Scott Hall asked: "What is the essential idea of our profession? What is that which inspires the medical man to do his best, not only in his own professional work, but his best for his profession? . . . I believe that the spirit that stimulates us is the spirit of altruism, and until the young medical man gets fired through and through with the spirit of altruism, I do not believe that his professional success will be up to its maximum." "The Peculiar Opportunity of the Medical Missionary," in *Proceedings of the Men's National Missionary Congress of the United States of America, Chicago, Illinois, May 3–6, 1910* (New York: Laymen's Missionary Movement, 1910),

pp. 395–96. The appropriation of altruism, a term coined by Auguste Comte, was indicative of the Christian effort to infuse it with religious purpose but with the broadest humanitarian appeal.

7. J. G. Kerr, *Medical Missions at Home and Abroad* (San Francisco: A. L. Bancroft, 1878), p. 3.

8. Ibid., p. 10.

9. A possibly unique study of the physical health of missionaries is by William G. Lennox, who was then on the faculty of Harvard Medical School. See *The Health and Turnover of Missionaries* (New York: Press of the Methodist Book Concern, 1933).

10. As popular as Schweitzer may have been during his lifetime and afterward, his life's work was as close to celebrity as it was to mission without becoming exclusively the former. One observer of Schweitzer remarked early on: "Schweitzer is highly endowed as an organizer, so that he is able to maintain his work independently by the aid of friends without the backing of missionary societies. This procedure is extraordinary to such an extent as to form neither norm nor example for others." Prof. Dr. Med. Olpp, "Medical Missions and Their International Relations," in *Modern Medical Missions: A Series of Papers Published by Order of the Federation of Societies for Medical Missions* (Burlington, Iowa: Lutheran Literary Board, 1932), p. 126.

11. See also J. H. Raymond, *History of the Long Island College Hospital and Its Graduates Together with The Hoagland Laboratory and The Polhemus Memorial Clinic* (Brooklyn, NY: Association of the Alumni, 1899); and James Macfarlane Winfield, "The Long Island College Hospital," *Long Island Medical Journal* 4, no. 7 (1910): 225–38.

12. See David Rosner, *A Once Charitable Enterprise: Hospitals and Health Care in Brooklyn and New York, 1885–1915* (Cambridge: Cambridge University Press, 1982), pp. 100–101.

13. Editorial, "Success in a Crowded Profession," *Medical Record* (New York) March 11, 1876, p. 175.

14. *Medical Record* (New York) March 19, 1887, p. 331.

15. Godkin, *Reflections and Comments*, p. 237.

16. For background to the rise of Protestant liberalism in the second half of the nineteenth century and early twentieth century, see William R. Hutchison, *The Modernist Impulse in American Protestantism* (Cambridge: Harvard University Press, 1976).

17. See, for example, Austin Flint (1812–1886), *An Address: Delivered to the Graduates of the Long Island College Hospital, Brooklyn, N.Y. at the Annual Commencement, on the Evening of July 24th, 1860* (Brooklyn: Wilton, 1860).

18. See the *Dictionary of American Biography*.

19. See Harriet Mott Stryker-Rodda, *Brooklyn and Long Island Sanitary Fair* (New York: Long Island Historical Society, 1964).

20. See Richard S. Storrs, *Foundation Truths of American Missions: An Address Delivered at the Annual Meeting of the American Board of Commissioners for Foreign Missions at New Haven, Conn., October 14, 1897* (Boston: The Board, 1897). Storrs had been president of the board the previous ten years.

21. See Helen H. Holcomb, *Men of Might in India Missions: The Leaders and Their Epochs, 1706–1899* (New York: Revell, 1901). The Scudder name endured in

missionary work in India well into the twentieth century, in particular, in the work of Ida Sophia Scudder (1870–1960), who graduated in 1899 from the Medical Department of Cornell University and spent much of her life in India. See Mary Pauline Jeffery, *Ida S. Scudder of Vellore: An Appreciation of Forty Years of Service in India* (Mysore City, S. India: Wesley Press, 1939).

22. Scudder later became secretary to the American Medical Missionary Society when it was organized in 1885 in Chicago. See *American Medical Missionary Society, Constitution with an Account of Its Organization and a Plea for Medical Missions* (Chicago: C. W. Magill, n.d.).

23. "Young Doctors," *Brooklyn Daily Eagle*, June 26, 1874.

24. "Long Island College Hospital," *Brooklyn Daily Eagle*, June 27, 1867.

25. Ibid.

26. In later years, Littlejohn published *Individualism: Its Growth and Tendencies, with Some Suggestions as to the Remedy for Its Evils* (New York: T. Whittaker, 1881).

27. "Long Island College Hospital," *Brooklyn Daily Eagle*, June 27, 1867.

28. Abram N. Littlejohn, *Conciones Ad Clerum, 1879–1880*, 3rd ed. (New York: Thomas Whittaker, 1881), p. 47.

29. Ibid., pp. 52–53.

30. Ibid., p. 77.

31. Littlejohn took up the question of the cure of souls again in adumbrated form in *The Christian Ministry at the Close of the Nineteenth Century, The Bishop Paddock Lectures, 1884* (New York: Thomas Whittaker, 1884), pp. 313–27.

32. "Doctors," *Brooklyn Daily Eagle*, June 28, 1878. See J. Wade Caurthers, *Octavius Brooks Frothingham, Gentle Radical* (University: University of Alabama Press, 1977).

33. Ibid. For a contemporaneous account of Frothingham's ideas, see Edmund C. Stedman, *Octavius Brooks Frothingham and the New Faith* (New York: Putnam's, 1876).

34. "Graduates," *Brooklyn Daily Eagle*, June 25, 1879. See also William A. Snively, "A Good Man's Death," in *Testimonies to the Supernatural* (New York: Thomas Whittaker, 1888), pp. 115–24.

35. The minister was the Reverend Charles H. Hall. "Doctors," *Brooklyn Daily Eagle*, June 20, 1883.

36. The minister was the Reverend Robert R. Meredith. "More Doctors," *Brooklyn Daily Eagle*, March 24, 1892.

37. "Doctors," *Brooklyn Daily Eagle*, June 24, 1880.

38. "Seventy-Two New Doctors," *Brooklyn Daily Eagle*, May 19, 1898, p. 7.

39. The minister was the Reverend Henry Van Dyke. "Diplomas," *Brooklyn Daily Eagle*, June 2, 1886, p. 2. Van Dyke (1852–1933) was the son of a physician. See his encomium to William Osler, "The Healing Gift," read at Johns Hopkins University on March 22, 1920, in *Camp-Fires and Guide-Posts: A Book of Essays and Excursions* (New York: Charles Scribner's, 1921), pp. 293–302.

40. *Medical Record*, April 1, 1872, p. 94.

41. Ibid.

42. Ibid.

43. For background see Aaron Ignatius Abell, *The Urban Impact on American Protestantism, 1865–1900* (Cambridge: Harvard University Press, 1943). On the role of the ministry more generally during this period, see Susan Curtis, *A Consuming Faith: The Social Gospel and Modern American Culture* (Baltimore: Johns Hopkins University Press, 1991).

44. See Clifford E. Clark, Jr., *Henry Ward Beecher: Spokesman for a Middle-Class America* (Urbana: University of Illinois Press, 1978).

45. "New Doctors," *Brooklyn Daily Eagle*, March 10, 1888.

46. "Graduates in Medicine," *Brooklyn Daily Eagle*, May 17, 1899, p. 7. For an excellent account of the competing images of progressivism at this time, including debates about the use of the term "personality" over and against "character," see Richard Wightman Fox, "The Culture of Liberal Protestant Progressivism, 1875–1925," *Journal of Interdisciplinary History* 23 (1993): 639–60. See also Warren I. Susman, "'Personality' and the Making of Twentieth-Century Culture," in *New Directions in American Intellectual History*, ed. John Higham and Paul K. Conkin (Baltimore: Johns Hopkins University Press, 1979), pp. 212–26.

47. See Kurt Danziger, *Constructing the Subject: Historical Origins of Psychological Research* (New York: Cambridge University Press, 1990).

48. An important work on the professionalization of psychology is JoAnne Brown, *The Definition of a Profession: The Authority of Metaphor in the History of Intelligence Testing, 1890–1930* (Princeton, NJ: Princeton University Press, 1992). Brown focuses specifically on the professionalization and commercialization of intelligence testing. In what follows, I can only suggest the need for a comparable history of vocational testing. Beneath the modern veil of class opportunity that has come to define life chances in the aggregate, a history of the search for the right "fit" between self and occupation remains to be written. See also Michael Sokal, ed., *Psychological Testing and American Society, 1890–1930* (New Brunswick, NJ: Rutgers University Press, 1987).

49. See Francis Greenwood Peabody, *Reminiscences of Present-Day Saints* (Boston: Houghton Mifflin, 1927), pp. 110–11.

50. Lysander S. Richards, *Vocophy [L. Voco, I Name; I Call] The New Profession. A System Enabling a Person to Name the Calling or Vocation One is Best Suited to Follow* (Marlboro, MA: Pratt Brothers, 1881). The book, in different form, had been previously serialized in the weekly *Boston Commonwealth* in 1879. On Richards, see John M. Brewer, *History of Vocational Guidance: Origins and Early Development* (New York: Harper and Brothers, 1942), pp. 44–45. For Richards's own brief account, see Lysander S. Richards, *Incidents in the Life and Times of Lysander S. Richards of Marshfield Hill, Mass., U.S.A., Up to the Age of Ninety, 1835–1925* (Boston: Rapid Service Press, 1925), pp. 45–46.

51. Ibid., p. 11.

52. Ibid., p. 28.

53. Ibid., pp. 11–12.

54. Ibid., p. 27, "the supreme law of the survival of the fittest."

55. Ibid., p. 98. Exhibiting the disinterest of a true science of vocophy, Richards listed as one of the sixty-one occupations, "Executioner": "Should have large destructiveness; must have no fear of death, and be devoid of any sympathy in witnessing

suffering in his fellow men. Although it is well to have a small, or perhaps a moderate, amount of brains, yet there is no pursuit that demands an organism more animalistic and so near akin to the brute as that of an executioner" (p. 92).

56. Max Weber, *The Protestant Ethic and the Spirit of Capitalism* (London: Routledge, 1992), p. 182.

57. On Parsons's life as a reformer, see Howard V. Davis, *Frank Parsons: Prophet, Innovator, Counselor* (Carbondale: University of Southern Illinois Press, 1969); and Arthur Mann, *Yankee Reformers in the Urban Age* (Cambridge: Harvard University Press, 1954). Mann remarks that Parsons "was attached to no religious denomination but his writings are saturated with Christian principles" (p. 126). For specific discussions of his role in the development of vocational guidance, see Frederick J. Allen, "The Rise of Modern Vocational Guidance and of the Vocational Counselor," in *Principles and Problems in Vocational Guidance: A Book of Readings*, ed. Frederick J. Allen (New York: McGraw-Hill, 1927); Brewer, *History of Vocational Guidance*; Girard T. Bryant, "The Growth and Development of the Vocational Guidance Movement in the United States, 1900–1930," Ph.D. diss., Washington University, St. Louis, 1963; Edmund G. Williamson, *Vocational Counseling: Some Historical, Philosophical, and Theoretical Perspectives* (New York: McGraw-Hill, 1965); and W. Richard Stephens, *Social Reform and the Origins of Vocational Guidance* (Washington, DC: Monograph of the National Vocational Guidance Association, 1970). For an excellent chronology of the history of vocational guidance, see Henry Borow, "Milestones: A Chronology of Notable Events in the History of Vocational Guidance," in *Man in a World at Work*, ed. Henry Borow (Boston: Houghton Mifflin, 1964), pp. 45–66.

58. Frank Parsons, *Choosing a Vocation* (Boston: Houghton Mifflin, 1909), pp. 4–5.

59. Ibid., p. 5.

60. Hugo Münsterberg, "Finding a Life Work," *McClure's Magazine*, February 1910, pp. 398–403.

61. See Matthew Hale, Jr., *Human Science and Social Order: Hugo Münsterberg and the Origins of Applied Psychology* (Philadelphia: Temple University Press, 1980), pp. 122–23.

62. Hugo Münsterberg, *Vocation and Learning* (St. Louis, MO: Lewis Publishing, 1910), p. 233.

63. For background, see Lancelot Law Whyte, *The Unconscious before Freud* (London: Tavistock, 1962).

64. Alfred T. Schofield, *Unconscious Therapeutics; or, The Personality of the Physician*, 2nd ed. (Philadelphia: P. Blakiston's, 1906), p. 22. The quote is taken from Maurice de Fleury, *Medicine and the Mind* (London: Downey, 1900), p. 372.

65. For an account of this force in nineteenth-century medical thought, see John Harley Warner, "Nature-Trusting Heresy': American Physicians and the Concept of the Healing Power of Nature in the 1850's and 1860's," in *Perspectives in American History*, vol. 11 (Cambridge: Charles Warren Center for Studies in American History, Harvard University, 1978), pp. 291–324.

66. Schofield, *Unconscious Therapeutics*, pp. 29–30.

67. Ibid., p. 33.

68. Ibid., pp. 50–51.

69. These works included D. W. Cathell's *The Physician Himself*; S. Weir Mitchell's *Doctors and Patients*; Ian Maclaren's *A Doctor of the Old School*; and Jukes De Styrap's *The Young Practitioner*.

70. Schofield, *Unconscious Therapeutics*, p. 98n.

71. Ibid., p. 99. Schofield recognized that the "idealism and platitudes that are poured forth" at the opening of medical school classes were nonetheless true, even though "the practical-minded student feels nauseated" by them (p. 103).

72. Ibid., p. 104.

73. Among the first to recognize such implications for the distinctiveness of modern life was the sociologist Georg Simmel. See his *The Philosophy of Money*, ed. David Frisby, trans. Tom Bottomore and David Frisby from a first draft by Kaethe Mengelberg, 2nd ed. (London: Routledge, 1990).

74. Schofield, ibid., pp. 106–7.

75. The most thorough account of Henderson's life and career is John Parascandola, "Lawrence J. Henderson and the Concept of Organized Systems," Ph.D. diss., University of Wisconsin, Madison, 1968.

76. Quoted in ibid., p. 26.

77. "Physician and Patient as a Social System," in *L. J. Henderson on the Social System: Selected Writings*, ed. Bernard Barber (Chicago: University of Chicago Press, 1970), p. 202. The essay was originally published in the *New England Journal of Medicine* 212 (1935): 819–23.

78. Ibid., p. 203.

79. Ibid.

80. Ibid., p. 208.

81. Ibid., p. 209n.

82. Ibid., pp. 209–11.

83. Charles McIntire, "The Importance of the Study of Medical Sociology," *Bulletin of the American Academy of Medicine* 1 (1894): 425. Quoted in Norman G. Hawkins, *Medical Sociology: Theory, Scope and Method* (Springfield, IL: Charles C Thomas, 1958), p. 19.

84. See James Peter Warbasse, *Three Voyages: The Story of an Inquiring Soul Exploring His Way Through Life and Living It as He Goes, Being Fragments of an Autobiography* (Superior, Wis.: Cooperative League of the U.S.A., 1956).

85. Hawkins, *Medical Sociology*, p. 19. See also Samuel W. Bloom, *The Word as Scalpel: A History of Medical Sociology* (New York: Oxford University Press, 2002).

86. James Peter Warbasse, *Medical Sociology: A Series of Observations Touching upon the Sociology of Health and the Relations of Medicine to Society* (New York: D. Appleton, 1909), p. 44.

87. Ibid., p. 45. Warbasse opened his discussion by referring to a friend who "preferred to suffer the physical ills entailed by tobacco than to sacrifice the pleasure of the fragrant plant. That is his affair" (p. 42).

88. Warbasse, *Medical Sociology*, p. 114.

89. Gerald Birney Smith, *Principles of Christian Living: A Handbook of Christian Ethics* (Chicago: University of Chicago Press, 1924), p. 133. Further expressions of Smith's theological liberalism can be found in his *Current Christian Thinking*

(Chicago: University of Chicago Press, 1928). Note in particular, chapter 10, "The Controversy over Evolution."

90. Henry Allen Moe, "The Doctor as Citizen," in *The Power of Freedom in Human Affairs* (Philadelphia: The American Philosophical Society and Princeton University Press, 1977), p. 54, 57. The essay first appeared in *Annals of Internal Medicine* 32, no. 2 (1950).

91. Joseph Garland, ed., *The Physician and His Practice* (Boston: Little, Brown, 1954), p. xi.

92. Ibid., p. 8.

93. See John P. McGovern and Chester R. Burns, *Humanism in Medicine* (Springfield, IL: Charles C Thomas, 1973).

94. Daniel C. Elkin, "A Case for the Study of the Humanities in the Making of a Doctor," *Annals of Surgery* 136, no. 3 (1952): 340. See Stanley Dorst, "Education for Professional Services," *Journal of Medical Education* 26 (1951): 269.

95. Elkin, "Study of the Humanities," p. 340.

96. Ibid., p. 343.

97. "Medicine and Religion Program Set," *JAMA* 188 (1964): 59.

98. Abraham Joshua Heschel, *The Insecurity of Freedom* (New York: Noonday Press, 1967), p. 34.

99. A specifically Jewish theological address to physicians' character does exist in various Jewish sources. My association of Heschel with what began as a Protestant tradition and became, in effect, a public tradition of addresses about physicians' character is intended to demonstrate the sociological rather than strictly theological import of his effort to speak to a larger audience that was diverse in religious background. His points were not intended exclusively for debate among Jews or Jewish physicians.

100. Ibid., p. 31.

101. Ibid., p. 36.

102. "Psychiatrist, Rabbi Agree on Importance of Warm Physician-Patient Relationship," *JAMA* 189 (1964): 27.

103. "MDs, Clergymen: Both Vital to 'Healing' Ministry," *JAMA* 193 (1965): 39.

104. Ibid., p. 40.

105. See Robert R. Huntley, "Epidemiology of Family Practice," *JAMA* 185 (1963): 175–78; and Robert J. Haggerty, "Etiology of Decline in General Practice," *JAMA* 185 (1963): 179–82.

106. "MDs, Clergymen," p. 40.

107. "'When Do You Pull the Plug?'" *JAMA* 205 (1968): 29.

CHAPTER 5   The Growth of Popular Distrust in Medicine

1. Kenneth S. Lynn, "Introduction to the Issue, 'The Professions,'" *Daedalus* 92 (1963): 647. See also Kenneth S. Lynn and the Editors of *Daedalus, The Professions in America* (Cambridge, MA: Houghton Mifflin, 1965).

2. James Coleman illustrates the broad decline in public confidence in major American institutions, including the professions, in chapter 5, "Relations of Trust," in *Foundations of Social Theory* (Cambridge: Harvard University Press, 1990), p. 95.

Coleman stipulates, in the case of medicine, that the degree of confidence is related to "whether to accept bad medical outcomes as unavoidable" (p. 97).

3. Writing in 1965, Ennio C. Rossi exemplified the growing problem of public perception of the physician's "impersonality." "Why Is the Medical Profession Estimable in the Individual but Not in the Generality?" *Perspectives in Biology and Medicine* 8, no. 2 (1965): 230–40.

4. The popular attacks on physicians and hospitals were based upon specific kinds of dissatisfaction with negligence and incompetence, malpractice and hospital care, and the lack of instruction in medical ethics in medical schools. See Howard R. and Martha E. Lewis, *The Medical Offenders* (New York: Simon and Schuster, 1970), esp. pp. 333–34. See also Fred J. Cook, *The Plot against the Patient* (Englewood Cliffs, NJ: Prentice-Hall, 1967).

5. *Wall Street Journal*, May 9, 1994, pp. B1, B3. The sociologist Marie R. Haug in 1977 anticipated the consequences of greater public accessibility to medical information: "Assuming that much of the expertise now controlled by professionals in medicine, law, and engineering can eventually be automated and that the public will learn methods of access, what will be the effect on professional power and authority, and thus on the concept of profession as an occupational category?" Marie R. Haug, "Computer Technology and the Obsolescence of the Concept of Profession," in *Work and Technology*, ed. Marie R. Haug and Jacques Dofny (Beverly Hills, CA: Sage, 1977), p. 225.

6. See Dianna B. Dutton with contributions by Thomas A. Preston and Nancy E. Pfund, *Worse Than the Disease: Pitfalls of Medical Progress* (Cambridge: Cambridge University Press, 1988).

7. In 1984, Paul Starr and Theodore Marmor cited several trends that they deemed significant in forecasting the future of medicine, among them the growth of professional classes due to expanded access to higher education, the "corporatizing" of medicine, and feminism. See "The United States: A Social Forecast," in *The End of an Illusion: The Future of Health Policy in Western Industrialized Nations*, ed. Jean de Kervasdoué, John R. Kimberly, and Victor G. Rodwin (Berkeley and Los Angeles: University of California Press, 1984), esp. pp. 247–48.

8. Eric J. Cassell, *Talking with Patients*, vol. 2: *Clinical Technique* (Cambridge: MIT Press, 1985), p. ix.

9. Between the concerns raised by Henderson and those raised by Cassell, a strong presence of psychological and psychoanalytic idealism prevailed in medical thinking about the doctor-patient relationship. For a useful illustration, see George H. Carter, "History Taking and Interviewing Technique," *Journal of Medical Education* 30, no. 6 (1955): 315–26. See further the Commonwealth Fund study, ed. Walter Bauer and Helen Leland Witmer, *Teaching Psychotherapeutic Medicine: An Experimental Course for General Physicians* (Cambridge: Harvard University Press, 1947).

10. Eric J. Cassell, *Talking with Patients*, vol. 1: *The Theory of Doctor-Patient Communication* (Cambridge: MIT Press, 1985), p. 1.

11. George Eliot recognized the contingency of Antigone's confrontation with Creon over the burial of Polynices, that the "turning point of the tragedy" was not the question of reverence for the dead but rather the problem of obedience to

authority itself. So it is the case with the nature of the physician-patient relationship, less the contingent factors of interactions at any moment in time, and more the general problem of authority inherent in profoundly asymmetrical encounters. See George Eliot, "The Antigone and Its Moral" (*Leader*, March 29, 1856, p. 306), in *Essays of George Eliot*, ed. Thomas Pinney (New York: Columbia University Press, 1963), pp. 261–65.

12. Cassell, *Talking with Patients*, 2:148. The question of the physician's responsibility for offering prognoses has been answered in recent years with a call for greater candor, notwithstanding Cassell's insight. See Nicholas A. Christakis, "The Bad News First," *New York Times*, August 24, 2007, p. A19.

13. Cassell, *Talking with Patients*, 2:157.

14. Elliot G. Mishler et al., *Social Contexts of Health, Illness, and Patient Care* (Cambridge: Cambridge University Press, 1981), p. 196.

15. One measure of Illich's critical influence was his appearance on National Public Radio to discuss the changing doctor-patient relationship and its effect on medical care, with Susan Stamberg, June 3, 1976, following the publication of *Medical Nemesis* in the United States.

16. Ivan Illich, *Medical Nemesis: The Expropriation of Health* (New York: Pantheon, 1976), p. 3.

17. Ibid., pp. 4, 6.

18. Ibid., pp. 8–9.

19. I examine McKeown's work in further detail in chapter 7.

20. Ibid., p. 29.

21. In his enthusiasm to find at least one example of medical intervention of which he approved, Illich cited the case of the Pap smear, which "has been proved: if the tests are given four times a year, early intervention for cervical cancer demonstrably increases the five-year survival rate" (ibid., p. 24). Actually, debates about the costs of such intervention as compared to the lives saved, based on the frequency of the test, have continued for decades. One important account is given in Louise B. Russell, *Educated Guesses: Making Policy about Medical Screening Tests* (Berkeley and Los Angeles: University of California Press, 1994); see, in particular, chapter 2.

22. See Renée C. Fox, "The Medicalization and Demedicalization of American Society," in *Essays in Medical Sociology: Journeys into the Field* (New York: Wiley, 1979), pp. 465–83.

23. Illich, *Medical Nemesis*, p. 33.

24. Ibid.

25. Ibid., p. 34.

26. Ibid., p. 35.

27. Ibid., p. 43 n. 13. Illich's dialogue with bioethics is muted by the polemical scope of his critique. The difficulty in placing him theologically then is less so now, in part because, like Ramsey, the real progress of medicine cannot be disassociated from what patients want whatever the moral or financial costs.

28. Ibid., p. 45.

29. Ibid., p. 46.

30. Paul Ramsey, *Ethics at the Edges of Life: Medical and Legal Intersections* (New Haven: Yale University Press, 1978.) Ramsey recognized the severity of the situation in which doctors had lost their autonomy as "moral entrepreneurs" (as they were recklessly defined by social scientists). Illich capitalized on this criticism of physicians, referring, for example, to the work of Howard Becker. See *Outsiders: Studies in the Sociology of Deviance* (New York: Free Press, 1963). Yet the cultural authority stripped from medicine would not eliminate the necessity of someone having to make life-and-death decisions. The persistent illusion, borne of social-scientific and lately bio-ethical hubris, has been that courts fill the vacuum created by medical defensiveness.

31. The absence of widespread national conflict over physician-assisted suicide and voluntary euthanasia is largely the result of lessons learned by the Supreme Court from the abortion controversy. Leaving states with the latitude to pass laws on end-of-life decisions, the Court avoided galvanizing national movements. See *Vacco, Attorney General of New York, et al. v. Quill et al.* (1997) and *Washington et al. v. Glucksberg et al.* (1997).

32. *New York Times Book Review*, May 2, 1976, p. 2. The editors provided the following caption line: "The 20th-century's leading Luddite turns to medicine."

33. Apparently the dismissal of Illich's arguments and approaches apply as well to his work on education. See David A. Gabbard, *Silencing Ivan Illich: A Foucauldian Analysis of Intellectual Exclusion* (San Francisco: Austin and Winfield, 1993).

34. Ibid. Two works cited by Geiger were René Dubos, *The Mirage of Health: Utopias, Progress, and Biological Change* (New York: Harper, 1959), and Rick J. Carlson, *The Limits of Medicine* (New York: Wiley, 1975). Illich wrote a foreword to Carlson's book.

35. See Illich's remarks on the reception of *Medical Nemesis* in Ivan Illich, "Twelve Years after *Medical Nemesis*: A Plea for Body History," in *In the Mirror of the Past: Lectures and Addresses, 1978–1990* (New York: Marion Boyars, 1992), pp. 211–17. See also Ivan Illich, *Ivan Illich in Conversation* (Concord, Ontario: Anansi, 1992).

36. Illich, *Medical Nemesis*, p. 127.

37. Ibid., p. 132.

38. On the "brokenness of existence" see Philip Rieff's examination of minimal and maximal culture in "Cooley and Culture," in *The Feeling Intellect: Selected Writings*, ed. Jonathan B. Imber (Chicago: University of Chicago Press, 1990), pp. 310–21. The failure of government-sponsored health care reform during the Clinton presidency has been the subject of numerous and well-publicized studies, all of which consider the failure of such reform to be a failure of politics. It is clearly much more than that.

39. For self-help guides in the 1990s alone, see Barbara M. Korsch, *The Intelligent Patient's Guide to the Doctor-Patient Relationship: Learning How to Talk So Your Doctor Will Listen* (New York: Oxford University Press, 1998); J. Alfred Jones, *Communicating with Your Doctor: Getting the Most Out of Health Care* (Cresskill, NJ: Hampton Press, 1995); Debra L. Roter and Judith A. Hall, *Doctors Talking with Patients: Improving Communication in Medical Visits* (Westport, CT: Auburn House, 1992); and Linus S. Geisler, *Doctor and Patient: A Partnership through Dialogue: New Ways of Mutual Understanding* (Frankfurt am Main: Pharma Verlag Frankfurt, 1991).

40. See Talcott Parsons, "Social Structure and Dynamic Process: The Case of Modern Medical Practice," in *The Social System* (New York: Free Press, 1951), pp. 428–79. Parsons further developed his perspectives on the physician-patient relation in response to his critics. See "The Sick Role and the Role of the Physician Reconsidered," *Millbank Memorial Fund Quarterly/Health and Society*, Summer 1975, pp. 257–78.

41. See, for example, Mizrahi, *Getting Rid of Patients*.

42. See Carol Hanisch, "The Personal is Political" (1970) in *Radical Feminism: A Documentary Reader*, ed. Barbara A. Crow (New York: New York University Press, 2000), pp. 113–16. Although now remembered as a radical feminist idea, Hanisch's formulation was remarkably tolerant, even quizzical in its approach to "apolitical" women. The emergence of the cliché conceals the ways in which radical feminist challenges were initially arguments internal to the Left. The triumph of feminism in matters of health suggests an important convergence between "women's" health and "public" health.

43. For an excellent historical summary, see Ellen S. More, *Restoring the Balance: Women Physicians and the Profession of Medicine, 1850–1995* (Cambridge: Harvard University Press, 1999).

44. New England Free Press originally published the book in 1971, and Simon and Schuster in 1973. See Boston Women's Health Book Collective, *Our Bodies, Ourselves: A Book by and for Women* (New York: Simon and Schuster, 1973). The 1973 edition was 276 pages. A second edition, published in 1976, was 383 pages. *The New Our Bodies, Ourselves*, published in 1984 was 647 pages. The twenty-fifth anniversary edition, published in 1992, was 751 pages. A 1998 edition, *Our Bodies, Ourselves for the New Century*, was 780 pages.

45. Boston Women's Health Book Collective, *Our Bodies, Ourselves* (1973), p. 1.

46. Candace West, *Routine Complications: Troubles with Talk between Doctors and Patients* (Bloomington: Indiana University Press, 1984), p. 11.

47. For overviews of social-scientific literature on the physician-patient relation since 1975, see West, *Routine Complications*, chap. 2; Howard Waitzkin, *The Politics of Medical Encounters: How Patients and Doctors Deal with Social Problems* (New Haven: Yale University Press, 1991), chap. 2; and L.M.L. Ong et al., "Doctor-Patient Communication: A Review of the Literature," *Social Science and Medicine* 40 (1995): 903–18.

48. Sue Fisher, *In the Patient's Best Interest: Women and the Politics of Medical Decisions* (New Brunswick, NJ: Rutgers University Press, 1986), p. 5.

49. Ibid., p. 6.

50. Ibid., p. 7.

51. For debates and studies on these matters, internal to the social sciences, see Sue Fisher and Alexandra Dundas Todd, eds., *The Social Organization of Doctor-Patient Communication* (Washington, DC: Center for Applied Linguistics, 1983); Sue Fisher, "Institutional Authority and the Structure of Discourse," *Discourse Processes* 7 (1984): 210–24; Eliot G. Mishler, *The Discourse of Medicine: Dialectics of Medical Interviews* (Norwood, NJ: Ablex, 1984); Sue Fisher and Alexandra Dundas Todd, eds., *Discourse and Institutional Authority: Medicine, Education, and Law* (Norwood, NJ: Ablex, 1986); Christian Heath, *Body Movement and Speech in Medical Interaction* (New York: Cambridge University Press, 1986); George Psathas, ed., *Interaction Competence* (Washington, DC: University Press of America, 1990); Paul ten Have, "Talk and Institution: A Reconsideration of the 'Asymmetry' of

Doctor-Patient Interaction," in *Talk and Social Structure: Studies in Ethnomethodology and Conversation Analysis*, ed. Deirdre Boden and Don H. Zimmerman (Berkeley and Los Angeles: University of California Press, 1991), pp. 138–63; Paul Atkinson, *Medical Talk and Medical Work* (Thousand Oaks, CA: Sage, 1995); and Nancy Ainsworth-Vaughn, *Claiming Power in Doctor-Patient Talk* (New York: Oxford University Press, 1998).

52. The implications of the absorption of social-scientific work into the practical work of physicians are illustrated in a literature written by physicians about physician-patient communication. For example, see the work of Frederic W. Platt, *Conversation Failure: Case Studies in Doctor-Patient Communication* (Tacoma, WA: Life Sciences Press, 1992) and *Conversation Repair: Case Studies in Doctor-Patient Communication* (Boston: Little, Brown, 1995).

53. In 1995, Fisher acknowledged the importance of the changing character of the physician-patient relationship, an acknowledgment that suggests that her research, like that of her many predecessors, should not be understood as cumulative in a scientific sense but as a reflection of the changing character of that relationship over time: "Has the situation changed? That is an empirical question without a ready answer. . . . Perhaps today there is a critical mass of women, especially women who identify as feminists . . . who can . . . fight to change the system. Perhaps they will change the ideology of clinical practice, or, at the least, perhaps as individual practitioners they will deal with patients differently, but this remains an open empirical question—a question that may organize my next research project." Sue Fisher, *Nursing Wounds: Nurse Practitioners, Doctors, Women Patients, and the Negotiation of Meaning* (New Brunswick, NJ: Rutgers University Press, 1995), p. 238.

54. In addition to works that address the sociolinguistic context of physician-patient interaction, see Diana Scully and Pauline Bart, "A Funny Thing Happened on the Way to the Orifice: Women in Gynecology Textbooks," *American Journal of Sociology* 78 (1973): 1045–50; Diana Scully, *Men Who Control Women's Health: The Miseducation of Obstetrician-Gynecologists* (1980; Williston, VT: Teachers College Press, 1994); and Emily Martin, *The Woman in the Body: A Cultural Analysis of Reproduction* (1987; Boston: Beacon Press, 2001).

55. Raymond Firth, "Acculturation in Relation to Concepts of Health and Disease," in *Medicine and Anthropology*, ed. Iago Galdston (New York: International Universities Press, 1959), p. 129.

56. Ibid., pp. 132, 142.

57. Consider, for example, Norman Cousins, *Anatomy of an Illness as Perceived by the Patient: Reflections on Healing and Regeneration* (New York: Norton, 1979). Although much of Cousins's influence was reflected in the importance of humor and "positive thinking" in illness, his message was also directed at the need for doctor-patient teamwork.

58. This is particularly the case in the work of the anthropologist Arthur Kleinman. See his *The Illness Narratives: Suffering, Healing, and the Human Condition* (New York: Basic Books, 1988).

59. Arthur W. Frank, *The Wounded Storyteller: Body, Illness, and Ethics* (Chicago: University of Chicago Press, 1995), pp. 146–47. See also Arthur W. Frank, *At the Will of the Body: Reflections on Illness* (Boston: Houghton Mifflin, 1991).

60. Frank, *The Wounded Storyteller*, p. 92.

61. Ibid., p. 96.

62. For the centrality of narrative in postmodernity, see George Steiner, *Grammars of Creation* (New Haven: Yale University Press, 2001); in bioethics in particular, see Hilde Lindemann Nelson, ed., *Stories and Their Limits: Narrative Approaches to Bioethics* (New York: Routledge, 1997), and Rita Charon and Martha Montello, *Stories Matter: The Role of Narrative in Medical Ethics* (New York: Routledge, 2002). These latter two books clearly reconstitute an earlier agenda of linking personal transformation with political purpose, less evident in Frank's work.

63. Arthur Frank, *The Wounded Storyteller*, p. 115.

64. Ibid., p. 116.

65. Ibid., p. 117.

66. Ibid., p. 175. See Renée C. Fox, *Experiment Perilous: Physicians and Patients Facing the Unknown* (1959; New Brunswick, NJ: Transaction, 1998). Fox's epilogue recounts the important changes in context of medical research, in which the physician-investigator becomes increasingly remote from the bedside. It is difficult to appreciate Frank's own quest outside the changed historical contexts of the physician-patient relationship.

67. Peter D. Kramer, *Listening to Prozac* (New York: Viking, 1993).

68. Sandra M. Gilbert, *Wrongful Death: A Medical Tragedy* (New York: Norton, 1995), p. 311.

69. Ibid., pp. 218–19.

70. Ibid., p. 219.

71. Ibid., pp. 289–90.

72. Lisa Alther, "American Tragedies," review of *Wrongful Death: A Medical Tragedy* and *Dreaming: Hard Luck and Good Times in America*, in *Women's Review of Books*, July 1995, p. 18.

73. On the utility of faith, Gilbert observed "we prayed, we begged, we meditated—and it did no good did it? There are things we may never do again. Never wear hamsa earrings. Never wear Puerto Rican healing beads or, maybe believe—if we ever did—in the protective efficacy of Buddhist services or Carmelite prayers or Orthodox Jewish meditations" (*Wrongful Death*, p. 341). Marta Buszewicz's review in the *Times Literary Supplement* expressed similar uncertainty about Gilbert's efforts: "It is hard to believe that this sort of adversarial process leads to a satisfactory outcome. . . . Sandra Gilbert describes the book as a tribute to her husband and an attempt to resolve some of the issues around his death. Whether it succeeds in this for the family, only they can tell." Marta Buszewicz, "The Cure that Wasn't," *TLS*, July 11, 1997, p. 29. Gilbert continued her own "quest" in Sandra M. Gilbert, *Death's Door: Modern Dying and the Ways We Grieve* (New York: Norton, 2006).

CHAPTER 6   The Evolution of Bioethics

1. The apparent complexities of characterizing what kind of era of medicine we are presently in is illustrated in Jacob S. Hacker and Theodore R. Marmor, "The Misleading Language of Managed Care," *Journal of Health Politics, Policy and Law* 24 (1999): 1033–43.

2. See Allan M. Brandt and Martha Gardner, "The Golden Age of Medicine?" in *Medicine in the 20th Century*, ed. Roger Cooter and John Pickstone (Amsterdam: Harwood Academic Publishers, 2000), pp. 21–37.

3. *JAMA* 143 (1950): 746. On the same page, announcement was made that the inauguration of the new president, Dr. Elmer L. Henderson, would be broadcast live for the first time on radio.

4. *Current Medical Digest*, October 1933, p. 9. At the time, the editors took pride in following "thirty of the leading journals of the world."

5. Social-science research on the physician's career during the 1950s and 1960s focused on physicians' socialization and on the quality of training. In the latter case, researchers examined empirically the factors that contributed to or interfered with the length of training of doctors. I speak here of a spiritual exhaustion in the meaning of the physician's career, not to indict that research in any way, but rather to place it in the context of the rising tide of normative research that would follow under the eventual rubric of bioethics. For empirical research on socialization at that time, see Robert K. Merton, George Reader, and Patricia L. Kendall, eds., *The Student-Physician: Introductory Studies in the Sociology of Medical Education* (Cambridge: Harvard University Press, 1957); Howard Becker et al., *Boys in White: Student Culture in Medical School* (1961; Rutgers, NJ: Transaction, 1997); and Renée C. Fox, "Is There a 'New' Medical Student? A Comparative View of Medical Socialization in the 1950s and the 1970s," in *Essays in Medical Sociology: Journeys into the Field* (New York: John Wiley, 1979), pp. 78–101. For empirical research on the quality of medical practice as determined by career-path choices, see Fremont J. Lyden, H. Jack Geiger, and Osler L. Peterson, *The Training of Good Physicians: Critical Factors in Career Choices* (Cambridge: Harvard University Press, 1968).

6. Grace Metalious, *Peyton Place* (1956; Boston: Northeastern University Press, 1999).

7. *Bantam Books, Inc. v. Sullivan*, 372 U.S. 58 (1963).

8. Ibid.

9. For a thorough appraisal of the social history of medicine, see Frank Huisman and John Harley Warner, eds., *Locating Medical History: The Stories and Their Meanings* (Baltimore: Johns Hopkins University Press, 2004). See also John C. Burnham, *How the Idea of Profession Changed the Writing of Medical History* (London: Wellcome Institute for the History of Medicine, 1998).

10. Thomas Henry Huxley, "On the Physical Basis of Life," in *Lay Sermons, Addresses, and Reviews* (New York: D. Appleton, 1871), p. 140. In the same volume of essays, Huxley is more forthright: "While as for the 'culte systématique de l"humanité,' I, in my blindness, could not distinguish it from sheer Popery, with M. Comte in the chair of St. Peter, and the names of most of the saints changed" ("The Scientific Aspects of Positivism," p. 149).

11. Hans Barth, *The Idea of Order: Contributions to a Philosophy of Politics*, trans. Ernest W. Hankamer and William M. Newell (Dordrecht: Reidel, 1960), p. 128.

12. F. A. Hayek, *The Counter-Revolution of Science: Studies on the Abuse of Reason* (Glencoe, Ill.: Free Press, 1952).

13. John H. Evans has documented in fascinating detail the role that bioethicists came to play in the shaping of bioethical debate with the increased role of the state in both organizing and rationalizing how this debate would take place. My interest here is to step back further in order to characterize the cultural and moral frameworks in which such usurpation became possible. See John H. Evans, *Playing God? Human Genetic Engineering and the Rationalization of Public Bioethical Debate* (Chicago: University of Chicago Press, 2002).

14. Daniel Callahan, *Abortion: Law, Choice, and Morality* (New York: Macmillan, 1970). Callahan dedicated his book to the Berrigan brothers, Daniel and Philip, and to Elizabeth Bartelme.

15. See John T. Noonan, *A Private Choice: Abortion in America in the Seventies* (New York: Free Press, 1979).

16. Kelly, *Emergence of Catholic Medical Ethics*.

17. Charles J. McFadden, *Medical Ethics*, 3rd ed. (Philadelphia: F. A. Davis, 1955), p. xiii.

18. Paul Tillich, "Moralisms and Morality from the Point of View of the Ethicist," in *Ministry and Medicine in Human Relations*, ed. Iago Galdston (New York: International Universities Press, 1955), p. 131. For an extensive theological discussion of Protestant and Roman Catholic approaches to ethics, see James M. Gustafson, *Protestant and Roman Catholic Ethics: Prospects for Rapprochement* (Chicago: University of Chicago Press, 1978). See also Tillich's further reflections on health in "The Meaning of Health," *Perspectives in Biology and Medicine* 5, no. 1 (1961): 92–100.

19. Stephen Toulmin, "How Medicine Saved the Life of Ethics," *Perspectives in Biology and Medicine* 25, no. 4 (1982): 736–50. See also a less noticed but equally important assessment by Richard M. Zaner, "Is 'Ethicist' Anything to Call a Philosopher?" *Human Studies* 7, no. 1 (1984): 71–90.

20. In a letter to the *New York Times* in 1994, R. Alta Charo and Daniel Wikler wrote: "All that bioethicists can offer is a somewhat less politically or emotionally charged, somewhat more dispassionate evaluation of our options. No doubt you will always be able to find one ethicist who considers a new development grotesque and another who wants to wait and see. But personal feelings about such innovations even from respected academics, do not reflect any rigorously derived consensus. We suggest the following pledge be taken by ethicists and the news media alike: No ethicist should be asked for a personal opinion. If asked, no personal opinion should be given. And if given, no personal opinion should be published. With issues so complicated, we cannot afford to let a small group of academics be a self-appointed, secular version of the Committee for the Defense of the Faith" (January 14, 1994, A28).

21. Veatch, "Diverging Traditions," pp. 121–32.

22. Ibid., p. 123.

23. Joseph Fletcher, *Morals and Medicine: The Moral Problems of: The Patient's Right to Know the Truth, Contraception, Artificial Insemination, Sterilization, Euthanasia* (Princeton, NJ: Princeton University Press, 1954), p. 6. Fletcher was an Episcopal priest whose work ushered in the era of "bioethics," a term adopted in part to move beyond the corruption of Protestant ethics as business ethics only as well as beyond the narrow and Catholic meanings associated with "pastoral" medicine.

24. Joseph Fletcher acknowledged as much: "As we often find in these matters of specific concrete moral questions, there is no Protestant discussion of surgery, autopsy, and other mutilative procedures—not even on the ethics of transplant donation." "Our Shameful Waste of Human Tissue: An Ethical Problem for the Living and the Dead," in *The Religious Situation: 1969*, ed. Donald R. Cutler (Boston: Beacon Press, 1969), p. 230.

25. See Frederick N. Dyer, *Champion of Women and the Unborn: Horatio Robinson Storer, M.D.* (Canton, MA: Science History Publication, 1999).

26. James C. Mohr, *Abortion in America: The Origins and Evolution of National Policy, 1800–1900* (New York: Oxford University Press, 1978).

27. A second meaning of "neologism," "a meaningless word coined by a psychotic," has its applicability as well, insofar as the broader institutional and cultural mandates of both sociology and bioethics cannot be easily defined or identified. See Andrew Wernick, *Auguste Comte and the Religion of Humanity: The Posttheistic Program of French Social Theory* (Cambridge: Cambridge University Press, 2001).

28. Van Rensselaer Potter, *Bioethics: Bridge to the Future* (Englewood Cliffs, NJ: Prentice-Hall, 1971). For an assessment of the word "bioethics," see Warren T. Reich, "The Word "Bioethics": Its Birth and the Legacies of Those Who Shaped It," *Kennedy Institute of Ethics Journal* 4 (1994): 319–35; and Warren T. Reich, "The Word 'Bioethics': The Struggle over Its Earliest Meanings," *Kennedy Institute of Ethics Journal* 5 (1995): 19–34. See also Robert Martensen, "The History of Bioethics: An Essay Review," *Journal of the History of Medicine* 56, no. 2 (2001): 168–75.

29. K. Danner Clouser, "Bioethics," in *Encyclopedia of Bioethics*, ed. Warren T. Reich (New York: Free Press, 1978), p. 118.

30. All quotations of "A Bioethical Creed for Individuals" come from Potter, *Bioethics*, inside cover.

31. Ibid., p. 73.

32. David J. Rothman, *Strangers at the Bedside: A History of How Law and Bioethics Transformed Medical Decision Making* (New York: Basic Books, 1991); Albert R. Jonsen, *The Birth of Bioethics* (New York: Oxford University Press, 1998); M. L. Tina Stevens, *Bioethics in America: Origins and Cultural Politics* (Baltimore: Johns Hopkins University Press, 2000).

33. Rothman, *Strangers at the Bedside*, p. 247.

34. See Eliot Freidson, *Professionalism Reborn: Theory, Prophecy, and Policy* (Chicago: University of Chicago Press, 1994). See also Samuel W. Bloom, "Professionalism in the Practice of Medicine," *Mount Sinai Journal of Medicine* 69, no. 6 (2002): 398–403; and Rosemary A. Stevens, "Themes in the History of Medical Professionalism," *Mount Sinai Journal of Medicine* 69, no. 6 (2002): 357–62.

35. See Nancy Howell Lee, *The Search for an Abortionist* (Chicago: University of Chicago Press, 1969). Howell, a sociologist, studied social networks and the differential access to abortion.

36. See Edward G. Andrew, *Conscience and Its Critics: Protestant Conscience, Enlightenment Reason, and Modern Subjectivity* (Toronto: University of Toronto Press, 2001). In his own time, Joseph Fletcher led one of the best-known debates implicating

antinomianism, which was then called "situation ethics." See Harvey Cox, *The Situation Ethics Debate* (Philadelphia: Westminster Press, 1968).

37. Two useful resources that examine the absence of religious ideas and thinking in much of contemporary bioethical thought are John F. Kilner, Nigel M. de S. Cameron, and David L. Schiedermayer, eds., *Bioethics and the Future of Medicine: A Christian Appraisal* (Grand Rapids, MI: Eerdmans, 1995); and Allen Verhey, *Religion and Medical Ethics: Looking Back, Looking Forward* (Grand Rapids, MI: Eerdmans, 1996). See also Gilbert Meilaender, *Bioethics: A Primer for Christians* (Grand Rapids, MI: Eerdmans, 1996); Leon R. Kass, *Life, Liberty and the Defense of Dignity: The Challenge for Bioethics* (San Francisco: Encounter Books, 2002); and Eric Cohen, "Conservative Bioethics and the Search for Wisdom," *Hastings Center Report* 36, no. 1 (2006): 44–56.

CHAPTER 7   Anxiety in the Age of Epidemiology

1. Stephen Spender, *Poems* (London: Faber and Faber, 1933), p. 41.

2. Daniel Patrick Moynihan recognized long ago the implications of studying traffic fatalities as nonrandom events, which are useful to understand statistically for the purposes of the improvement of public policy based on such understanding. See Daniel Patrick Moynihan, "The War against the Automobile," *Public Interest*, Spring 1966, pp. 10–26.

3. Concerns about "the masses," exemplified in such classic writings as Gustav Le Bon's *The Crowd: A Study of the Popular Mind* (1896) and Ortega y Gasset's *The Revolt of the Masses* (1930) were expressed in opposition to social conformism. These kinds of elite anxieties presaged cultural criticisms of "dumbing down," for example. Those elites who once expressed alarm about overpopulation, or who today embrace the broad mandates of environmentalism, now promote a scientifically informed anxiety about human-created (i.e., "mass") dangers to the earth's environment.

4. The remarkable increase in public anxieties about nuclear war, and their rapid disappearance, is exemplified in such works as Ruth Adams and Susan Cullen, eds., *The Final Epidemic: Physicians and Scientists on Nuclear War* (Chicago: Educational Foundation for Nuclear Science, 1981), and Spencer R. Weart, *Nuclear Fear: A History of Images* (Cambridge: Harvard University Press, 1988).

5. A comprehensive history of modern epidemiology has yet to be written. An excellent place to begin is Mervyn Susser, *Causal Thinking in the Health Sciences* (New York: Oxford University Press, 1973), as well as Mervyn Susser, "Epidemiology in the United States after World War II: The Evolution of Technique," *Epidemiologic Reviews* 7 (1985): 147–77. See also Jay S. Kaufman, "Looking Back on 'Causal Thinking in the Health Sciences,'" *Annual Review of Public Health* 21 (May 2000): 101–19; and Mark Parascandola, "Epidemiology: Second-Rate Science?" *Public Health Reports* 113, no. 4 (1998): 312–20. For an excellent textbook introduction, see Paul D. Stolley and Tamar Lasky, *Investigating Disease Patterns: The Science of Epidemiology* (New York: Scientific American Library, 1995). See also William G. Rothstein, *Public Health and the Risk Factor: A History of an Uneven Medical Revolution* (Rochester, NY: University of Rochester, 2003).

6. See Thomas McKeown, *The Role of Medicine: Dream, Mirage, or Nemesis?* 2nd ed. (Princeton, NJ: Princeton University Press, 1979).

7. McKeown's arguments became the source for considerable debate, in particular, among quantitative historians of a new generation. See his *The Modern Rise of Population* (New York: Academic Press, 1976) and *The Origins of Human Disease* (Oxford: Basil Blackwell, 1988). See also Dorothy Porter, "The History of Public Health: Current Themes and Approaches," *Hygiea Internationalis* 1, no. 1 (1999): 9–21; and John Colgrove, "The McKeown Thesis: A Historical Controversy and Its Enduring Influence," in *American Journal of Public Health* 92 (2002): 725–29.

8. The *Journal of Chronic Diseases*, for example, was launched in 1955. See "The Changing Role of Chronic Disease," (pp. 86–87) which estimated that approximately four million people were suffering from serious chronic illness. *Journal of Chronic Diseases* 1 (January 1955).

9. Mrs. H. M. Plunkett, *Women, Plumbers, and Doctors; or, Household Sanitation* (New York: D. Appleton, 1885). See James H. Cassedy, "The Flamboyant Colonel Waring: An Anticontagionist Holds the American Stage in the Age of Pasteur and Koch," *Bulletin of the History of Medicine* 36 (1962): 163–76.

10. See Constance A. Nathanson, "Disease as Social Change: Toward a Theory of Public Health," *Population and Development Review* 22 (1996): 609–37.

11. Henry E. Sigerist, "Living under the Shadow," in *When Doctors are Patients*, ed. Max Pinner and Benjamin F. Miller (New York: Norton, 1952), p. 3.

12. For a little noticed but excellent overview of the "worried well" see Arthur J. Barsky, *Worried Sick: Our Troubled Quest for Wellness* (Boston: Little, Brown, 1988).

13. Jonathan R. Cole, "Dietary Cholesterol and Heart Disease: The Construction of a Medical 'Fact,'" in *Surveying Social Life: Papers in Honor of Herbert H. Hyman*, ed. Hubert J. O'Gorman (Middletown, CT: Wesleyan University Press, 1988), pp. 437–66.

14. McKeown, *The Role of Medicine*, pp. 135, 145, and 151. If such a revitalization has occurred, it is probably best understood at present as the renewed emphasis in medical education on what is called "bedside manner," which now invokes more than a half century of research on physician-patient communication.

15. See, for example, Russell, *Educated Guesses*.

16. See Sally Satel, "ADD Overdose," *Wall Street Journal*, July 23, 2003, p. A14.

17. Mark Twain, *The Adventures of Tom Sawyer* (New York: Harper and Brothers, 1903), pp. 126–27.

18. Theodor Adorno noted: "Nowadays it is altogether problematical to oppose mere opinion in the name of truth, because a fatal elective affinity has been established between the former and reality, which in turn proves useful to the stubborn rigidity of opinion. Certainly the opinion of the fool who moves her bed around her bedroom in order to shield herself from the danger of evil rays is pathogenic. But the risk of exposure in a radioactively contaminated world has grown so great that the anxiety is belatedly honored by the same faculty of reason that eschews its psychotic character. The objective world is approaching the image persecution mania renders of it." Theodor W. Adorno, "Opinion Delusion Society," in *Critical Models: Interventions and Catchwords*, trans. Henry W. Pickford (New York: Columbia University Press, 1998), p. 119.

19. The sociological literature on "risk" is extensive. An excellent overview is Iain Wilkinson, *Anxiety in a Risk Society* (New York: Routledge, 2001). For other

important statements, see Graham Burchell, Colin Gordon, and Peter Miller, eds., *The Foucault Effect: Studies in Governmentality* (Chicago: University of Chicago Press, 1991); Ulrich Beck, *Risk Society: Towards a New Modernity* (Thousand Oaks, CA: Sage, 1992); and Deborah Lupton, *Risk* (New York: Routledge, 1999).

20. No informed reader can afford to ignore the following works: Allan M. Brandt, "The Cigarette, Risk, and American Culture," *Daedalus* 119 (1990): 155–76; Allan M. Brandt, *The Cigarette Century: The Rise, Fall, and Deadly Persistence of the Product That Defined America* (New York: Basic Books, 2007); Lester Breslow, "Some Sequels to the Surgeon General's Report on Smoking and Health Thirty Years Later," *Annals of Epidemiology* 6 (1996): 372–75; John C. Burnham, "American Physicians and Tobacco Use: Two Surgeons General, 1929 and 1964," *Bulletin of the History of Medicine* 63 (1989): 1–31; Johannes Clemmesen, "Lung Cancer from Smoking: Delays and Attitudes, 1912–1965," *American Journal of Industrial Medicine* 23 (1993): 941–53; Richard Doll, "Uncovering the Effects of Smoking: Historical Perspective," *Statistical Methods in Medical Research* 7 (1998): 87–117; Richard Doll, "The First Reports on Smoking and Lung Cancer," in *Ashes to Ashes: The History of Smoking and Health*, ed. S. Lock, L. A. Reynolds and E. M. Tansey (Amsterdam: Rodopi, 1998), pp. 130–42; Michael J. McFarlane, "Evolution of the Epidemiology of Lung Cancer: A Twentieth Century Phenomenon," chapter 9 in *Lung Cancer: The Evolution of Concepts*, ed. John G. Gruhn and Steven T. Rosen, vol. 1 (New York: Field and Wood, 1989), pp. 219–39; Alton Ochsner, "My First Recognition of the Relationship of Smoking and Lung Cancer," *Preventive Medicine* 2 (1973): 611–14; John Parascandola, "The Surgeons General and Smoking," *Public Health Reports* 112 (1997): 440–42; Mark Parascandola, "Cigarettes and the US Public Health Service in the 1950s," *American Journal of Public Health* 91 (2001): 196–205; Stanley Joel Reiser, "Smoking and Health: The Congress and Causality," in *Knowledge and Power: Essays on Science and Government*, ed. Sanford A. Lakoff (New York: Free Press, 1966), pp. 293–311; Jesse L. Steinfeld, "Smoking and Lung Cancer: A Milestone in Awareness" (a commentary on E. L. Wynder and E. A. Graham, "Tobacco Smoking as a Possible Risk Factor in Bronchiogenic Carcinoma: A Study of 684 Proved Cases"), *JAMA* 253 (1985): 2995–97; Paul D. Stolley, "When Genius Errs: R. A. Fisher and the Lung Cancer Controversy," *American Journal of Epidemiology* 133 (1991): 416–26; Jan P. Vandenbroucke, "Those Who Were Wrong," *American Journal of Epidemiology* 130 (1989): 3–5; Colin White, "Research on Smoking and Lung Cancer: A Landmark in the History of Chronic Disease Epidemiology," *Yale Journal of Biology and Medicine* 63 (1990): 29–46; Ernst L. Wynder, "Tobacco as a Cause of Lung Cancer: Some Reflections," *American Journal of Epidemiology* 146 (1997): 687–94.

21. See David J. Rothman, "The Fielding H. Garrison Lecture: Serving Clio and Client: The Historian as Expert Witness," *Bulletin of the History of Medicine* 77 (2003): 25–44; and Jonathan D. Martin, "Historians at the Gate: Accommodating Expert Historical Testimony in Federal Courts," *New York University Law Review* 78 (2003): 1518–49. See also Colin Talley, Howard I. Kushner, and Claire E. Sterk, "Lung Cancer, Chronic Disease Epidemiology, and Medicine, 1948–1964," *Journal of the History of Medicine and Allied Sciences* 59, no. 3 (2004): 329–74; Allan M. Brandt, "From Analysis to Advocacy: Crossing Boundaries as a Historian of Health Policy," in Huisman

and Warner, *Locating Medical History*, pp. 460–84; and Robert N. Proctor, "'Everyone Knew but No One Had Proof': Tobacco Industry Use of Medical History Expertise in US Courts, 1990–2002," *Tobacco Control* 15, no. 6 (2006): iv117–iv125.

22. "Lung cancer accounts for more deaths than any other malignancy. Although the number of new cases in the United States is about the same as breast and prostate cancer, the number of deaths caused by lung cancer far exceeds those of the other two. Although screening is recommended for breast and prostate cancer, there are no such recommendations for lung cancer. This is surprising, because it is well documented that early diagnosis in all three results in higher cure rates than later, symptom-prompted diagnosis." Claudia I. Henschke, preface to "Lung Cancer," *Radiologic Clinics of North America* 38, no. 3 (2000): 452.

23. See, for example, Richard Kluger, *Ashes to Ashes: America's Hundred-Year Cigarette War, the Public Health, and the Unabashed Triumph of Philip Morris* (New York: Alfred A. Knopf, 1996); Cassandra Tate, *Cigarette Wars: The Triumph of "The Little White Slaver"* (New York: Oxford University Press, 1999); and Brandt, *The Cigarette Century*.

24. See Richard Klein, *Cigarettes Are Sublime* (Durham, NC: Duke University Press, 1993).

25. See Ronald J. Troyer and Gerald E. Markle, *Cigarettes: The Battle over Smoking* (New Brunswick, NJ: Rutgers University Press, 1983), and Jacob Sullum, *For Your Own Good: The Anti-smoking Crusade and the Tyranny of Public Health* (New York: Free Press, 1998).

26. One way to appreciate this difference is to compare the strategy of litigation, which is more recent, with earlier attempts to persuade smokers to quit. See Richard A. Daynard, "Tobacco Liability Litigation as a Cancer Control Strategy," *Journal of the National Cancer Institute* 80, no. 1 (1988): 9–13. See also Peter D. Jacobson and Kenneth E. Warner, "Litigation and Public Health Policy Making: The Case of Tobacco Control," *Journal of Health Politics, Policy and Law* 24 (1999): 769–804.

27. See Allan M. Brandt, "The Rise and Fall of the Cigarette: A Brief History of the Antismoking Movement in the United States," in *Advancing Health in Developing Countries: The Role of Social Research*, ed. Lincoln C. Chen, Arthur Kleinman, and Norma C. Ware (New York: Auburn House, 1992), pp. 59–77.

28. Alton Ochsner and Michael DeBakey, "Symposium on Cancer, Primary Pulmonary Malignancy, Treatment by Total Pneumonectomy, Analysis of 79 Collected Cases and Presentation of 7 Personal Cases," *Surgery, Gynecology, and Obstetrics* 68 (1939): 435. A similar effort to link smoking with health was published a year earlier by Raymond Pearl, whose interest was not lung cancer but rather longevity—the three greatest inhibitors of longevity were smoking, alcohol, and hard labor. See Raymond Pearl, "Tobacco Smoking and Longevity," *Science* 87, no. 2253 (1938): 216–17.

29. Among the various factors implicated in the causes of increased lung cancer were use of tobacco; exposure to pollutants such as automobile exhaust, dust and fumes; industrial pollution; air pollution from oil and coal furnaces; tars used in road construction; late sequelae of influenza and tuberculosis; occupation; radiation; and heredity. The apparent increase was attributed to better diagnosis; improved histological examination; and increased longevity of the population. See the first five

editions (1931, 1935, 1940, 1944, 1950) of William Boyd, *The Pathology of Internal Diseases* (Philadelphia: Lea and Febiger). See also William Boyd, *Lectures in Pathology* (Lawrence: University Extension Division, University of Kansas, 1939), p. 4: "Is the recent increase real? . . . The great majority of writers believe that the increase is real. I feel that it is only apparent. Neither side can prove their point. It becomes a matter of probability." And see Paul W. Schafer, *Pathology of General Surgery* (Chicago: University of Chicago Press, 1950), p. 219: "Little is known of its etiology, though many possible factors have been considered. Most of these are presumed to cause a chronic irritation of the respiratory membranes, and they include atmospheric pollution by tobacco smoke, exhaust gases, coal-tar products, and related substances, as well as the chronic inflammatory changes associated with lung abscess, tuberculosis, silicosis, bronchiectasis, and chronic bronchitis. Little evidence exists to incriminate any of the above causative factors." Finally, Richard Doll observed: "The enormous increase in mortality recorded since 1911 is, however, not all real. In part it is an artifact due to the improved methods of diagnosis that resulted from the successive introduction of chest x-rays, bronchoscopy, and open chest surgery, and the introduction of effective methods of treatment for pneumonia after the sulphonamide series of drugs began to be developed in 1936. . . . How much of the early increase in the mortality attributed to lung cancer was spurious and due to these changes and how much was real was debated hotly for many years." Richard Doll, "Major Epidemics of the 20th Century: From Coronary Thrombosis to AIDS," *Journal of the Royal Statistical Society*, ser. A (General), 150, no. 4 (1987): 377.

30. Alexander Gilliam, chief of the Epidemiology Section at the National Cancer Institute, wrote in 1955: "The International Lists of Causes of Death did not separately list cancer of the lung and pleura, or even cancer of the respiratory system as a whole, until the Fourth Revision,—first used in 1930. . . . It was not until the Fifth revision came into use in 1939 that deaths which physicians charged to bronchogenic cancer were separately identified in official statistics. . . . These changes in medical and in tabulation practices in an expanding Death Registration Area therefore make it impossible to determine the exact trend in this country of mortality attributed on death certificates to what is generally included as cancer of the lung." Alexander G. Gilliam, "Some Aspects of the Lung Cancer Problem," *Military Medicine* 116, no. 3 (1955): 164. It is clear now that the German researchers were ahead of American and British scientists on establishing a link between smoking and disease, but their findings were reported during the period of the Third Reich and thus received no attention. See Robert N. Proctor, "The Nazi War against Tobacco: Ideology, Evidence, and Possible Cancer," *Bulletin of the History of Medicine* 71 (1997): 435–88. See also Richard Doll, "Commentary: Long Cancer and Tobacco Consumption," *International Journal of Epidemiology* 30, no. 1 (2001): 30–31. Doll's commentary refers to an article published in Germany in 1943 (and translated for the first time in the same issue of the *International Journal of Epidemiology*) linking smoking and lung cancer.

31. Alton Ochsner and Michael DeBakey, "Carcinoma of the Lung," *Archives of Surgery* 42, no. 2 (1941): 221.

32. John Wilds and Ira Harkey, Alton Ochsner, *Surgeon of the South* (Baton Rouge: Louisiana State University Press, 1990), p. 177.

33. Ochsner and his associates published various case study reports throughout the 1940s, sometimes citing the association between carcinoma and tobacco production and smoking. In later reports, based always on a review of clinical cases, they were less persuaded by the evidence. See Alton Ochsner and Michael DeBakey, "Primary Carcinoma of the Lung," *New Orleans Medical and Surgical Journal* 93, no. 8 (1941): 387–95; Alton Ochsner, J. Leonard Dixon, and Michael DeBakey, "Primary Bronchiogenic Carcinoma: An Analysis of 190 Cases, 58 of Which Were Successfully Treated by Pneumonectomy, with a Review of the Literature," *Clinics* 3 (1945):1187–1245; Alton Ochsner, J. Leonard Dixon, and Michael DeBakey, "Primary Bronchiogenic Carcinoma," *Diseases of the Chest* 11, no. 2 (1945): 97–129. Two articles that acknowledged implicitly the limits of generalization from clinical observation were Alton Ochsner, Michael E. DeBakey, and Leonard Dixon, "Primary Pulmonary Malignancy Treated by Resection, An Analysis of 129 Cases," *Annals of Surgery* 125, no. 5 (1947): 522–40: "In the 129 resected cases no factor was found which might bear a significant relationship to the occurrence of the disease. Neither occupation nor smoking habits, which some reports, including our own, have stressed as of possible etiologic significance, seemed of any special significance in this particular series" (p. 525); and Alton Ochsner, Michael E. DeBakey, and Irving M. Richman, "Bronchiogenic Carcinoma," *Southern Surgeon* 14, no. 8 (1948): 595–604: "Although we were previously aware of the opinion that the chronic irritation resulting from excessive cigarette smoking was a factor, this cannot be proved. However, the fact there is a parallelism between the number of cigarettes sold in the United States and the increased incidence of bronchiogenic carcinoma is interesting" (p. 596).

34. U.S. Department of Health and Human Services, *Reducing Tobacco Use: A Report of the Surgeon General* (Washington, DC: U.S. Department of Health and Human Services, Centers for Disease Control and Prevention, National Center for Chronic Disease Prevention and Health Promotion, Office of Smoking and Health, 2000), p. 38. The quotation "an anti-smoking enthusiast" is from Burnham, "Physicians and Tobacco Use," p. 18. Further evidence of Ochsner's religious motivations is found in his "The Death of a Smoker," released in the Great Sermon series, Word Records, Waco, Texas, in the 1960s. The phonograph record also included a transcript of his talk.

35. See John C. Burnham, *Bad Habits: Drinking, Smoking, Taking Drugs, Gambling, Sexual Misbehavior, and Swearing in American History* (New York: New York University Press, 1993).

36. Wynder's own account provides one of the best introductions to his multiple contributions. Ernst L. Wynder, "The Past, Present, and Future of the Prevention of Lung Cancer," *Cancer Epidemiology Biomarkers and Prevention* 7, no. 9 (1998): 735–48.

37. There are many useful accounts of these developments, the best by Doll and Hill themselves, already cited in note 20. See also Richard Doll, "Sir Austin Bradford Hill and the Progress of Medicine," *British Medical Journal* 305 (1992): 1521–26; and Richard Doll, "Sir Austin Bradford Hill: A Personal View of His Contribution to Epidemiology," *Journal of the Royal Statistical Society*, ser. A (Statistics in Society), 158, no. 1 (1995): 155–63. Hill's own contributions to statistical thinking are best

exemplified in A. Bradford Hill, "Observation and Experiment," *New England Journal of Medicine* 248 (1953): 995–1001; and Sir Austin Bradford Hill, "The Environment and Disease: Association or Causation?" (President's Address Section of Occupational Medicine), *Proceedings of the Royal Society of Medicine* 58 (May 1965): 295–300. And see the entire issue of *Statistics in Medicine* 1, no. 4 (1984), which includes a bibliography of Hill's work.

38. Doll provides an overview of the methodological virtues and problems with both retrospective and prospective studies in Richard Doll, "Retrospective and Prospective Studies," in *Medical Surveys and Clinical Trials*, ed. L. J. Witts, 2nd ed.(London: Oxford University Press, 1964), pp. 71–98.

39. It is interesting to note that animal studies of the toxic effects of alcohol on living tissue were conducted in the late nineteenth century but were unsuccessful in establishing a link between alcohol and cirrhosis of the liver. See Thomas S. Chen and Peter S. Chen, *Understanding the Liver: A History* (Westport, CT: Greenwood, 1984), p. 132.

40. Ernest L. Wynder, Evarts A. Graham, and Adele B. Croninger, "Experimental Production of Carcinoma with Cigarette Tar," *Cancer Research* 13 (1953): 855–64. See also Ernest L. Wynder and Dietrich Hoffman, *Tobacco and Tobacco Smoke: Studies in Experimental Carcinogenesis* (New York: Academic Press, 1967). During this period, far and away the most serious criticism of such studies was by the chief pathologist of the National Cancer Institute, Harold Stewart. See Harold L. Stewart and Katherine M. Herrold, "A Critique of Experiments on Attempts to Induce Cancer with Tobacco Derivative," *Bulletin de L'Institut International de Statistique* 39 (1962): 457–77. Richard Doll observed, "To cancer research workers the obstacle was the failure to have identified any known carcinogen in smoke and the lack of firm evidence that tobacco smoke could produce lung cancer in experimental animals, while physicians had no understanding of the power and validity of large-scale case-control studies in the investigation of non-infectious disease" ("First Reports on Smoking," p. 136). More recent debates over cancer risk with respect to experimental carcinogenesis in particular are presented in detail in D. A. Freedman and H. Zeisel, "From Mouse-to-Man: The Quantitative Assessment of Cancer Risks," *Statistical Science* 3, no. 1 (1988): 3–28.

41. Wynder's reputation in light of present-day tobacco litigation has been challenged because he held out for a "safer" cigarette. See Nicole Fields and S. Chapman, "Chasing Ernst L. Wynder: 40 Years of Philip Morris' Efforts to Influence a Leading Scientist," *Journal of Epidemiology and Community Health* 57 (2003): 571–78. See also Ernst L. Wynder, "Some Concepts of the Less Harmful Cigarette," in *A Safe Cigarette?* ed. Gio B. Gori and Fred G. Bock (Cold Spring Harbor, NY: Cold Spring Harbor Laboratory, 1980), pp. 3–12.

42. On the first twenty years of NCI, see Michael B. Shimkin, "As Memory Serves—an Informal History of the National Cancer Institute, 1937–57," *Journal of the National Cancer Institute* 59, no. 2 (suppl.) (1977): 559–600. For background on ACS, see Victor A. Triolo and Michael B. Shimkin, "The American Cancer Society and Cancer Research Origins and Organization: 1913–1943," *Cancer Research* 29 (1969): 1615–40.

43. See James T. Patterson, *The Dread Disease: Cancer and Modern American Culture* (Cambridge: Harvard University Press, 1987).

44. E. Cuyler Hammond and Daniel Horn, "Tobacco and Lung Cancer," in *Cancer of the Lung (Endemiology), A Symposium*, ed. J. Clemmesen (Paris: C.I.O.M.S., 1953), pp. 81–85.

45. E. Cuyler Hammond, "The Place of Tobacco in the Etiology of Lung Cancer," in *CA, A Bulletin of Cancer Progress*, March 1954, p. 49.

46. Ibid., p. 52.

47. Around the same time as controversy began to grow about cigarettes, economic assessments of the costs of traffic accidents were already becoming important in guiding public safety campaigns. See D. J. Reynolds, "The Cost of Road Accidents," *Journal of the Royal Statistical Society*, ser. A (General), part 4 (1956): 393–408.

48. *New York Times*, June 5, 1957, p. 1.

49. Ibid., p. 25.

50. From the standpoint of technical matters pertaining to the research design and results of prospective studies, Sir Richard Doll observed in 1984, "If Hammond and Horn's article ["Smoking and Death Rates: Report on 44 Months of Follow-up of 187,783 Men," part 1, "Total Mortality," *JAMA* 166 (1958): 1159–72; part 2, "Death rates by cause," *JAMA* 166 (1958): 1294–1308] is to be criticized at all, and it would be unrealistic to think that any article covering such a vast and important field would not be open to some criticism, it is that the authors failed to discuss the extent to which the excess mortality observed in the different categories of smoker was actually due to the habit and how far it might be possible to explain it by other factors associated with it, such as alcohol consumption, an extrovert personality, or a modified diet. These possibilities would have opened up a wide field of debate, and the authors were perhaps wise in leaving it for readers to assess them for themselves, or it would have been impossible to keep the article within the limits that would be acceptable to an editor. Even now, alternative explanations for some of the excess rates observed have not been fully disposed of, but the mass of other evidence, that has been collected makes it clear that if they do play a part it is one that is synergistic with smoking (as in the case of alcohol) or is relatively small." Richard Doll, "Smoking and Death Rates," *JAMA* 251 (1984): 2857.

51. David M. Spain, "The Duty of the Physician towards His Patients in Regard to Cigarette Smoking," *CA*, March–April 1959, p. 62.

52. "Lung Cancer Prevention and the Physician," *CA*, March–April 1960, p. 54.

53. Howard C. Taylor, "Physicians and Cigarette Smoking," *CA*, January–February 1963, p. 43. Taylor also observed that "The vast majority of physicians, however, have with respect to this problem claimed the layman's privilege of ignorance. 'We are not cancer researchers or specialists in the diseases of the heart or chest.' 'We do not have any opinion because we haven't bothered to study the evidence'" (p. 43).

54. Thomas G. Harvey, "Is This the Negligent Physician?" *CA*, March–April 1963, p. 75.

55. In 1975, Dr. Richard C. Bates proposed that medical school admissions committees not accept applicants who smoked. In 1983, he insisted that "Philosophically, then, a physician who smokes is marketing a product, health preservation, that he

does not buy and use himself. He is in the position of a policeman who breaks the law; a clergyman who sins; an accountant who over-draws his checking account; a banker who goes bankrupt, or a Ford dealer who drives Chevrolets." "Doctors Who Smoke," *New York State Journal of Medicine* 83 (1983): 1294. This issue of the *New York State Journal of Medicine* was devoted in its entirety to "The World Cigarette Pandemic."

56. See History of Cancer Control Project, UCLA School of Public Health, principal researcher and writer Larry Agran, *A History of Cancer Control in the United States, 1946–1971*, vol. 1: *A History of Scientific and Technical Advances in Cancer Control* (Washington, DC: Dept. of Health, Education, and Welfare, Public Health Service, National Institutes of Health, National Cancer Institute, Division of Cancer Control and Rehabilitation, 1978), chap. 3, "Tobaccogenic Cancer," pp. 169–95.

57. See Hill, "The Environment and Disease."

58. "The plausibility of the causal hypothesis is assessed, not in terms of the results of one particular study or a 'crucial experiment,' but in terms of the totality of available biologic evidence." Abraham M. Lillienfeld, "'On the Methodology of Investigations of Etiologic Factors in Chronic Diseases'"—Some Comments," p. 46, which follows J. Yerushalmy, and Carroll E. Palmer, "On the Methodology of Investigations of Etiologic Factors in Chronic Diseases," *Journal of Chronic Diseases* 10 (July 1959): 27–46.

59. Physicians' opinions about abortion in the heyday of the liberalization of abortion laws were interestingly more "conservative" the more likely they might be personally faced with a request to perform one. See Imber, *Abortion and Private Practice*, pp. 24–30.

60. "Professional Briefs," *Medical Economics* 42 (1965): 218.

61. Joseph Gusfield, "The Social Symbolism of Smoking and Health," in *Smoking Policy: Law, Politics, and Culture*, ed. Robert L. Rabin and Stephen D. Sugarman (New York: Oxford University Press, 1993), esp. pp. 54–55.

62. See K. A. Brownlee, "A Review of 'Smoking and Health," *Journal of the American Statistical Association* 60 (1965): 722–39. A great deal more could be written about the relatively few "hold-outs" not persuaded by the cumulating evidence against cigarettes. As one of the leading clinical epidemiologists, Alvan R. Feinstein, remarked about one of them, P.R.J. Burch, "Regardless of whether or not one agrees with Burch's conclusions, he displays admirable courage in being willing to raise public questions about an epidemiological doctrine that has become so firmly entrenched as to seem almost like a religious dogma. With a professional home in medical physics, Professor Burch may not risk being burnt at an epidemiological stake, but his heresy will surely be thoroughly denounced." P.R.J. Burch, "Smoking and Lung Cancer: The Problem of Inferring Cause," *Journal of the Royal Statistical Society* 141 no. 4 (1978): 437–77 (includes discussion, pp. 458–77), p. 468. To appreciate Burch's reputation, it is only necessary to see that he engaged in exchanges with Richard Doll and Abraham Lillienfeld, both leading researchers and highly respected leaders in epidemiology. See P.R.J. Burch, "Does Smoking Cause Lung Cancer?" *New Scientist*, February 21, 1974, pp. 458–63; along with Richard Doll, "Smoking, Lung Cancer and Occam's Razor" *New Scientist*, February 21, 1974, pp. 463–67. See

also P.R.J. Burch, "The Surgeon-General's 'Epidemiologic Criteria for Causality': A Critique," *Journal of Chronic Diseases* 36 (1983): 821–36; along with Abraham M. Lillienfeld. "The Surgeon General's Epidemiologic Criteria for Causality: A Criticism of Burch's Critique. *Journal of Chronic Diseases* 36 (1983): 837–45; and P.R.J. Burch. "The Surgeon-General's 'Epidemiologic Criteria for Causality': Reply to Lillienfeld," *Journal of Chronic Diseases* 37 (1984): 148–57.

63. For example, such matters as masturbation and circumcision, as a result of medical and social epidemiology scrutiny, are no longer exclusively condemned or approved in religious and moral terms. See Allan M. Brandt and Paul Rozin, eds., *Morality and Health* (New York: Routledge, 1997).

64. John Passmore, *The Perfectibility of Man* (London: Duckworth, 1970), p. 174n.

65. Ibid., p. 276. Carl Elliott, in much of his work, has substantially borne out Passmore's insight, in turn indebted to Freud. See *Better Than Well: American Medicine Meets the American Dream* (New York: Norton, 2003). See also Carl Elliott, *A Philosophical Disease: Bioethics, Culture and Identity* (New York: Routledge, 1998).

66. See Dutton, *Worse Than the Disease*.

67. Roberta J Apfel and Susan M. Fisher, *To Do No Harm: DES and the Dilemmas of Modern Medicine* (New Haven: Yale University Press, 1985).

68. See Michael D. Green, *Bendectin and Birth Defects: The Challenges of Mass Toxic Substances Litigation* (Philadelphia: University of Pennsylvania Press, 1996); and Joseph Sanders, *Bendectin on Trial: A Study of Mass Tort Litigation* (Ann Arbor: University of Michigan Press, 1998).

69. With regard to general health, among the early but now largely dismissed contenders was coffee. See Brian MacMahon and Takashi Sugimura, eds., *Coffee and Health* (Cold Springs Harbor, NY: Cold Spring Harbor Laboratory, 1984). But research into the refinement of associations between coffee and health has produced numerous other studies, such as Jørn Olsen, Kim Overvad, and Grethe Frische, "Coffee Consumption, Birthweight, and Reproductive Failures," *Epidemiology* 2, no. 5 (1991): 370–74. For accounts and critiques of health promotion and the regulation of "lifestyle," see Michael S. Goldstein, *The Health Movement: Promoting Fitness in America* (New York: Twayne, 1992); Deborah Lupton, *The Imperative of Health: Public Health and the Regulated Body* (Thousand Oaks, CA: Sage, 1995); and Michael Fitzpatrick, *The Tyranny of Health: Doctors and the Regulation of Lifestyle* (New York: Routledge, 2001).

70. Alvan R. Feinstein, "Scientific Standards in Epidemiologic Studies of the Menace of Daily Life," *Science* 242, no. 4883 (1988): 1257–63.

71. Ibid., p. 1262.

72. For a classic account of the historical development of clinical research, see J. P. Bull, "The Historical Development of Clinical Therapeutic Trials," *Journal of Chronic Diseases* 10 (September 1959): 218–48.

73. Letters, *Science* 243, Issue 4896 (1989): 1255.

74. Ibid., p. 1256.

75. Ibid.

76. Taubes has written in the tradition of scientific muckraking that has provoked enthusiastic supporters and critics. See his *Nobel Dreams: Power, Deceit, and*

the Ultimate Experiment (New York: Random House, 1987), and *Bad Science: The Short Life and Weird Times of Cold Fusion* (New York: Random House, 1993).

77. Gary Taubes, "Epidemiology Faces Its Limits," *Science* 269, no. 5221 (1995): 164–65, 167–69.

78. The growth of the phenomenon of reporting of risks in medical journals is examined by John-Arne Skolbekken, "The Risk Epidemic in Medical Journals," *Social Science and Medicine* 40, no. 3 (1995): 291–305. And see David B. Resnik, "Ethical Dilemmas in Communicating Medical Information to the Public," *Health Policy* 55 (2001): 129–49. In one study of the reporting of medical news, the authors concluded that "editors need to be familiar with the context of medical research and be sensitive to the presence of special interest groups competing for a voice in the direction of the medical profession." Edward Caudill and Paul Ashdown, "The *New England Journal of Medicine* as News Source," *Journalism Quarterly* 66 (1989): 462. See also Suzan M. DiBella, Anthony J. Ferri, and Allan B. Padderud, "Scientists' Reasons for Consenting to Mass Media Interviews: A National Survey," *Journalism Quarterly* 68 (1991): 740–49.

79. See Irwin D. Bross, "Why Proof of Safety Is Much More Difficult Than Proof of Hazard," *Biometrics* 41 (1985): 785–93. See also Steven P. Millard, "Proof of Safety vs Proof of Hazard," *Biometrics* 43 (1987): 719–24, along with Bross's response, pp. 724–25.

80. Mervyn Susser has described the origins of this uncertainty in the rise of public health, in alliance with the state, during the nineteenth century: "Its originality was to attack disease and poverty in the community at large at their perceived source in the environment. Previously the positive pursuit of health had found a place in the teachings of Galen, and those who followed him, at an individual level only. The pursuit of community health at the population level was something new, and the assumption of state responsibility for maintaining community health was equally so (if one puts aside the acute emergencies of plague and other epidemics)." Mervyn Susser, "Ethical Components in the Definition of Health," *International Journal of Health Services* 4 (1974): 545.

81. The letter was signed by Walter Willett, Sander Greenland, Brian MacMahon, Dimitrios Trichopoulos, Ken Rothman, David Thomas, Michael Thun, and Noel Weiss. *Science* 269, no. 5229 (1995): 1325–26.

82. "Perhaps the decline of both magic and religion in the modern Western world, coupled with the human need for meaningful accounts, particularly of misfortunes, has led to modern Western hypersensitivities to the principal moral doctrine of doing no harm to others. With the expansion of epidemiological research and identification of risk factors, there are opportunities for exquisite subtleties" Paul Rozin, "The Process of Moralization," *Psychological Science* 10, no. 3 (1999): 220.

83. The faith in equality that inspires certain segments of contemporary epidemiology is based on the following observation: "The lower one is situated in the social hierarchy, as defined by work, lodging, education, income, or whatever, the lower one's probability of staying in good health and the lower one's life expectancy. This is the most frequent and most pervasive of all the observations made in the history of public health research (Haan, Kaplan, and Syme, 1989)." Quoted in Marc

Renaud, "The Future: Hygeia versus Panakeia?" in *Why Are Some People Healthy and Others Not? The Determinants of Health of Populations*, ed. Robert G. Evans, Morris L. Barer, and Theodore R. Marmor (New York: Aldine de Gruyter, 1994), p. 322. See M. N. Haan, G. A. Kaplan, and S. L. Syme, "Socioeconomic Status and Health: Old Observations and New Thoughts," in *Pathways to Health: The Role of Social Factors*, ed. J. P. Bunker, D. S. Gomby, and B. H. Kehere (Menlo Park, CA: Henry J. Kaiser Family Foundation, 1989), pp. 76–138. The documentation of inequalities in the provision of health services has rapidly become one of the defining features of contemporary social epidemiology. The increase in medical screening, a form of social monitoring, has produced massive amounts of data, presenting significant problems of cost for public health policy. Even as such screening promises to identify more and more people with disease, the expense incurred in finding everyone with disease seems likely only to increase as more and more diseases become identifiable over time. Finally, it is important to see that the calls for greater "equity" in health care come from the same end of the political spectrum where numerous dissenting traditions about the virtues of medical progress have long resided. The sheer enthusiasm of the liberal politics that drove the efforts of health care reform (e.g., plans for greater equity in the delivery of services) during the first Clinton administration helped to conceal numerous forms of other dissatisfactions with technological medicine, including objections to technology and medicalization per se, instead of the problem of social equity.

CHAPTER 8   Trust and Mortality

1. The epigram is attributed to Callicter and Nicarchus. The translation used here, by H. Wellesley, appears in John Booth, ed., *Epigrams, Ancient and Modern* (London: Longmans, Green, 1865), p. 3. The following translation is given in Norman Douglas, *Birds and Beasts of the Greek Anthology* (New York: J. Cape and H. Smith, 1929): "Feeling slightly feverish, I happened to remember the name of Doctor Pheidon; and straight-way died" (p. 198), and quoted in Herbert Silvette, *The Doctor on the Stage: Medicine and Medical Men in Seventeenth-Century England* (Knoxville: University of Tennessee Press, 1967), p. 246. For the original Greek, see Hermann Beckby, ed., *Anthologia Graeca* (Munich: Ernst Heimeran, 1957), xi.118, p. 604. A more literal translation might be, "Phidon did not give me a clyster or lay hands on me, but when I had a fever, I thought of his name and died." My thanks to Mary R. Lefkowitz and Sir Hugh Lloyd-Jones. See also *Satire and Caricature in Medical History*, Historical Series, 4th supplement (Yonkers, NY: New York Pharmacal Association et al., 1928); and Andreas Weber, *Tableau de la Caricature Médicale depuis les Origines jusqu'à Nos Jours* (Paris: Hippocrate, 1936).

2. H. Bunker Wright and Monroe K. Spears, eds., *The Literary Works of Matthew Prior*, vol. 1 (Oxford: Clarendon Press, 1959), p. 410. Prior also wrote, "You tell your doctor, that y'are ill / And what does he, but write a bill." Quoted in Dorothy Porter and Roy Porter, *Patient's Progress: Doctors and Doctoring in Eighteenth-Century England* (Stanford, CA: Stanford University Press, 1989), p. 57. A long tradition of aphorisms specific to medical treatment also exists. See Sir Humphry Rolleston, "Medical Aphorisms Chiefly in English," *Bulletin of the History of Medicine*, 10 (1941): 544–67.

3. "To Doctor James Craik," September 8, 1789, in *The Writings of George Washington* (Washington, DC: USGPO, 1939), 30:396.

4. Ibid., "To James McHenry," p. 351.

5. See John C. Burnham, "American Medicine's Golden Age: What Happened to It?" *Science* 215 (1982): 1474–79. For a more recent account, taking this theme to heart and to task, see Brandt and Gardner, "Golden Age of Medicine?"

6. Burnham, "American Medicine's Golden Age," p. 1476. Burnham's account lays out important elements of what I examine here, including his discussion of the physician's "sacredotal role."

7. Osler's canonization as a medical saint has been assured in recent years by the publication of the proceedings of the American Osler Society. See Jeremiah A. Barondess, John P. McGovern, Charles G. Roland, eds., *The Persisting Osler: Selected Transactions of the First Ten Years of the American Osler Society* (Baltimore: University Park Press, 1985); and Jeremiah A. Barondess and Charles G. Roland, eds., *The Persisting Osler II: Selected Transactions of the American Osler Society, 1981–1990* (Malabar, FL: Krieger, 1994). Fifteen years after his death, Osler's reputation was still so highly regarded that David Israel Macht subtitled his study of the Jewish physician, Moses Maimonides, "The William Osler of Mediaeval Arabic and Hebrew Medicine." See *Bulletin of the Institute of the History of Medicine* 3, no. 7 (1935): 585–98. See also Wilburt C. Davison, "The Basis of Sir William Osler's Influence on Medicine," *Annals of Allergy* 27 (August 1969): 366–72.

8. See W. Bruce Fye, M.D., "William Osler's Departure from North America: The Price of Success," reprinted from the *New England Journal of Medicine* 320 (1989):1425, in Barondess and Roland, *The Persisting Osler II*, pp. 245–57.

9. Harvey Cushing, *The Life of Sir William Osler*, 2 vols. (Oxford: Clarendon Press, 1925), 1:664–74.

10. N. John Hall, *Anthony Trollope: A Biography* (Oxford: Clarendon Press, 1991), p. 485. Hall refers to Robert Tracy, *Trollope's Later Novels* (Berkeley and Los Angeles: University of California Press, 1978), p. 285. See *Massinger, Middleton, and Rowley, The Excellent Comedy Called, The Old Law, or, A New Way to Please You* (London: Printed for Edward Archer, 1656). See also Bradford A. Booth, *Anthony Trollope: Aspects of His Life and Art* (Bloomington: Indiana University Press, 1958), p. 129.

11. Anthony Trollope, *The Fixed Period* (1882; New York: Penguin, 1993), p. 39.

12. Ibid., p. 176.

13. Tracy, *Trollope's Later Novels*, p. 287. See Donald Smalley, ed., *Trollope: The Critical Heritage* (London: Routledge and Kegan Paul, 1969), pp. 487–92.

14. Hall, *Anthony Trollope*, p. 487.

15. See David Skilton, "The Fixed Period: Anthony Trollope's Novel of 1980," *Studies in the Literary Imagination* 6 (Fall 1973): 46.

16. In fact, Trollope's proposed means of departure was not chloroform. "As to the actual mode of transition, there had been many discussions held by the executive in President Square, and it had at last been decided that certain veins should be opened while the departing one should, under the influence of morphine, be gently entranced with a warm bath. I, as president of the empire, had agreed to use the

lancet in the first two or three cases, thereby intending to increase the honors conferred" (*The Fixed Period*, pp. 39–40).

17. William Osler, "The Fixed Period," in *Aequanimitas*, pp. 381–83.

18. *New York Times*, February 27, 1905, p. 1. For accounts of this episode, see Henry R. Viets, "William Osler and 'The Fixed Period,'" *Bulletin of the History of Medicine* 36 (1962): 368–70; Steven L. Berk, M.D., "Sir William Osler, Ageism, and 'The Fixed Period': A Secret Revealed," *Journal of the American Gerontological Society* 37 (1989): 263–66, reprinted in Barondess and Roland, *The Persisting Osler II*, pp. 297–301; Michael Bliss, *William Osler: A Life in Medicine* (New York: Oxford University Press, 1999), pp. 321–28.

19. William Osler, preface to *Aequanimitas*, p. viii. An early biographer of Osler noted that his convictions about such matters were deeply self-referential, attributing their strength to his own early maturity. See Edith Gittings Reid, *The Great Physician: A Short Life of Sir William Osler* (London: Oxford University Press, 1931), pp. 174–77.

20. See David B. Hogan, "Sir William Osler: Fixed Terms, Fixed Ideas, and 'Fixed Period,'" *Annals of the Royal College of Physicians and Surgeons of Canada* 28, no. 1 (1995): 25–29.

21. See Eliot Freidson, *Professionalism: The Third Logic* (Chicago: University of Chicago Press, 2001).

22. See George Ritzer and David Walczak, "Rationalization and the Deprofessionalization of Physicians," *Social Forces* 67, no. 1 (1988): 1–21. Bernhard J. Stern already noted a trend in the increase of salaried physicians between the late 1920s and early 1940s (*American Medical Practice*, p. 100).

23. See Burnham, *Idea of Profession*. See also Arthur Isak Applbaum, *Ethics for Adversaries: The Morality of Roles in Public and Professional Life* (Princeton, NJ: Princeton University Press, 1999), esp. chap. 3, "Doctor, Schmoctor: Practice Positivism and Its Complications," pp. 45–60.

24. Anyone who doubts O'Connor's special concern for these matters need only consult her concurring opinion in *Washington, et al, Petitioners 96–110 v. Harold Glucksberg et al.* and *Dennis C. Vacco, Attorney General of New York, et al., Petitioners 95–1858 v. Timothy E. Quill et al.*: "Death will be different for each of us. For many, the last days will be spent in physical pain and perhaps the despair that accompanies physical deterioration and a loss of control of basic bodily and mental functions. . . . Every one of us at some point may be affected by our own or a family member's terminal illness." See Susan M. Behuniak, *A Caring Jurisprudence: Listening to Patients at the Supreme Court* (Lanham, MD: Rowman and Littlefield, 1999).

25. James T. Stephens and Edward LeRoy Long, Jr., *The Christian as a Doctor* (New York: Association Press, 1960), p. 54. See *JAMA* 171:16 (December 19, 1959): p. 147.

26. Stephens and Long, *Christian as Doctor*, p. 55. See "Old Fashioned Doctors Disliked, Poll Shows," *New York Times*, December 30, 1958, p. 20.

27. Marilyn Chase, "Health Journal," *Wall Street Journal*, September 23, 1996, p. B1. See Janice Hopkins Tanne, "The Best Doctors in America," *American Health*, March 1996, pp. 61–88. The phenomenon of "best lists" in medicine is not reserved to physicians. See *U.S. News and World Report*, September 2, 1996, "America's Top HMOs: The First Rigorous Assessment of Quality, State by State."

28. *Wall Street Journal*, September 23, 1996, p. B1.

29. Charles L. Bosk, *Forgive and Remember*, p. 192.

30. Peter Sloterdijk, *The Critique of Cynical Reason* , trans. Michael Eldred (1983; London: Verso, 1988), p. 267.

31. Max Weber, "Science as a Vocation," in *From Max Weber: Essays in Sociology*, ed. and trans. H. H. Gerth and C. Wright Mills (London: Routlege and Kegan Paul), p. 144.

32. A report on Julie De Rossi, whose death in an accident at the age of forty-four resulted in the donation of her organs and tissues to a federally regulated, non-profit organ and tissue procurement center in Houston, came to light as the result of the donation of her Achilles' tendon for use in a surgery to repair the left knee of the top-paid player in the National Football League, Carson Palmer. See "Unlikely Support System for Bengals' Palmer," *New York Times*, August 9, 2006. In contrast, a more obviously sordid account of the "tissue-processing" industry came to light because of whose body was "surgically plundered." See Michael Brick, "Alistair Cooke's Bones Were Stolen for Implantation, His Family Says," *New York Times*, December 23, 2005, p. A23. Cooke's daughter, Susan Cooke Kittredge, later wrote an op-ed, "Black Shrouds and Black Markets," *New York Times*, March 5, 2006, sec. 4, p. 15.

33. The debate on how to reduce the scarcity of organs for transplant is examined well by Sally Satel, "Supply, Demand, and Kidney Transplants," *Policy Review* 144 (August–September 2007): 59–69.

34. See L. A. Siminoff, R. M. Arnold, A. L. Caplan, B. A. Virnig, and D. L. Seltzer. "Public Policy Governing Organ and Tissue Procurement in the United States: Results from the National Organ and Tissue Procurement Study," *Annals of Internal Medicine* 123, no. 1 (1995): 10–17.

35. An earlier generation, less taken up by the progress of litigation and the public exposure in the media, used such terms as "sanctity" and "sacredness," which have altogether disappeared from the discourse of mainstream bioethics. See *Life or Death: Ethics and Options* (Seattle: University of Washington Press, 1968), with essays by Edward Shils, Norman St. John-Stevas, Paul Ramsey, P. B. Medawar, Henry K. Beecher, and Abraham Kaplan. See also David Daube, "Sanctity of Life," *Proceedings of the Royal Society of Medicine*, vol. 60 (London, 1967), pp. 1245–40, reprinted in *All Heal: A Medical and Social Miscellany* (London: Heinemann Medical Books for the Royal Society of Medicine, 1971), pp. 135–45.

36. See Edwin Rembert Dubose, Jr., "The Illusion of Trust: A Phenomenological and Theological Investigation of the Medical Profession's Fiduciary Commitment," Ph.D. diss., Rice University, 1990. See also Bradford H. Gray, "Trust and Trustworthy Care in the Managed Care Era" *Health Affairs* 16, no. 1 (1997): 34–49.

37. Gilbert Meilander, *The Nature of Suffering and the Goals of Medicine*, by Eric J. Cassell, *Commentary*, April 1992, p. 60.

38. See Elliott, *Better Than Well*.

39. Sigmund Freud, *Civilization and Its Discontents*, in *The Standard Edition of the Complete Psychological Works of Sigmund Freud* (London: Hogarth Press, 1961), 21:90–91.

40. Friedrich Nietzsche, *Twilight of the Idols or How to Philosophize with a Hammer* (New York: Penguin, 1968), p. 88.

41. William Edward Hartpole Lecky, *The Map of Life: Conduct and Character* (New York: Longmans, Green, 1899), pp. 340–41. In 1923, John Galsworthy wrote: "Curious, by the way, that we should have a prayer against sudden death; and if our Litany were to be revised, suffrage would convert it. Most of us would now prefer to have our lives blown out as a man blows out a candle; choose to burn steadily to a swift last, instead of with a flickering sorrowful dwindling of our flames into darkness that we can see creeping round us. 'To sudden death, not premature, O Fate, deliver us!' would run our prayer." "Burning Leaves," in *In Castles in Spain and Other Screeds* (New York: Scribner's, 1927), p. 188.

42. James, *Varieties of Religious Experience*, pp. 239–40.

43. See Herbert Spiegelberg, "'Accident of Birth': A Non-utilitarian Motif in Mill's Philosophy," *Journal of the History of Ideas* 22 (1961): 135–46, reprinted in *Steppingstones Toward an Ethics for Fellow Existers: Essays, 1944–1984* (Dordrecht: Martinus Nijhoff, 1986), pp. 107–30.

44. Bernard Shaw, *Doctors' Delusions, Crude Criminology, and Sham Education* (London: Constable, 1932), p. 1.

45. See Tom Verducci and Lester Monson, "What Happened to Ted Williams?" *Sports Illustrated*, August 8, 2003, pp. 66–73.

46. Information about both facilities can be found at their respective websites: http://www.alcor.org/ and http://www.cryonics.org/refs.html.

47. http://www.cryonics.org/whatsnew.html.

48. "A Cold Calculus Leads Cryonauts to Put Assets on Ice," *Wall Street Journal*, January 21–22, 2006, A1, A7.

49. See Lewis D. Solomon, *The Quest for Human Longevity: Science, Business, and Public Policy* (New Brunswick, NJ: Transaction, 2006).

50. See Stephen G. Post and Robert H. Binstock, eds., *The Fountain of Youth: Cultural, Scientific, and Ethical Perspectives on a Biomedical Goal* (New York: Oxford University Press, 2004).

51. See Sidney Perkowitz, *Digital People: From Bionic Humans to Androids* (Washington, DC: Joseph Henry Press, National Academies Press, 2004).

52. The resonance of the desire to please one's mother with the latest news from the Cryonics Institute about sons cryopreserving their mothers should not go unobserved.

53. See Leon Kass, "Mortality," in *Powers that Make us Human: The Foundations of Medical Ethics*, ed. Kenneth Vaux (Urbana: University of Illinois Press, 1985), pp. 7–27. See also Daniel Callahan, "The Desire for Eternal Life: Scientific versus Religious Visions: The 2002–03 Ingersoll Lecture," *Harvard Divinity School Bulletin* 31, no. 2 (2003). On Spielberg's films, see Lester D. Friedman, *Citizen Spielberg* (Urbana: University of Illinois Press, 2006).

54. Julius B. Poppinga, letter to the editor, *New York Times*, June 13, 1994, p. A14.

55. See Herbert Hendin, *Seduced by Death: Doctors, Patients, and Assisted Suicide* (New York: Norton, 1998). See also Kathleen M. Foley and Herbert Hendin, eds.,

The Case against Assisted Suicide: For the Right to End-of-Life Care (Baltimore: Johns Hopkins University Press, 2004).

56. See Jonathan B. Imber, "Abortion Policy and Medical Practice," in *Society* 27, no. 5 (1990): 27–34, reprinted in *Human Sexuality* 91–92, annual editions (16th ed.), ed. by Ollie Pocs, pp. 28–35. The resistance to abortion was undermined as well not simply by the emergence of far from fail-proof forms of contraception but also because new possibilities in the creation of life posed new dilemmas for jurists over the meaning of the acts that precede such creation. Before in vitro fertilization, there was artificial insemination by husband, along with artificial insemination by donor (AID). As Immanuel Jakobovits pointed out, in 1921 the Canadian Supreme Court said that AID constituted adultery and was therefore against the law. The prohibition against adultery has stood in contrast to the routinization of its violation in biomedical progress for nearly a century. Religious prohibitions once informed the practice of technical innovation, but those prohibitions eventually became "religious" in ways that are now so deeply taken for granted that resistance to medical and technical advance, particularly in the case of abortion, is interpreted as entirely based on religious belief. See Jakobovits, *Jewish Medical Ethics*, p. 244–45.

57. Ramsey, *Ethics at Edges*, p. 42.

Close Encounters of the Third Kind (film), 191

Cold War, 102

Cole, Jonathan R., 147

collectivism, 193

coma, 179, 188

commencement addresses. *See* addresses, sermons, and eulogies

commercialism, 99–100

communitarians, 179

competence, xi, xviii, 73, 87, 118, 130, 131, 177

Comte, Auguste, 59, 74, 134, 139

conscience, 23, 31–32, 33, 38, 41–42, 130, 131, 138, 160, 177

consciousness-raising, 119

consumer/consumer consciousness, xviii, 114, 122, 151, 169, 177, 215n14

contraception, 22, 133

Cousins, Norman, 243n57

Cowling, Maurice, 226n14

Craik, James, 168

craniotomy, 28, 29, 31, 34–35, 36, 37–38, 39, 40, 136

creationism, 48

Cruzan, Nancy, 116

cryonics, 186–88

cultural consensus, 133–34

cultural repression, 194–97

Cushing, Harvey, *The Life of Sir William Osler,* 171

cyborgs, 190

Darwin, Charles, *On the Origin of Species by Means of Natural Selection,* 46

Dassel, William, 26

death/mortality, 148; acknowledgement of, 181; anxiety about, 64; certainty about, 184; debates over, 141; and dignity, 189; and medical education, 170; Nietzsche on, 182–83; Potter on, 139; and rights, 189, 193; and science fiction, 190–91; and technology, 189; usefulness of, 179. *See also* end-of-life care

DeBakey, Michael, 152–53

de Fleury, Maurice, *Medicine and the Mind,* 85

democracy, 33, 78, 124, 142, 184, 194

Dennis, James S., 66

de Rochemont, Louis, *M.D.—the U.S. Doctor,* 131

diagnosis, 109, 118, 148, 152, 160, 162, 190

diagnostic testing, 149

Dickens, Charles, *Bleak House,* 44

disease(s): acute *vs.* chronic, 169; of affluence, 147, 149; causation of, 184; environmental determinants of, 114; and epidemiology, 147, 163, 166, 184; McKeown on, 114, 146; of poverty, 146, 147; and science *vs.* prayer, 50–60; and tobacco use, 150–55; and Warbasse, 93–94. *See also* illness; patients

divine positive law, 135

DNA analysis, xiii

Doll, Richard, 154, 251n29, 254n40, 255n50

Dorst, Stanley Elwood, "A Case for the Study of the Humanities in the Making of a Doctor," 98

Draper, John W., *History of the Conflict between Religion and Science,* 47

Durkin, Joseph T., 36

duty, 6, 37, 38, 44, 97, 140

Edward, Prince of Wales, 51–52

egalitarianism, 80

Eliot, George, 239n11

Elkin, Daniel C., 98

Emerson, Ralph Waldo, 32

end-of-life care, xii, xiii, 22, 116, 117, 148, 169, 178–80, 188–90, 194. *See also* death/mortality

Enlightenment, 136, 143

environment, 114, 184

epidemiology, 94, 145, 184; and anxiety, 149–50; and bioethics, 140; and cause-effect relationships, 161; and class, 228n35; development of, xi, xiv; and disease, 147, 163, 166, 184; and environment, 184; and iatrogenic harms, 108; and managed care, 177; and morality, 161; and prayer-gauge debate, 53, 55, 57, 59; research funding for, 165; and tobacco use, 150, 151, 154, 160, 161, 162–63; and women's health, 163

illness: anxiety about, 64; chronic, 147, 161; narrative of, 123–25; and prayer-gauge debate, 55; psychosomatic, 169; terminal, 148; as vocation, 123. *See also* disease(s); health; patients

immortality, 190–91

immunization, 145, 146

individualism, 32, 33, 36, 80, 138, 191, 194

Innocent X, 23

Jacksonianism, 33

Jakobovits, Immanuel, 264n56

James, William, 62, 194; *The Varieties of Religious Experience,* 63, 183–84

Jellett, John Hewitt, 57–60; *The Efficacy of Prayer,* 58

Jesus Christ, 75

Jews, xiii, xiv, 9

Johns Hopkins University Medical School, 15

Jonsen, Albert R., 141; *The Birth of Bioethics,* 140

Judaism, 24

Kafka, Franz, 1

Kant, Immanuel, 136

Kass, Edward H., 164, 165

Kelly, David F., 23–24; *The Emergence of Roman Catholic Medical Ethics in North America,* 135

Kerr, J. G., 66–67

Kevorkian, Jack, 116, 175

Kierkegaard, Søren, "The Present Age," 144

Kim, Stephan S., 49

Kimball, Bruce, 216n15

Klarmann, Andrew, 41

Koch, Robert, 160

Kramer, Peter D., *Listening to Prozac,* 126

Lasagna, Louis, 4–5

law, 3, 24, 27, 38, 43, 48, 141–42, 169, 179. *See also* litigation

Le Baron, Samuel, 177

Le Bon, Gustav, *The Crowd,* 248n3

Lecky, William Edward Hartpole: *History of European Morals,* 183; *History of Rationalism,* 183

Lewis, C. S., 192

life, extension of, xiii, xix

Lillienfeld, Abraham M., 256nn58, 62

litigation, 126–29, 130, 141. *See also* law; malpractice

Littlejohn, Abram Newkirk, 70–73, 79

Long, Jr., Edward LeRoy, *The Christian as a Doctor,* 176

Long Island College Hospital, 67–78, 210–11

lung cancer, 151–53, 159–60, 164

Luther, Martin, 18

Macgowan, Daniel J., "The Claims of the Missionary Enterprise on the Medical Profession," 66

Magnien, Alphonse, 36–37

malpractice, 101, 111, 114, 126, 130. *See also* litigation

managed care, xi, 102, 136, 177, 196. *See also* medical care/health care

Mantle, Mickey, 179–80

Marmor, Theodore, 239n7

Marxism, 113, 119

Massinger, Philip, *The Old Law,* 171

materialism, 70, 71, 85, 99

McCosh, James, 60–61

McFadden, Charles J., *Medical Ethics,* 135

McGinley, Laurie, "Breast Cancer Patients Get More Assertive by Doing Research and Asking Questions," 108

McHenry, James, 168

McHugh, John Ambrose, 41

McIntire, Charles, 92

McKeown, Thomas, 114, 148, 155; *The Role of Medicine,* 145–46

McLeod, Thomas B., 75

Medicaid, 103, 118

medical care/health care, 118, 119; access to, 54, 162; and bureaucracies, 169, 177; consumers of, 122; cost of, 148, 162, 185; demand for higher levels of, 114; effectiveness of, 114; inequities in, 141;

medical care/health care (*cont.*)
reform of, 177; and technology, 107. *See also* managed care

medical economics, 131, 133

medical education, xi, 245n5; Boardman on, 10; and character, 103; and codes of professionalism, 33; and death, 170; and humanities, 98–99; and Münsterberg, 84; pastoral role in, 148; and physicians as caring *vs.* curing, 97–99; and professionalism, 14–15; qualifications for, 79; Schofield on, 86; and science, xviii; and trust, 95. *See also* professional training

medical ethics, xi–xii, 23, 25, 31, 32. *See also* bioethics; morality

medical etiquette. *See under* physicians

medicalization, 116

medical missionaries, 66–67, 70. *See also* physicians

medical profession, 67, 68, 69, 71, 74, 131, 141. *See also* medicine; physicians; professions

medical specialties, 114, 176–77

Medicare, 103, 118

medication/drugs, 126, 163, 192

medicine: alternative, 64, 148; autonomy of, 169; and bioethics, 139; commerce of, 95; corporate, 175, 176; defensive, 148; distrust in, 107–29; enhancement, 148–49; for-profit, 196; golden age of, 168–69, 170, 175; as indifferent to suffering, 179; interests of, 121; as moral enterprise, 115; negative publicity about, 107; and other professions, 79; redemptive dimension of, 7–8; and religion, 95, 103, 113; and science, 74, 88, 102, 178; social context of, 112, 113; and society, 94; technical *vs.* contractual understanding of, 181; as vocation, 14, 85; as vocation *vs.* career, 96–97. *See also* medical profession; physicians

Meilander, Gilbert, 180–81

Mendes, Frederick de Sola, 62–63

Menninger, William C., 99, 100

Metalious, Grace, *Peyton Place*, 132

middle class, 82, 118

Middleton, Thomas, *The Old Law*, 171

Mill, John Stuart, *Autobiography*, 162

Mishler, Eliot, 112, 113

missions, 33, 65–67, 123

Moe, Henry Allen, 96

Mohr, James, 138

morality: Beecher on, 76–77; and Busey, 33–34, 37, 38, 39, 40; Catholic, 33; and epidemiology, 161, 166; Illich on, 115; and pastoral medicine, 136–37; and physician-patient relationship, 5; and physicians, 196; Protestant, 33; and rights, 142; Schofield on, 87; and technology, 162; and tobacco use, 154, 161; and Warbasse, 93. *See also* bioethics; medical ethics

Mott, Lucretia, 9

Moynihan, Daniel Patrick, 248n2

multivocal clinical ethic, 123

Münsterberg, Hugo, 89; "Finding a Life Work," 83–84; *Vocation and Learning*, 84

narratives, 122–26

National Cancer Institute (NCI), 156

natural law, 23, 40, 41, 135–36

Nazis, 183

Newman, John Henry, 186

Nietzsche, Friedrich, 182–83, 193

1960s, 95, 99, 102, 103, 107–8, 112, 131, 132, 168, 169

Noonan, John T., 134, 135

obstetrics, 28, 31, 34–35, 39

Ochsner, Alton, 151–53

O'Connor, Sandra Day, 176

office, 18, 19, 73, 78, 130

organ donation, 179–80

Ortega y Gasset, José, *The Revolt of the Masses*, 248n3

Osgood, Samuel, 13

Osler, William, 170–71, 172–75, 178; *Æquanimitas*, 174; "The Fixed Period," 171; "Vocation in Medicine and Nursing," 22, 23

Ovid, 7

Papanicolaou, George N., 157

Pap smear, 156, 160

Pareto, Vilfredo, 89

Parker, Joel, 16–19

Parker, Theodore, 32

Parsons, Frank, 82–83, 95; *Choosing a Vocation,* 83

Parsons, Talcott, 120; *The Social System,* 117–18

Passmore, John, *The Perfectibility of Man,* 162

pastoral counseling, 192

pastoral medicine, 22–25, 37, 41, 95, 131, 136–37, 138

patienthood, vocation of, 125

patients: acute *vs.* nonspecific and chronic symptoms in, 118; as artifacts of test results, 190; autonomy of, 140, 182–86; changing population of, 118; and competence *vs.* manner, 177; as consumers, xviii, 114, 122, 151, 169, 177, 215n14; dignity and rights of, 110; duty to, 6; empowerment of, 107, 108, 118, 122, 123; financial means of, 118; Illich on, 116; and narratives, 122–26; personal vigilance of, 108; responsibility of, 118–19, 121; rights of, 180; self-care by, 148; and sick role, 117, 118; subjectivity of, 109; and tobacco use, 160; wishes of, 189. *See also* disease(s); illness; women's health movement

Pearl, Raymond, 251n28

Percival, Thomas, *Medical Ethics,* 6

Pernick, Martin, 29

Peyton Place (film), 132

Philadelphia, 9, 10, 16, 20, 44, 68, 70, 208–9

physician-patient relationship: Annis on, 101; and authority, 110; call to transform, 119; and character, xv, 5; communication in, 108, 109–12; confidentiality in, 42, 91; evolution of, 180; expectations in, 110; Henderson on, 88–91; Heschel on, 100, 101; and moral authority, 16; and morality, 5; mutual dependency in, 180; mutual responsibility in, 94; as personal, mutually-informed encounter, 118;

psychological aspects of, 85–91; reciprocity in, 6; Schofield on, 85–87, 89–90; and social science, 117; and sociology, 141; and suffering, 180–81; trust in, xviii–xix, 5; and women's health movement, xiv

physicians: absence of publicity about, 95–96; accountability of, 102–3, 140; affective neutrality of, 117; as arrogant, xiii, 101, 114; authority of, 41, 45, 87, 90–91, 94, 95–96, 103, 110, 111, 123, 130, 169; autonomy of, 38, 41, 94, 175; and bioethics, 139; as caring *vs.* competent, 73; as caring *vs.* curing, 97–99, 117–18, 169; and Catholic priests, 29–30; and changing population of patients, 118; Chapin on, 43–44; and Christianity, 102; and chronic illness, 161; and clergy, 13–15, 16, 17–20, 43–44, 45–46, 60, 64, 66, 67–73, 74, 75, 80, 81, 154; and collegialism, 15; competence of, xi, xviii, 73, 87, 118, 130, 131; and competence *vs.* manner, 177; consolation from, 19–20; and corporations, 175; demeanor of, 130, 177; and environmental determinants of health, 114; and expertise *vs.* care, 177; failures of, 168; generalist, 176–77; in golden age of medicine, 169; impaired, xii, 72, 75, 213n2; as impersonal, 101; as indifferent, 97, 101, 118, 141; and inebriation, 75; as judgmental and noninformative, 120; and medical etiquette, 23, 25, 137–38; monitoring by, 155; as moral guides, 18–19; as non-judgmental, 74–75, 91; persona of, 64, 86–87, 120, 140; popular perception of, 118; and profit motive, 117; proletarianization of, 175; publicized as caring and competent, 131; responsibility of, 8–9, 118, 120; socialization of, 141, 245n5; and society, 79, 87–89, 91, 98; specialist, 114, 176–77; spiritual counsel of, 16; and suicide, xiii, 170, 178, 179, 183, 193, 194, 241n31; and tobacco use, 160; truth-telling by, 110–11; and vocational counseling, 81. *See also* iatrogenesis; medical missionaries; medical profession; medicine

placebo effect, 169

Plato, *Dialogues,* 186
Plunkett, H. M., *Women, Plumbers, and Doctors,* 146
Poppinga, Julius B., 193, 195
Porter, Roy, 219n41
positivism, 59, 134, 139
posttraumatic syndromes, 125
Potter, Van Rensselaer, *Bioethics,* 139–40
prayer-gauge debate, 52–63, 172. *See also* religion
prevention, 5, 51–52, 53, 57, 114, 140, 146, 150, 155, 156, 166, 184
Price, William, 172
Prior, Matthew, 167
professionalism: and accountability, 78; and authority, 87; and Busey, 31–32, 36, 38; and Capellmann, 31; and career choice, 82; and Catholicism, 94; and character, 78–79; and clergy, 94; codes of, 33; cultural expectations of, xi; Kimball on, 216n15; and medical education, 14–15; and moral authority, 94; and Parsons, 118; and personality, 78; and Protestantism, 23, 25, 41, 94, 137–38; and social science, 95; and vocation, 12–21
professional training, 22, 78, 79, 89, 95. *See also* medical education
professions: as corporate enterprises, xv; corporate power of, 141; distrust of, 107; dominance of, xviii, 122; and Protestantism, 130; trust in, 65–66; veneration of, 69; and vocational counseling, 80–81. *See also* medical profession
prognosis, probabilistic, 150, 151
progress, 192, 193
Progressive Era, 82, 83, 94
Prohibition, 32, 154, 158
prosthetic god, 181, 191, 193
Protestant clergy, 9, 10, 21, 24, 25, 32, 41, 68, 69
Protestantism, 107; and abortion, 23, 25, 138, 142; and American Medical Association, 137; and authority, 40, 41, 78, 137–38; and Busey, 31–32, 36, 37, 41; and Catholic pastoral medicine, 138; and character, xiii,

xviii, 95, 130, 133; and conscience, 23, 33; and duty, 37; and Fisher, 121; and Henderson, 88, 91; inheritance from, 130, 132; and materialism, 99; and medical etiquette, 137–38; and medical missions, 66; and morality, 33; and natural law, 135–36; and office, 78, 130; and Parsons, 117, 118; and professionalism, 23, 25, 41, 94, 137–38; and professions, 130; and responsibility, 8–9; and science, 7–8, 41; and Smith, 94; and social reform, 32–33; and virtues of hard work, 83; and vocation, 6–12, 22, 23, 75, 80, 138; and Warbasse, 92
psychoanalysis, 45, 85, 90, 119, 192, 239n9
psychology, 79, 80, 84, 85–87, 89–91, 92, 239n9
public health, 65; and Beadle, 20–21; and Beecher, 76, 77; and disease prevention, 155; and environmental determinants *vs.* physicians' interventions, 114; and epidemiology, 145; and gun control, 184; and Henderson, 91; rise of, 258n80; and Smith, 94; and social improvement, 146; and tobacco use, 151, 155, 160; and utilitarianism, 147; and Warbasse, 93–94
Puritanism, 32

Quinlan, Karen Ann, 116, 180, 189
Quintard, Charles T., 9, 12–13

Ramsey, Paul, 115–16; *Ethics at the Edges of Life,* 196
Reiser, Stanley Joel, 109
religion, 33, 143; absolutist claims in, 47; and American Medical Association, 99–103; and bioethics, xiii, 103, 134–35; Boardman on, 10, 11; and Busey, 32, 36; and cause-effect relationships, 51; and Comte, 134; and epidemiology, 166; and medicine, 95, 103, 113; and Ochsner, 153–54; Rusk on, 102; and science, xiv, 44–49, 52; and self-help movements, 123; and superstition, 63; and Tyndall, 49. *See also* faith; prayer-gauge debate
religious pluralism, 33

religious toleration, 47

Rhode Island Commission, 132–33

Richards, Lysander Salmon, 83, 95; *Vocophy [L. Voco, I Name; I Call] The New Profession,* 80

Rieff, Philip, 241n38

rights, 110, 142, 180, 189, 193

right-to-life doctrine, 27, 37, 195

Roe v. Wade, 138

The Romish Intrigue: Frémont a Catholic!! (pamphlet), 34

Rosenkrantz, Barbara Gutmann, 15

Rothman, David J., *Strangers at the Bedside,* 140

Rowley, William, *The Old Law,* 171

Rusk, Howard A., 101–2

Ryan, Michael, 6

sanitary science, 146

Schafer, Paul W., 251n29

Schiavo, Terri, 116, 188, 189

Schofield, Alfred Taylor, 89, 92, 95, 111; *Unconscious Therapeutics,* 85–87, 90

Schweitzer, Albert, 67, 96

science, xi; and abortion, 27, 28; accountability to, 15; and associations, 164, 166; authority of, 72; and autonomy of medicine, 169; Bayless on, 43; Boardman on, 10–11; and Busey, 31, 32, 38, 41; and Capellmann, 27, 28; and Catholicism, 33; and cause-effect relationships, xiv, 51, 52, 57, 58, 59, 63, 164; and faith, 43–64; interventions by, 145; James on, 62; Littlejohn on, 71; and medical education, xviii; and medicine, 74, 88, 102, 178; and Parson, 117; and prayer, 49–63; progress in, 107, 130; and Protestantism, 7–8, 23, 41; and reason, 72; and religion, xiv, 44–49, 52; role of, xiv; and skepticism, 58; and tobacco use, 151, 154; verification in, 62; and Weber, 178, 179

science fiction, 190–91

Scopes trial, 48

Scudder, Henry Martyn, 70

Scudder, Jared Waterbury, 70

Scudder, John (father), 70

Scudder, John (son), 70

secularism, 48, 49

Selbie, W. B., 231n70

self-help/self-help movements, 107, 117, 123, 125, 126

Semmelweis, Ignaz, 165

sentiments, theory of, 89–90

sermons. *See* addresses, sermons, and eulogies

sexuality, 93–94, 195

sexual sterilization, 136

shame, 194, 195

Shapiro, Samuel, 164, 165

Shaw, George Bernard, *The Doctor's Dilemma,* 185

Shrady, George F., 68–69

Sigerist, Henry E., 147

Simmel, Georg, 220n60

Sloterdijk, Peter, 178, 179

Smith, Gerald Birney, 94

Smoking and Health (report of the Surgeon General), 151, 160, 161

Snively, William A., 74–75

social class, 58

social context, 112, 113

social improvement, 146

social problems, 77, 93

social reform, 32–33

social science, 92, 95, 107, 112, 117, 119, 143. *See also* anthropology; sociology

society: advanced industrial, 113; and Illich, 113; and medicine, 94; and physician-patient relationship, 180; and physicians, 79, 87–89, 91, 98; purpose in, 83

sociology, xvii, 89, 92–95, 121, 133–34, 141, 142, 143, 175, 191. *See also* social science

Sophocles, *Antigone,* 110

Spain, David, 159

The Spectator, 53–55

Spencer, Herbert, 92

Spender, Stephen, "The Funeral," 144

Spielberg, Steven, 191

Stanley, Arthur Penrhyn, 51

Starr, Paul, 239n7

statistics, 55–56, 57, 58, 64, 144, 151, 156, 157, 159, 161, 164, 230n52

stem-cell research, xiii, 142, 179, 195

Stephens, James T., *The Christian as a Doctor,* 176

Stevens, M. L. Tina, *Bioethics in America,* 140

Stewart, Harold, 254n40

Storrs, Richard Salter, 70

suffering/pain, 71, 75, 102; alleviation of, 78; Boardman on, 11, 16; and communication, 123; Illich on, 113, 116–17; indifference to, 194; James on, 183; medicine as indifferent to, 179; and physician-patient relationship, 86, 180–81; Potter on, 139; spiritual and physical, 78

suicide, 174–75; and hope, 193; Nietzsche on, 182–83; physician-assisted, xiii, 170, 178, 179, 183, 193, 194, 241n31. *See also* euthanasia

Supreme Court, 132–33, 142, 189, 241n31

Susser, Mervyn, 258n80

Talmage, Thomas De Witt, 76, 77–78

Taubes, Gary, 165–66

Taylor, Howard C., 255n53

technology, xii, 107, 109, 130, 162, 181, 188, 195

Temkin, Owsei, xvii

Terry, Luther, 160

theocracy, 32, 33

Thompson, Henry, 52–53, 172

Thompson, Hugh Miller, 61

Thompson, W. Burns, 66

Tillich, Paul, 135–36, 142

tobacco growers, 156

tobacco product manufacturers, xiv, 150, 156, 161

tobacco use, xiv, 150–64

Tocqueville, Alexis de, 33

Toulmin, Stephen, 136

Townsend, Stephen, 21

Tracy, Robert, 171

Trollope, Anthony, *The Fixed Period,* 171–72, 173, 174, 175

trust: and American Medical Association, 131; and authority of physicians, 111; Bayless on, 43; and confidentiality issue, 42; cultural expectations of, xi, 140; decline of, xii–xiii, xviii–xix, 107–29, 169, 175, 176; as emotional buffer, 148; and Gilbert, 126, 128; in golden age of medicine, 168–69; Henderson on, 91; in individual *vs.* profession, 65–66, 167–70, 181; and medical education, 95; and medical profession, 114; in physician-patient relationship, xviii–xix, 5; and physician's communication skills, xv; and prayer-gauge debate, 52; and professionalism, 15; in professional training, 79; and public health, 76; and righteousness, 7; rise of, xviii; Schofield on, 86, 87, 92; shallowness of, 193; and technology, 181

truth, 110–11, 127, 128

Turner, Frank M., 47, 49–63

Twain, Mark, 68; *The Adventures of Tom Sawyer,* 149

Tyndall, John, 49, 51, 231n68; "Apology for the Belfast Address," 46–47; and prayer-gauge debate, 52, 53, 57, 59, 60, 61, 62, 63, 64, 172

unconscious, 85–86, 89–90

Unitarianism, 32

universities, 48, 95, 136, 147

University of Pennsylvania, 9, 10, 20

Utilitarians, 179

Veatch, Robert, "Diverging Traditions," 137, 222n17

vocation, 107; and career, 131–32; changing ideas about, 82; and Elkin, 98; Henderson on, 88; illness and disability as, 123; and individualistic psychology, 80; Littlejohn on, 71; medicine as, 14, 85, 96–97; and Parson, 117; of patienthood, 125; and professionalism, 12–21; and Protestantism, 6–12, 22, 23, 75, 80, 138; and technical *vs.* contractual understanding of medicine, 181; as term, 82. *See also* career

vocational guidance, 79–84